P9-DCI-826

Treating Addicted Survivors of Trauma

Treating Addicted Survivors of Trauma

KATIE EVANS
J. MICHAEL SULLIVAN

THE GUILFORD PRESS
New York   London

© 1995 The Guilford Press
A Division of Guilford Publications, Inc.
72 Spring Street, New York, NY 10012

All rights reserved

No part of this book may be reproduced, stored in a retrieval system, or transmitted, in any form or by any means, electronic, mechanical, photocopying, microfilming, recording, or otherwise, without written permission from the Publisher.

Printed in the United States of America

This book is printed on acid-free paper.

Last digit is print number: 9 8 7 6 5 4 3 2

Library of Congress Cataloging-in-Publication Data
Evans, Katie.
    Treating addicted survivors of trauma / by Katie Evans and
    J. Michael Sullivan.
        p.   cm.
    Includes bibliographical references and index.
    ISBN 0-89862-306-5.   ISBN 0-89862-324-3 (pbk.)
    1. Substance abuse—Treatment.   2. Adult child abuse
victims—Rehabilitation.   I. Sullivan, J. Michael.
II. Title.
RC564.E85 1995
616.85′82239—dc20   94-31708
                                                  CIP

Preface

✧

Who Is the Victim Now?

I feel so ashamed, I am so nasty, I feel so dirty.
You've degraded my strength, left me feeling so totally weak and worthless.
I don't want to open my eyes, my body turns ice cold and endless miles of
    numbness.
Please don't feel emotion, I don't want to open my eyes.
I feel you standing above me, I open my eyes and see nothing but bloody
    walls and terror.
He pushes his hell and anger in and out of my entity,
He weaves through out everything and lives with in me.
He erupts his anger into me.
I am his garbage can where he throws his hate.
I cry with relief it is over at least for tonight,
I guess life isn't the fairy tale that I wanted it to be,
Nobody believes me, nobody will ever believe me.
I fall asleep in the tub.
I dream that I am in a black room.
You too are asleep in this room.
Whirlpools of hate fall upon you as I see you sleeping.
A rifle hangs on a nail on the wall. It screams your name
The room turns white as the bullet races through the air.
The blood gushes out of you like a waterfall,
That single split second in slow motion as I watched you melt away.
I hear the sound of my own loud laughter.
Hurdles of murderous laughter getting louder and louder echoing
    throughout our souls.
In the end, in the very end, who is the victim now?

RACHEL, age 16

A young woman who is both an addict and a survivor in dual recovery
wrote this poem. We will be sharing her story and poetry with you
throughout this book. We have included other survivors' poetry as well.
The survivors we see often possess tremendous artistic talents, which they,
as well as we, are proud to share with you.

    Our goal in writing this book is to provide readers with an easy to understand, practical, and integrated overview for treating survivors of childhood trauma who are also chemically dependent. There are many excellent books dedicated to the treatment of survivors of childhood abuse and other forms of trauma, and we have referenced many of these in this text. This book's unique focus is its concentration on the treatment of survivors with alcohol and drug problems. We hope that students and professionals who are newcomers to this field will learn a great deal from reading this book. To help our readers understand the material we present, we define and illustrate key concepts and procedures and provide a basic introduction to fundamental issues of theory, diagnosis, and treatment before discussing more advanced concepts critical to treating the addicted survivor. We hope that more experienced professionals will find the basic material a useful review and our integration and extension of this material a stimulus to their creativity.

We feel that this book fills an important gap in the existing literature on how to treat clients who present with these coexisting issues. Recent years have seen tremendous growth in the ability of professionals to successfully treat the person with either a history of childhood abuse or chemical dependency. Unfortunately, many treatment professionals have not had the tools or training to treat the client who is both a survivor of abuse and dependent on chemicals. This was certainly true for us when we started in this field. It also appears to be true for the professionals we meet in the workshops we have conducted.

For a variety of reasons, the field of alcohol and drug counseling became divorced from the field of mental health some time ago. Many mental health professionals have had limited training and experience in the assessment and treatment of substance abuse disorders, and many alcohol and drug counselors have had only minimal training in mental health issues. Moreover, most professionals in these fields have had little training in the effective treatment of clients with both sets of issues, including those with substance use disorders who are survivors of abuse. The organization of school training programs, clinics and hospitals, and state licensing departments and the regulations of various third-party payers also reflect this split between mental health and chemical dependency.

Chemically dependent survivors can often be difficult to treat. They typically present with a high acuity level and are crisis prone and at high risk for relapse. Simultaneously confronting the denial of their addiction and supporting their recovery from abuse requires that clinicians engage in a delicate balancing act. This work can be both rewarding and draining.

The model we share with you in these pages is one we have developed over time in our own clinical practice. This model incorporates the concepts of many fine clinicians as well as the results of the many hours we have spent discovering what seems to work best with our own clients. We are continuously revising our ideas and in this book present a distillation of what we think and do today. Readers familiar with our previous writing will see that while we have modified our strategies and tactics, we continue to adhere to the same treatment philosophy. This philosophy emphasizes combining mental health paradigms with disease models of addiction and combining psychotherapeutic techniques with 12-step recovery practices. Our goal has always been the development of a truly integrated and practical recovery model for individuals suffering from both a psychiatric disorder and a substance use disorder.

We have tended to be more inclusive than exclusive in our review of the literature on survivors of abuse and on the conditions and consequences of such abuse. We have looked for, and found, common themes useful for working with substance-dependent survivors of childhood abuse across a variety of sources. We believe, for example, that both research on Vietnam veterans with posttraumatic stress disorder and articles on adult children of alcoholics' (ACOA) issues can enrich our understanding of abusive processes. We also see underlying similarities between incest survivors and persons suffering from borderline personality disorder, between trance phenomena and posttraumatic stress disorder, and between mental health and 12-step recovery models.

A word about terminology is in order at this point. We use the word *survivor* deliberately. This strategy, consistent with common practice in the field, is aimed at simultaneously acknowledging the reality of the abuse while empowering and validating the client. Our intention is not to reduce clients to a category when we use this language. We do believe, however, that having a label that names a key aspect of their experience helps clients begin to transcend their fate and heal. We have found that the hundreds of survivors we treated over the years possessed courage and strength. The term *survivor* helps both therapist and client to emphasize these assets.

We use the phrase *substance use disorder,* and its variants, to describe individuals suffering negative consequences from their use of chemicals. This is an umbrella term to describe a range of behaviors, from abuse of chemicals to full-blown substance dependence.

Although it is not technically correct—but is consistent with the recovery literature—we also use the terms *alcoholic* and *addict* somewhat interchangeably.

Finally, this book was going to press just as or the fourth edition of the American Psychiatric Association's *Diagnostic and Statistical Manual of Mental Disorders* (DSM-IV) was published. Consequently, readers will find the DSM-IV cited in the following chapters.

Our hope is that this book will provide readers with increased comfort and competence in assessing and treating chemically dependent survivors who have a variety of presenting problems. To this end, our general objectives include the following: (1) providing an overview of various types of childhood abuse and other traumas, of moderating variables, and of the range of effects such abuse produces; (2) discussing the disease of addiction and its treatment; (3) exploring ways to identify substance-dependent survivors and assess their treatment needs; (4) presenting an integrated model of treatment to help organize, direct, and plan treatment that is specific and practical and that provides for simultaneously treating both addiction and survivor issues; (5) addressing special issues that arise in treating chemically affected adolescent survivors as well as issues related to working with significant others; (6) discussing and illustrating specific treatment, strategy, and tactics; and (7) exploring the personal concerns and issues that this work creates for professionals.

We believe that this book has a number of strengths. These include the presentation of a systematic model for treating survivors, the integration of 12-step and mental health approaches, and the provision of detailed, concrete treatment interventions and strategies. While our emphasis is on survivors of childhood trauma, we believe the material is also applicable to survivors of trauma experienced in adulthood. We strongly encourage readers to obtain appropriate training and supervision before applying the procedures we describe.

We have included clinical examples to illustrate our concepts. These case examples always represent composites of several clients and, in order to protect our clients' confidentiality, contain no identifying information. Any resemblance to one person or family is coincidental. We have always obtained clients' permission to use any specific written material.

Our beliefs, approaches, and practices spring from a number of sources. Katie Evans, CADCII, NCACII, is a drug and alcohol counselor who is board certified nationally and in Oregon. She is in the process of completing her Ph.D. in psychology. Evans worked for 7 years for child protective services in the state of Oregon, investigating child abuse and neglect cases and providing counseling for survivors and their families. She has also served as counselor and program director for inpatient and outpatient dual diagnosis programs for adults and adolescents and has developed dual diagnosis programs for nationwide health care companies. Evans has an active private practice of both adult and adolescent survivors in recovery from addiction. She has maintained a program of continuous sobriety from chemical dependency since 1983 and is also in recovery as a child of an alcoholic and as a survivor of rape.

J. Michael Sullivan, Ph.D., is a licensed clinical psychologist who has worked in both inpatient and outpatient settings; with both adults and adolescents; and with both single and dually diagnosed survivors, as well as with other dually diagnosed clients. He has also served as program director and consultant in a variety of settings. Sullivan is in active recovery from childhood sexual abuse from a clergy member.

Both of us are certified hypnotherapists. We give workshops across the country on dual diagnosis issues and on treatment of resistant populations, and we publish articles and books in these areas. Finally, we have reviewed a great deal of the professional literature and have tried to incorporate this into our practice and this book.

We invite reader feedback and comments. We can be reached at our clinic in Beaverton, Oregon, at (503) 644-1984. You can write to us at this address: Evans and Sullivan Clinic, 9670 S.W. Beaverton-Hillsdale Hwy., Beaverton, Oregon 97005. We would also be happy to send you more information about our workshops, consultation, or our other publications.

Acknowledgments

✦

We wish to thank those family members who have supported us through the many hours we needed to write this book: Craig, Casey, Callie, Kathy, and Pat. Their understanding, love, and patience made this book possible. We want to thank Ms. Shirley Kimmel, who guided us to a further understanding of survivor recovery. And a special thanks to Frank Fitzpatrick and the Attleboro survivors group.

Contents

Chapter 9
Addicted Survivors in Their Families, at Work, and in Therapy Groups
225

Afterword
The Dragon Dies, the Child Survives
254

Appendix
263

Index
275

Treating Addicted Survivors of Trauma

Philosophy of Treatment

I Drank to Their Diseases

They pretended that there was nothing wrong,
Their lies stole my trust.
They said that they were "normal."
I felt insane.
They said, "We love you,"
I was alone.
I used alcohol to kill the pain.
It made me a liar.
I drank to feel "normal,"
I became insane.
I cried, "Please love me!"
I was still alone.

— KATHERINE, age 40

We will begin by discussing five central assumptions underlying our treatment approach:

1. A large proportion of the seriously troubled clients seen in any clinical setting have a history of childhood trauma. Taking this fact and the impact of the trauma into account significantly enhances treatment.

2. Successful treatment of the trauma must include safely working through the memories of the abuse in an experiential way but only after the clinician and client have laid a base of safety and skills.

3. Substance abuse or dependence is an important part of the clinical picture for a substantial proportion of survivors of childhood abuse, and unless treatment deals with the chemical abuse or addiction, treatment of the person's survivor issues will most likely be ineffective.

1

Conversely, treating only the addiction of individuals with serious survivor symptoms is also likely to be unsuccessful.

4. The disease model of addiction and the use of 12-step practices offer a productive approach for treating the addicted survivor.

5. Any treatment model for clients who are survivors of childhood abuse and who are substance dependent must be integrated and must address the synergism of addiction and trauma. The model must blend mental health and chemical dependency treatment approaches in a way that provides for treating both problems simultaneously and in a comprehensive fashion. A "first-this-problem-then-that" or a "two track" model is less likely to be effective than an integrated one.

CHILDHOOD TRAUMA AND ITS ROLE IN PSYCHOLOGICAL DIFFICULTIES

Recent years have witnessed a growing appreciation of the role of childhood abuse as a causative factor in many mental health difficulties. Surveys have demonstrated that the experience of childhood sexual abuse is common, approaching rates of 1 in 4 for women and 1 in 7 for men in the general American population (1). The same surveys have indicated that a substantial proportion of survivors (in the case of women, up to a third) have never told anyone of the abuse. Comparable studies of the incidence and prevalence of physical and emotional abuse do not exist, but clinical experience suggests that the rates for these are even higher. Studies of psychiatric inpatients have consistently demonstrated both very high rates of childhood physical or sexual abuse and a strong positive correlation between a background of such experiences and serious mental and emotional problems later in life (2, 3). Similar studies with outpatients and with persons not in treatment have shown similar trends (4, 5, 6).

Most of the available research literature has focused primarily on sexual abuse, with physical abuse being studied to a lesser extent. A few investigators, however, have explored the impact of other kinds of abuse on functioning. For example, psychological abuse and neglect and a negative home atmosphere also appear to contribute to psychological difficulties later in life (7, 8). Physical neglect, emotional withdrawal, and inconsistency in parenting (or caretaking), as well as a history of childhood separations, are also frequently found among individuals seeking mental health services and are correlated with a variety of psychiatric difficulties (9, 10). This correlation occurs in persons seeking treatment as well as in members of the general population (11).

These findings raise questions about how we define abuse. Certainly, daily beatings or the experience of childhood incest is traumatic. However, childhood experiences with parents who are consistently angry or critical or who constantly belittle and demean also leave scars. And what about the overweight girl whose father made fun of her weight, made "mooing" sounds when she wore shorts or a bathing suit, and predicted that she would never have a boyfriend because of her weight (while her mother offered her cookies when she was upset)? This example, taken from the history of a client we treated who had an eating disorder, illustrates that abuse can take forms that are less obviously traumatic than incest but that are still damaging. Moreover, abuse can result not only from what *did* happen but also from what *did not*. Experiencing ongoing neglect, "underparenting," or little emotional validation and support also has a negative impact. Finally, not only is abuse by emotional and physical abandonment traumatic in itself, but it usually exacerbates the effects of "active" abuse such as incest or physical abuse. Many clients whom we have treated experienced their mother's denial of their sexual abuse ("You're lying!") as more damaging than the actual abuse itself. This particular observation of ours agrees with the available research (12).

Individuals with a history of childhood abuse generally show a variety of mental, emotional, and behavioral difficulties, either at the time of the abuse or later in life. These *difficulties* can include chronic and high levels of depression and anxiety; multiple somatic complaints with a psychological basis; flashbacks, intrusive memories, emotional numbing, and amnesia's high rates of self-defeating behaviors such as suicide attempts and relationships with abusive persons; and interpersonal difficulties such as isolation, emotional detachment, and difficulty trusting others. Survivors can qualify for a variety of *diagnoses*, which can include major depression, various kinds of anxiety disorders, personality disorders, and even (anxiety-based) attention-deficit disorder (13). Experts have attempted to define a common survivor *syndrome* without success because of the variety of symptoms and problems survivors experience. Survivors often have a "disguised presentation," with the common factor of childhood abuse underlying an array of different presenting symptoms and complaints (14).

Understanding that many of our clients have a history of childhood abuse and using this frame to shape treatment holds a number of strengths. Rather than focusing on a multitude of shifting symptoms and diverse presenting problems, we can, instead, deal with core issues and make our interventions more efficient. To enrich and expand our therapeutic approaches, we can adapt conceptual notions and treatment tactics from various bodies of literature, including that on Vietnam veterans with posttraumatic stress disorder, on adult rape survivors and other victims of trauma, and on child development. We can also gain increased insight into and compassion for manifestations of client "resistance," such as outbursts of anger in a session, failure to engage in a therapeutic alliance, and extensive use of denial. Rather than seeing these clients as "difficult," we can see them as hurting and as playing out in our treatment relationship the abuse that other authority figures have inflicted on them. By respecting the impact of trauma on survivors' lives and by validating their experience, we can support survivors instead of retraumatizing them. For any number of reasons, seeing clients with a history of childhood trauma as sharing common issues and responding to similar treatment approaches, and not as a collection of unrelated syndromes, appears to be helpful in our clinical work.

Recent writing surrounding the controversy of "false memory syndrome" has, among other things, certainly pointed to the pitfalls of seeing mental health clients *only* as survivors *even when* they present at intake with no memories of childhood abuse (15). Certainly, there are clients who are reacting to current stresses or who suffer from diseases, such as schizophrenia or bipolar disorder, that have a large genetic component. Certainly, there are difficulties with defining abuse so widely that any stressor experienced in the past is seen as traumatic, thereby trivializing the concept. Certainly, there must be factors that make a difference among clients with a history of abuse. Otherwise, we would not need all of our various diagnostic categories, we would be able to identify a common syndrome, and we would never meet individuals who managed to survive trauma relatively unscathed.

Nonetheless, these facts remain: The majority of children do not experience serious abuse of either the traumatic or the abandoning kind. Those who do experience such abuse appear to be at risk for significant mental, emotional, and behavioral difficulties. Many of the clients we and other professionals see in our practices appear to be survivors of childhood abuse. Most survivors recall at least something of their childhood trauma at intake and are not generally unduly influenced to have false memories. Research on the parameters of childhood abuse (see Chapter 4) can account for some of the differences in presentation among clients who are survivors. And the treatment model we present in Chapters 6 and 7 does allow a way of organizing individual differences among survivors into core themes and treatment categories, a process that we feel makes treatment more effective and efficient.

WORKING THROUGH ABUSE SAFELY

If, how, and when survivors should work through memories of the abuse is somewhat controversial. There are three possible positions: (1) clients do not ever need to work through memories of the abuse; (2) clients must always immediately discuss the abuse and work it through; and (3) clients will have a better treatment outcome if they work through the memories of the abuse, but the clinician must time and titrate this to be effective. We support the third position.

The available literature and our own experience support the value of the third stance. "Active" abuse is traumatic. The theoretical models of trauma responses available in the literature all postulate the value of some sort of reexperiencing of the trauma (16). Psychodynamic thinking emphasizes the ego's use of maladaptive defenses to handle the overwhelming emotional stimulation of the trauma and the resultant need to master the original traumatic situation. Behavioral models use classical conditioning paradigms that support the need to decondition responses through exposure to conditioned stimuli. Even biochemical models focusing on the neurological changes that occur in response to trauma include a role for both medication *and* reexposure in the treatment of such trauma.

The clinical literature almost universally advocates the need to provide clients with a combination of (1) some form of reexposure to and working through of the memory of the original traumatic abuse, (2) social support, and (3) instruction in the learning of new coping skills. The clinical literature also emphasizes either enhancing coping skills prior to working through the abuse or limiting the exposure to manageable doses, or matching the two sets of interventions to the client's current presentation (16). Whether this is viewed as assisting clients to stay in the middle between the extremes of overwhelming flooding and frozen emotional numbing (17) or as assisting them to work at their "affective edge" in order to reexperience painful memories without triggering denial or dissociation (18), the emphasis is on a balanced approach that meets clients where they are in terms of their clinical status and that combines both here-and-now work with efforts to reprocess the past. The available treatment evaluation research suggests that coping skills training has value in the short run and that exposure and working through have value in the long run (19).

While effective treatment requires that survivors ultimately work through traumatic memories, clients sometimes present us with the opposite problem: They come to therapy with suspicions of having been abused and with clinical symptoms that are often associated with a history of abuse but with no specific memories or other hard data to support their suspicions (e.g., siblings revealing that they had been abused), and they want to work to uncover their memories "right now!" In these cases our job is to slow down the client, without communicating rejection and invalidation, and to maintain a balance between being open to the possibility that abuse has occurred and harboring suspicions of being led on a wild goose chase. In other cases clients come to us flooding and overwhelmed by memories. The clinical task in these cases is to prevent clients from drowning and to teach them titration and coping skills. Failing to provide clients with a proper foundation of social support and acquired coping skills while thoughtlessly and relentlessly encouraging them to work through their memories "no matter what" only retraumatizes clients or keeps the experience so dissociated that they gain no benefit.

Treatment of the addicted survivor complicates this issue of what needs to happen first even further. Many recovery experts point out the futility of attempting insight-oriented psychotherapy with someone who is still drinking or using drugs. They may even suggest (or sometimes insist) that the addicted survivor achieve a minimum of a year of abstinence prior to beginning any survivor work. There are others, from the survivor school of therapy, who view chemical use as secondary to the trauma work; these experts believe that survivors are self-medicating their tremendous pain and that once the pain is abreacted, they no longer have a need for chemical use. We respond to these concerns with a both/and, not an either/or attitude. We believe that clinicians cannot ignore painful periods of flooding and suicidal ideation and suggest that abstinence and working an addiction recovery program alone is not the solution. If they feel unable to cope one day at a time with their trauma-based symptoms, survivors may begin to doubt that recovery can work for them.

THE ADDICTED SURVIVOR

The available data suggest that individuals with a psychiatric disorder are at increased risk for having a substance abuse disorder. Epidemiological studies in the United States have reported prevalence rates for chemical abuse and dependency (including alcohol) of 7% in the general community (20). An individual with a past or current psychiatric disorder has a substantially increased risk for substance abuse disorder. The risk is at least double for those with affective and anxiety disorders and is often higher for other psychiatric disorders (21, 22).

A history of childhood sexual and physical abuse is often associated with increased risk of substance use disorder, with some research indicating that trauma involving physical abuse is a particular risk factor (23). Individuals suffering from borderline personality disorder constitute the most thoroughly researched group of survivors. Typically, those suffering from this disorder have experienced emotional neglect and inconsistent parenting as well as serious physical and sexual abuse (4, 9, 24). They are at substantially increased risk of getting into trouble with drugs and alcohol (25, 26). A recent study of women in a chemical dependency treatment center in South Carolina reported that 80% of the women entering treatment for addiction had a history of sexual abuse and that 32% had been abused before the age of 11 (49).

Clinical and research data (27) consistently show a high correlation between parents having a substance abuse disorder (especially fathers) and physical and sexual abuse directed toward their children. Survivors would thus appear to have a genetic vulnerability to developing chemical dependency as well as familial modeling of substance abuse. In addition, survivors have higher rates of either "acting-in" symptoms, such as depression and social withdrawal, or "acting-out" symptoms, such as aggressive behavior and promiscuity, than members of the general population. Using chemicals not only provides an opportunity to obtain relief from the distressing negative emotional states associated with "acting in" but also satisfies the high need for excitement, immediate gratification, and defiance of authority commonly found among acting-out clients.

Many survivors constantly feel a profound sense of loneliness and alienation from others. To satisfy their need to belong, a need common to all people, survivors—with their shattered self-esteem, fears, and unmet needs for connection—are at extremely high risk for gravitating toward the most readily available forms of social support: the crowd at the local tavern and drug-using party people.

Furthermore, current traumatic experiences are extremely common for individuals who abuse chemicals. These include accidents as well as physical and sexual assaults. In our clinical experience, survivors of childhood sexual abuse, especially when chemically dependent, tend to have multiple traumatic sexual experiences in their current lives. We have heard many accounts from both our adolescent and adult female clients of having been raped at a party by a drunken partner who assumed they were promiscuous because they were drinking and would not take no for an answer. Even more troubling are the frequent accounts of gang rapes that we hear from many of the young women we treat, again revealing the attitude common in our society that men are entitled to have sex with a drunken female. Young women are increasingly gang raped in their initiation into gangs or as part of being a "good time for the sect."

Survivors who have a substance use disorder have "double trouble" in comparison to survivors who do not. Substance use disorders by definition entail negative consequences because of the substance abuse (27). Survivors then experience two sets of difficulties. Substance abuse and dependency also interact to exacerbate the psychiatric symptoms survivors have, increasing the frequency and intensity of such symptoms as disabling levels of anxiety and depression (28). High rates of substance use also appear to be associated with an increased rate of other difficulties, such as suicide attempts (7, 29). Survivors with chemical use problems find themselves in a vicious and accelerating circle of pain and problems.

This "double trouble" also extends to the manner in which substance use disorders can thwart treatment efforts. As discussed in more detail in Chapter 4, denial is a cardinal feature of chemical use disorders. Denial encompasses a set of attitudes based on the individual's belief that he or she does not have a problem and that treatment is not necessary. Survivors with acting-out defenses often show denial about the need to focus on themselves and take responsibility for their part in their difficulties. They excuse their behavior and blame others to an extent that is dysfunctional. Even acting-in survivors often have denial about their childhood abuse. Survivors of either variety who are also in trouble with substances often have double denial and, consequently, have decreased motivation for treatment. Most individuals do not enter therapy, with its painful work and investment of time, energy, and money, because they want to. They generally seek treatment and stay in therapy because they have to, either because of external pressures or internal distress. Chemical use increases the likelihood that survivors will resist external pressures, denying they have a problem, and dilutes their motivation for therapy by temporarily reducing their internal distress. Finally, successful treatment of abuse involves reexposure and reexperiencing of uncomfortable emotions, as we have discussed in the previous section. Mood-altering chemicals can block the reexperiencing of anxiety and other negative emotions necessary for depth treatment of the abuse and can reinforce the patterns of emotional and behavioral avoidance typically found among survivors (28, 30).

The implications of the preceding discussion are clear. Clinicians must be ready to identify, assess, and treat substance use disorders when working with survivors. Survivors are at increased risk for substance abuse, which in turn increases the risk of additional trauma. Exploration of substance use patterns when assessing survivors for treatment needs is crucial, and if any doubt about an individual's chemical use exists, abstinence is indicated.

MODELS FOR TREATING ADDICTION
AND ALCOHOLISM

Clinicians attempting to treat survivors with a substance use disorder face the task of selecting a treatment approach or combination of approaches that will address the chemical abuse. Several different approaches for treating substance abuse and dependence exist. Unfortunately, no strong consensus exists among professionals about the best approach in general or with a particular client. While the 12-step recovery model for treating chemical dependence is probably the most widely accepted approach among addiction specialists, this acceptance is not universal.

Moral Model

The moral model views substance abuse as a sign of sin, a character defect, bad behavior, and/or as a legal matter only. Society, for the most part, continues to hold this stance, as does the typical client. The moral model suggests that the remedy for chemical dependency is taking the pledge, trying harder, or going to jail. The expression *falling off the wagon* illustrates the idea that the drunk has fallen from some previous height (or at least a height considered to be higher than acute intoxication). The "accountability" notion is a variant of the moral model in which the substance abuser is seen as needing to be more responsible and less weak willed. To date, the results of this approach seem unimpressive, and in the case of survivors filled with more than enough shame and guilt it is more likely to be harmful than helpful. In addition, anyone who has treated alcoholics and addicts knows that they are anything but weak willed—they are, in fact, paragons of self-will. For the most part, professionals have abandoned the moral model of substance abuse disorder but sometimes moralize more or less overtly in practice.

Mental Health Models

Traditional mental health approaches view the person's problems with chemicals as a symptom of or response to a psychiatric disorder or family dysfunction (31, 32). Whether seen as self-medication, a sign of personality disorder, or a response to an out-of-kilter family, this "symptom of something else" view suggests that using applicable mental health interventions for the "underlying" problem is all that is needed to get a person clean and sober. According to this model, treating those problems of survivors that stem from their childhood abuse is probably sufficient for eliminating the chemical use disorder. A popular variant of this view is the belief that chemically dependent individuals are self-medicating their emotional pain. While "relief" use of chemicals is often part of the use pattern of many addicts and alcoholics (including addicted survivors), we believe this is a symptom of the disease of addiction and not its cause.

Education Models

Other approaches focus on the chemical dependency as an independent problem in its own right. Educational approaches, either alone or in combination with other types of intervention, are commonly used. In the education model of treatment clinicians attempt to motivate their clients to moderate or stop their substance use by providing them with information (33). Lectures and reading material about chemicals and their negative consequences, perhaps supplemented by objective and detailed feedback about the client's own personal symptoms and problems via X rays, psychological testing, and the concerns of significant others, are standard components of this approach. Persons in the early stages of getting in trouble with chemicals often benefit from an educational approach (34).

Behavioral Models

Behavioral therapies are another set of approaches used for individuals with substance use disorders. Aversive conditioning (in which the sight, smell, and taste of alcohol is paired with a noxious stimulus such as electric shock or chemically induced vomiting) attempts to promote avoidance of chemicals through a classic behavioral approach (35). Some skills training approaches attempt to train clients to control their drinking. Examples of such interventions include having individuals keep a written journal to increase their awareness of their drinking pattern, encouraging them to substitute slower drinking rates, and arranging for rewards for their success in modifying their use of chemicals (36). Using medications—for example, disulfiram (Antabuse), to produce an aversive reaction to alcohol; methadone, to block withdrawal symptoms and any euphoric affect from opiate use; benzodiazepines, for managing alcohol withdrawal; and antidepressants, for cocaine withdrawal symptoms—represent clinical tactics designed to, among other things, promote abstinence by decreasing the rewards of substance use and the unpleasant effects of eliminating intake of the chemical (37, 38).

Contingency management tactics have received more attention recently and show treatment outcomes suggesting some value for these approaches (39). In general, these procedures involve random urinalysis to detect chemical use and the provision of concrete awards and penalties (e.g., involving money) to reinforce abstinence. Defining contingencies more broadly, therapists may attempt to reinforce abstinence by improving the client's job status, empowering family members to discourage use or risk loss of relationship, or increasing alternative recreational opportunities. Another variant within the behavioral framework is a more cognitive–behavioral approach (40). Clinicians using this approach attempt to make clients more aware of problematic thinking patterns associated with substance use and to teach them to substitute more productive ones.

The strengths of these behavioral approaches typically involve a commitment to an empirical evaluation of results. In addition, chemically dependent clients will sometimes accept these approaches when they will not accept the 12-step recovery approach. Critics of these approaches point out that while clients may decrease their use of particular substance, such as cocaine, seasoned clients often go on to accelerate their use of other substances. Another criticism frequently heard is that unless chemically dependent persons make significant and substantial life-style changes across the board, they are likely to relapse after treatment.

The Disease Model of Addiction and the 12-Step Recovery Model

The disease process model of addiction, coupled with a 12-step recovery approach, is currently one of the most influential and widely used models employed by alcohol and drug counselors. This recovery model has two key assumptions and four essential treatment tactics. The first assumption is that chemical dependency is a disease, one for which there is no cure but whose progression can be arrested by abstinence from all mood-altering chemicals. The second assumption is that a chemically dependent individual must not only abstain from mood-altering substances but also complete a program of recovery to repair the personal and social consequences of addiction and to prevent a relapse. Studies of controlled drinking approaches that show high rates of relapse and continued and accelerating life problems due to drinking (including deaths) provide support for the need for abstinence (41). The treatment tactics of a 12-step recovery program involve (1) attending 12-step support group meetings; (2) "working" the 12 steps of Alcoholics Anonymous (AA); (3) having a sponsor, or personal guide, for help with working the steps; and (4) developing an enhanced sense of spirituality (42).

We draw heavily from the disease model of addiction and from the 12-step recovery approach in our work with survivors. We find these notions and tactics useful for several different reasons. Survivors have enormous amounts of shame, are socially alienated, and have a wide variety of psychosocial problems, including those involving issues of powerlessness and control. Abstinence is an appropriate goal for survivors who are chemically dependent and would appear to be a reasonable goal even for survivors who abuse chemicals, given their risk for addiction and the detrimental effect of chemicals on treatment. The concept of chemical dependency as a disease provides a helpful way to talk to survivors about what their problem is and what they need to do. It minimizes shame and helps to shift the focus away from the "blame game" to an emphasis on taking positive action to get healthy (43). The 12-step slogan "Not bad getting good, but sick getting well" captures the spirit of this perspective. Moreover, the 12-step program provides a readily available source of social support. Through meetings and the adjunct recreational activities that AA groups typically sponsor, this "second family" or circle of understanding friends provides survivors with the kind of supportive experiences that were previously lacking to them and also supports the therapeutic process. Working the 12 steps provides a structured approach to dealing with denial; confronting distorted notions of control, hopelessness, and shame; and developing healthy attitudes that decrease the chances of relapse. A sponsor can provide additional and special support for the survivor, and attention to spiritual issues can help survivors deal with questions of faith, hope, and the meaning of their experience, questions that plague survivors. The 12-step approach provides ongoing, long-term encouragement of a new and different life-style. Finally, similar 12-step meetings are also available for other family members.

We acknowledge that simply using chemicals does not necessarily mean that a person is addicted and needs full-scale alcohol and drug treatment. We are aware of the fact that the notion that chemical dependency is a disease is controversial and has its critics (44). We know that the emphasis on spirituality found in 12-step approaches is especially controversial (41). We also appreciate that other approaches have generated useful treatment tactics and are pragmatic enough to borrow from them and to apply 12-step notions flexibly. We have used educational methods that were enough to promote abstinence in survivors who were clearly using alcohol to self-medicate, and we have encouraged the use of Antabuse in survivors who had trouble with impulsive drinking. We have had clients evaluated for antidepressant medication not only when careful evaluation suggested an endogenous depression but also when cocaine withdrawal symptoms were intense and prolonged. We use urine-drug screens, set up behavior contracts, teach refusal skills, conduct family counseling, and refer clients for vocational assistance and training. We also understand that precisely because the 12-step program addresses core issues, survivors will also need therapeutic assistance to embrace this approach. For example, for hypersensitive survivors to openly share in a 12-step meeting often takes preparation. We have seen standard applications of "step work" fail (and even backfire) often enough to have developed written material that modifies this process by taking into account issues particular to survivors and thus helps them work the steps. And we understand that no one approach has proven vastly superior to all others and that, given individual differences, no one approach is likely to ever suit all clients.

The 12-step approach is consistent with other models of changing addictive behavior (45) and, nonetheless, we have found the 12-step approach to recovery very helpful when working with chemically dependent survivors. This approach is the primary source for strategies targeting the substance dependence of our survivor clients. Our experience has shown that the 12-step recovery approach provides a comprehensive and clinically rich basis for helping survivors who cannot just say no to chemicals in spite of being advised/educated to moderate/stop their intake. We do modify the 12-step recovery approach and combine it with other interventions when this is appropriate and when the core of the 12-step approach can be maintained. We will reserve a detailed discussion of our application of these notions for later chapters.

THE NEED FOR AN INTEGRATED MODEL

We and other writers in the area of "dual diagnosis" have consistently argued for an integrated treatment approach for clients suffering from substance abuse disorders and coexisting psychiatric disorders (46, 47). Not only does the treatment need to address both illnesses simultaneously, but it must weave the treatment together in order to address the intertwined reality of these two fused conditions.

Survivors with chemical use problems certainly have dual diagnoses, and any model for treating these clients should have certain characteristics to be effective. There are two key characteristics that we feel are necessary for the success of a treatment program for chemically dependent survivors: The program must be comprehensive and coordinated.

A comprehensive model is one that adopts a broad clinical perspective that blends both mental health and substance dependence treatment modalities. A successful blend takes seriously the notion that these disorders are coexisting, independent illnesses worthy of equal attention; it recognizes that the substance abuse disorder did not cause (although it may exacerbate) the survivor's psychiatric difficulties and vice versa. These separate illnesses exhibit a synergism that requires that they receive simultaneous treatment. The clinician should not wait for survivors to achieve abstinence before starting treatment for their abuse-related difficulties. The reverse holds equally true. This is not to say that survivors should be confronting their abuser during detox! As detailed in later chapters, a strong foundation laid in early recovery is necessary before any "advanced" work is done.

Traditional mental health and substance dependence approaches tend to have points of view that differ from this "dual" view. Both these viewpoints make great use of the primary–secondary distinction. The strong form of this distinction is that one of these disorders is "primary," that it is the cause of the other; it is believed that treating the primary disorder automatically addresses the "secondary" one. The weaker form of the primary–secondary distinction gives treatment priority to the emergent problem by focusing on this "primary" one first. Only after a significant period of psychiatric stability (if the mental health problem is considered the primary one) or abstinence (if the chemical dependence is considered primary) does the other issue, the "secondary" one, merit attention.

The primary–secondary distinction tends to ignore several important issues. While survivors appear to be at higher risk for chemical dependency, many survivors are not chemically dependent and many chemically dependent persons are not survivors, suggesting at least somewhat independent processes. There is also, as noted earlier, a synergism between survivors' psychiatric and substance abuse disorders. Having both disorders seems to intensify the symptoms and problems of each disorder. For example, prolonged substance abuse increases symptoms of depression and anxiety (29) and many suicide attempts and other self-destructive behaviors occur while individuals are intoxicated. In addition, survivors are unlikely to achieve prolonged periods of stability in either area unless they receive simultaneous treatment for their coexisting disorders. Survivors are very unlikely to attain psychiatric stability if the substance abuse is continuing. Conversely, they are unlikely to achieve significant periods of abstinence if their coexisting psychiatric disorder is untreated. Survivors, for example, are at higher risk for relapse after alcohol and drug treatment than "singly" diagnosed chemically dependent people (48).

The second key characteristic of an integrated model, the approach be coordinated, entails focusing on *common* issues in the two disorders and using *comprehensive* interventions whenever possible. Survivors, especially those dependent on chemicals, present with a vast array of symptoms and problems, which could lead clinicians to attempt to implement a vast array of interventions. For example, a clinician may ask himself or herself, "Do I focus on the severe anxiety, the drinking, or the current abusive relationship that this client is in?" Without a coordinated approach that provides a focus, clinicians run the risk of chasing after too many problems and of inundating clients with too many interventions. Both parties can come to feel overwhelmed, and the treatment can exhaust the time and resources available. Compounding this problem is the fact that service delivery systems tend to focus on either the psychiatric disorder or the chemical dependency. Besides promoting primary–secondary thinking, this fragmentation repeats survivors' experience in their family and, at worst, can present conflicting models to survivors, which adds to their sense of feeling "crazy."

A coordinated model also takes into account the need to *blend* elements of mental health and chemical dependence treatment approaches if dual treatment is to work. Examination of mental health and recovery treatment models reveals many points of convergence that can serve as bridges. Both, for example, use the notion of syndromes, emphasize social support, strive for insight and acceptance of their life problems, provide for practice of communication and other skills, and make use of structured counseling and therapy interventions. Referring a client to a divorce recovery group or an AA group in each case involves the objective of providing social support. In addition to emphasizing commonalities, blending the two approaches requires unifying positions on several points that often produce conflict. Some of these key flash points are psychotropic medications, spirituality, and labeling (calling oneself an alcoholic/addict and survivor).

The rest of this book discusses the issues that blending raises in much greater detail. The next chapter presents the extended story of one of our clients. This case history illustrates the impact of severe childhood abuse and the process of recovery of a chemically dependent survivor who is getting well, one day at a time.

REFERENCES

1. Crewdson, J. (1988). *By silence betrayed: Sexual abuse of children in America.* Boston: Little, Brown.
2. Jacobson, A., & Richardson, B. (1987). Assault experiences of 100 psychiatric inpatients: Evidence of the need for routine inquiry. *American Journal of Psychiatry, 144,* 908–913.
3. Bryer, J. B., Bernadette, A. N., Miller, J. B., et al. (1987). Childhood sexual and physical abuse as factors in adult psychiatric illness. *American Journal of Psychiatry, 144,* 1426–1430.
4. Harman, S., Finn, S. E., & Leon, G. U. (1987). Sexual abuse experiences in a clinical population: Comparisons of familial and nonfamilial abuse. *Psychotherapy, 24*(2), 154–159.
5. Haratera, S., Alexander, P. C., & Neimeyer, R. A. (1988). Long-term efforts of incestuous child abuse in college women: Social adjustment, social cognition and family characteristics. *Journal of Consulting and Clinical Psychology, 51*(1), 5–8.
6. Briere, J., & Runitz, M. (1988). Symptomatology associated with sexual victimization in a nonclinical adult sample. *Child Abuse and Neglect, 12,* 51–59.
7. Sanders, B., & Geolas, M. H. (1991). Dissociation and childhood trauma in psychologically disturbed adolescents. *American Journal of Psychiatry, 148*(1), 50–54.

8. Zanarini, M. C., & Gunderson, T. B. (1987). Childhood abuse common in borderline personality. *Clinical Psychiatry News, 6*, 1.
9. Jarmas, A. L., & Kazak, A. E. (1992). Young adult children of alcoholic fathers: Depressive experiences, coping styles and family systems. *Journal of Consulting and Clinical Psychology, 60*(2), 244–251.
10. Braver, M., Bumberry, J., Greene, K., et al. (1992). Childhood abuse and current psychological functioning in a university counseling center population. *Journal of Counseling Psychology, 39*(22), 252–257.
11. Carmen, E. H. (1984). Victims of violence and psychiatric illness. *American Journal of Psychiatry, 141*, 378–383.
12. Gold, E. (1986). Long-term effects of sexual victimization in childhood: An attributional approach. *Journal of Consulting and Clinical Psychology, 54*(4), 471–475.
13. Terr, L. C. (1991). Childhood traumas: An outline and overview. *American Journal of Psychiatry, 148*(1), 10–20.
14. Gelinas, D. (1983). The persisting negative effects of incest. *Psychiatry, 46*, 312–332.
15. Yapko, M. D. (1994). *Suggestions of abuse: True and false memories of childhood sexual trauma.* New York: Simon & Schuster.
16. Fairbank, J. A., & Nicholson, R. A. (1987). Theoretical and empirical issues in the treatment of post-traumatic stress disorder in Vietnam veterans. *Journal of Clinical Psychology, 43*(1), 44–55.
17. Horowitz, M. J. (1973). Phase-oriented treatment of stress response syndromes. *American Journal of Psychotherapy, 27*, 505–515.
18. Cornell, W. F., & Oleo, K. A. (1991). Integrating affect in treatment with adult survivors of physical and sexual abuse. *American Journal of Orthopsychiatry, 61*(1), 59–69.
19. Foa, B. E., Rothbaum, B. O., Riggs, D. S., & Murdock, T. B. (1991). Treatment of post-traumatic stress disorder in rape victims: A comparison between cognitive–behavioral procedures and counseling. *Journal of Consulting and Clinical Psychology, 59*(5), 715–723.
20. Myers, J. K., Weissman, M. M., Tischler, G. L., et al. (1984). Six-month prevalence of psychiatric disorders in three communities. *Archives of General Psychiatry, 41*, 959–967.
21. Christies, K. A., Burke, J. D., Regner, D. A., et al. (1988). Epidemiologic evidence for early onset of mental disorders and higher risk of drug abuse in young adults. *American Journal of Psychiatry, 148*(8), 971–975.
22. Luthar, G. G., Anton, S. F., Merikangas, K. R., et al. (1992). Vulnerability to substance abuse and psychopathology among siblings of opiate abusers. *Journal of Nervous and Mental Disease, 180*(3), 153–161.
23. Brown, G. R., & Anderson, B. (1991). Psychiatric morbidity in adult inpatients with childhood histories of sexual and physical abuse. *American Journal of Psychiatry, 148*, 55–61.
24. Gartner, A. F., & Gartner, J. (1988). Borderline pathology in post-incest female adolescents. *The Menninger Bulletin, 52*, 101–115.
25. Nace, E. P. (1987). *The treatment of alcoholism.* New York: Brunner/Mazel.

26. American Psychiatric Association. (1994). *Diagnostic and statistical manual of mental disorders* (4th ed.). Washington, DC: Author.
27. Frick, P. J., Lahey, B. B., Loeber, R., et al. (1992). Familial risk factors for oppositional defiant disorder and conduct disorder: Parental psychopathology and maternal parenting. *Journal of Consulting and Clinical Psychology, 60*(1), 49–55.
28. Kranzler, H. K., & Liebowitz, N. R. (1988). Anxiety and depression in substance abuse. *Medical Clinics of North America, 72*(4), 867–885.
29. Shuckit, M. A. (1985). The clinical implications of primary diagnostic groups among alcoholics. *Archives of General Psychiatry, 42,* 1043–1049.
30. Bibb, J. L., & Chambless, D. L. (1986). Alcohol use and abuse among diagnosed agoraphobics. *Behaviour Research and Therapy, 24,* 49–58.
31. Institute of Medicine. (1987). Psychopathology related to alcohol abuse. In *Causes and consequences of alcohol problems* (pp. 133–151). Washington, DC: National Academy Press.
32. Khantzian, E. (1985). The self-medication hypothesis of addictive disorders: Focus on heroin and cocaine dependence. *American Journal of Psychiatry, 142,* 1256–1264.
33. Chick, J., Lloyd, G., & Crombie, E. (1980). *Early identification of the problem drinker.* Washington, DC: National Institute of Alcohol Abuse and Alcoholism.
34. Miller, W. R. (1985). Motivation for treatment: A review with special emphasis on alcoholism. *Psychiatric Bulletin, 48*(1), 84–1007.
35. Miller, W. R., & Hester, R. K. (1980). Treating the problem drinker: Modern approaches. In W. R. Miller (Ed.), *The addictive behaviors: Treatment of alcoholism, drug abuses, smoking and obesity* (pp. 111–141). Oxford, UK: Pergamon Press.
36. Miller, W. R., & Munoz, R. F. (1982). *How to control your drinking* (2nd ed.). Albuquerque, NM: University of New Mexico Press.
37. Shuckit, M. A. (1984). *Drugs and alcohol abuse: A clinical guide to diagnosis and treatment.* New York: Plenum Press.
38. Kleber, N. D., Gowin, F. N., Washton, A. M., et al. (Eds.). (1987). *Cocaine: A clinician's handbook.* New York: Guilford Press.
39. Higgins, S. T., Delaney, D. D., Budney, A. J., et al. (1991). A behavioral approach to achieving initial cocaine abstinence. *American Journal of Psychiatry, 148*(9), 1218–1224.
40. Walker, R. (1992). Substance abuse and B-cluster disorders II: Treatment recommendations. *Journal of Psychoactive Drugs, 24*(3), 233–241.
41. Christopher, J. (1992). *SOS sobriety.* Buffalo, NY: Prometheus Books.
42. Alcoholics Anonymous World Services. (1976). *Alcoholics Anonymous.* New York: Author.
43. Stone, A. M. (1992). The role of shame in post-traumatic stress disorder. *American Journal of Orthopsychiatry, 62*(1), 131–136.
44. Walters, G. D. (1992). Drug-seeking behavior: Disease or lifestyle? *Professional Psychology: Research and Practice, 23*(2), 139–145.
45. Prochaska, J. O., DiClemente, C. C., & Noncross, J. C. (1992). In search of

how people change: An application to addictive behaviors. *American Psychologist, 47*(9), 1102–1114.

46. Evans, K., & Sullivan, J. M. (1990). *Dual diagnosis: Counseling the mentally ill substance abuser.* New York: Guilford Press.
47. Polcin, D. L. (1992). Issues in the treatment of dual diagnosis clients who have chronic mental illness. *Professional Psychology: Research and Practice, 23*(1), 30–37.
48. Nace, E. P., Saxon, J. J., & Shore, N. (1986). Borderline personality disorder and alcoholism treatment: A one year follow-up study. *Journal of Studies on Alcoholism, 47,* 196–260.
49. Grice, D. E., Brady, K. T., Dustan, L. R., et al. (1994). PTSD, victimization and substance abuse. *American Journal of Psychiatry.* Manuscript submitted for publication.

CHAPTER 2

Rachel's Story

✧

The Black Hole

Living to sleep, laughing to fight back tears,
I feel so misplaced here as if something is not right.
I laugh, what is the meaning in anything and everything?
If I kill myself I will die to find what?
My holiness is dead for they took it from me,
I am trapped in this black hole forever.
I use to try to break free, but now I have let go,
I am falling still deeper.
I begin to laugh, I laugh so loud,
I do not know why I am laughing
I just laugh in the face of life.
Behind my laugh is a big hidden tear.
I once had a God, something to believe in, but now there is
    nothing! I cling to my loud barbaric laugh.
So come on and laugh with me, laugh really loud! Scream!
Laugh with me!

—RACHEL, age 14

Rachel was a 14-year-old girl at the time she was referred to us by a school counselor. She was suspected of having smoked marijuana at school with some other adolescents, and during a search of her locker school officials found an empty beer bottle. School policy required that a drug and alcohol evaluation be done under such circumstances, and so Rachel was referred to us.

During the initial assessment it became clear that Rachel had not only a drug and alcohol problem but also significant survivor issues related to a long history of sexual and physical abuse. In her first interview Rachel was dressed in a highly seductive manner: She wore a very skimpy blouse and a tight micro-miniskirt with black fishnet stockings. She did not wear a bra, and her makeup—black eyeliner, purple lipstick, and lip liner—was applied heavily. She looked very much like a young woman who was trying to merchandise herself as a sexual object. At the same time, Rachel's emotional presentation left an impression far different from that made by her attire. In the interview she sat huddled over, folded into herself, and she tended to talk in a soft, childlike voice when Katie interviewed her alone. When her mother later joined the interview, Rachel assumed a surly adolescent attitude, arguing with her mother about each and every minute detail of her situation.

In addition to her singular behavior and dress, Rachel exhibited a somewhat unusual thinking style. She tended to bounce between the concrete thinking of a young child or someone suffering from schizophrenia to a more intellectual, insightful, and adult mode of thinking. There was also a strong psychotic flavor to her discussions: She reported seeing bloody daggers and frightening scenes at times. She also vacillated between being quite closed off and suspicious to the point of paranoia and being overly compliant and too self-revealing.

At the time of intake, Rachel was drinking and using chemicals on a nearly daily basis. She was in constant conflict with her mother, and her school performance was poor. She suffered from mood swings, lapses in concentration, anxiety, depression, and outbursts of anger. She also had clear memories of experiencing substantial childhood abuse. We developed an outpatient plan for her treatment.

In the pages that follow is the story of Rachel's life, trauma, strength, and recovery. We have provided as many details of this case as we can without breaching the confidentiality of Rachel and her family members. We also have Rachel's and her mother's permission to present this material. We have changed some of the facts to protect her identity (e.g., *Rachel* is a pseudonym).

Readers may find the graphic detail of Rachel's story rough going. If you should become overwhelmed or feel unsafe, put down the book or skip this chapter. You will not miss any significant information about our treatment approach. Our goal is not to titillate or traumatize but to illustrate in concrete detail the subject matter of this book. In particular, we focus on the early stages of Rachel's dual recovery from substance dependence and trauma because the early therapy work is often the most difficult for us and for other counselors.

Rachel never knew her father. He and her mother divorced when she was an infant. Rachel never received birthday cards from her father but did occasionally get a note from her father's sister, who notified Rachel of her father's death when Rachel was 11 years old.

Rachel's mother was living in a commune at the time of Rachel's birth in the '70s. The commune embraced many "alternative" beliefs, including those regarding promiscuous sexual relations and the heavy use of mood- and mind-altering chemicals. All adults in the commune were "family members" who shared resources, child care duties, and so forth. To complicate matters further, sexual partners were fairly polygamous, and there was a free exchange of sexual favors between adults. Commune members believed that people should "make love in front of children, as they make war and fight in front of children." Thus, Rachel observed numerous adults having sex, including her mother, who had sex with her partner while Rachel was awake and in the same bed. Rachel found all these "mommies and daddies" confusing.

Rachel also witnessed her mother's addictive use of cocaine and was able to recall an incident in which her mother had overdosed: Her mother sat on the floor rocking, urinating on herself, and crying out, "Please, please can't someone help me; please, Rachel, help me; I am going to die!" Rachel had flashbacks of this scene for many years. She also remembered being frightened at night. It was "against the rules" to get up and go to the bathroom or to make any noise. Rachel recalled urinating in the closet into a pair of her own shoes in desperation one night because she "couldn't hold it any longer" and her mother was too impaired from drugs and alcohol to take her to the bathroom located outside their sleeping quarters.

When Rachel was 2½ years old her mother left the commune and went first to live with her own mother and then to a small apartment. Rachel's mother located day care for her daughter through a "friend of a commune brother" so that she could begin to work. She believed that Rachel was in good hands at a Christian day-care center.

From ages 2 to 4 and on a near-daily basis Rachel was fondled, sodomized, and forced to preform oral sex by a male teacher who owned the day-care center and worked there. With amazing clarity Rachel was able to recount the first time he approached her sexually. (When she first told us this story, Rachel was dissociated and spoke in a flat, emotionless tone of voice as if she were reciting a list of spelling words.) Rachel recalled that the "teacher" asked her if he could "touch her privates" and "lick her privates." She was very frightened and cried when this happened. She told the teacher that what he wanted her to do was "naughty" and that she did not want to do it because she would get into trouble with her mommy. The teacher told the little girl that what he was showing her was one of the "lessons" that he needed to teach her at school. He told her, "All little girls learn these lessons about touching other people in special ways." He explained that he was just trying to do his job, adding that if she told her mother about these "lessons," he would have to kill her for being a "bad girl" who did not want to learn at school and for making such a "fuss" about learning. And if she died, he continued, he would have to kill her mommy also because her mommy would be too ashamed at having such a bad daughter and too sad at her death to go on living.

Rachel complied with her "teacher's" demands in order to live and to save her mother's life. Rachel was cooperative with her abuser and did what she was told, trying hard to be a strong and "good" little girl so that she could make her mother happy and so that she could live safely. Rachel had assumed the role of protector of her mother at the age of 3 and, understandably, believed that she was literally responsible not only for her own life but for her mother's.

Rachel was full of fear and tension. She hated her special "lessons." Rachel never told her mother—or anyone else—about the abuse because of the threats her offender had made. She did try to protect herself indirectly by complaining about having "tummy aches" and playing sick to avoid going to school. But because Rachel's mother was a single parent and needed to go to work to pay the bills, the little girl's ploy did not meet with much success; her mother insisted that she go to the day-care center. It was only later, when she was in treatment, that Rachel finally told her mother why she had not liked going there.

The abuser's double-bind message made her mother a part of the abuse scenario in Rachel's mind. A child's natural tendency to believe parents are all-knowing and all-powerful reinforced this message. Rachel felt in a double bind toward her mother as well: Although she felt that she had to protect her mother, she also came to seriously and deeply mistrust her.

Among her bad memories, Rachel had recalled that her abuser would tell her that her vaginal area tasted like "butterscotch." Rachel soon began avoiding butterscotch; she became violently ill when butterscotch pudding was served in school or when she saw butterscotch topping being served in a restaurant. When asked by her mother what was wrong, Rachel simply stated, "Butterscotch makes me sick." Rachel learned at a very young age that it is not always safe to tell the truth. (Our own secondary traumatic response to Rachel's experience is that neither of us can enjoy the taste of butterscotch. This has not, of course, made our lives unmanageable, but our reaction does demonstrate the secondary trauma that this work can cause professionals.)

When Rachel was 4 her mother moved to the Pacific Northwest. Unfortunately, a new type of abuse—at the hands of her mother's new boyfriend—replaced the abuse of the day-care center. Since Rachel's new "daddy" did not work during the day, he took care of her while her mother worked to support the three of them. On a nearly daily basis this boyfriend would force Rachel to have oral sex with him and would attempt to penetrate her rectally. This pulled Rachel's mother into an abusive dynamic once again. The little girl thought, now more than ever, that her mother really did know about the abuse and that the abusers somehow had her mother's permission to hurt her.

We want to deal with some questions about Rachel's mother and her role at this point. Did she know what her child was experiencing? Was she dissociated? Too trusting? Too busy making a living and too tired to notice? Rachel's mother admitted to us her past drug use and to Rachel's experience in the commune. She sincerely denied knowing of her daughter's subsequent experiences and was devastated when she learned how much the child had suffered.

The continued violation of Rachel's trust and respect for her mother, the only consistent figure in her life, laid the foundation for her distrust of all authority figures, a reaction that was exacerbated in adolescence. Rachel was extremely rebellious at the time of her admission to our outpatient program.

Rachel first took drugs and alcohol at age 7; a teenage girl who baby-sat Rachel thought it was "cool" to get the child high. During the early part of her treatment Rachel, who was proud of having begun her drug abuse at a younger age than her peers, would describe this baby-sitter in a positive light. This attitude naturally changed once she began to understand her own addiction and work her own recovery program. Rachel reported that when she began to use drugs and alcohol, she felt the incredible pain and burden of her young life diminish for the first time ever. The impression this made on her, this power of chemicals, cannot be overstated. Rachel felt that she had, at long last, finally found a "friend" who would help her ease her pain; when she was under the influence of chemicals, she found a measure of peace and some respite from the pain that pierced her insides.

Rachel never really felt that she fitted in with children her own age. During the abuse at the day care center, Rachel was given a "priestess" status; this incited jealousy and envy in other children and prevented the formation of friendships. Rachel was actually very shy and often depressed. After school she sought the solitude and safety of her room and the magical set of friends in the "pretend world" she developed through her vivid fantasy life. In her pretend world, the children had all the power and the adults took good care of them and spent all their time meeting the children's every want and need. Rachel had the fantasy that her father would one day drive up to her house in a shiny, expensive new car; would shower her with armfuls of gifts just for her; and would take her to a Disneyland-type life free of pain and poverty. The smaller the amount of money her mother was able to earn, the more elaborate was her fantasy about what an important person her father was and how much he really loved her. Rachel began to imagine that her mother was jealous that her father loved her more and that her mother was trying to keep her away from her father. She would write her father special letters and draw him beautiful pictures, but she had no address to send them to. She told us,

"I saved my gifts for Daddy so that when he did come he could see them all!"

A world of make-believe built on a foundation of fragmentation, dissociation, and chemically induced trance states was a natural breeding ground for paranoid thinking. These fearful thoughts such as "life is a lie" or "all men want you for is sex" made Rachel hold back and avoid mingling with children her own age and trusting adults. By age 10 she was beginning to experience severe problems with her peers at school. She was shy, frightened, hurt, and ill clothed (as a single parent on a minimum wage job, Rachel's mother could not provide her daughter with the kind of clothing worn by her classmates). Although she was shabbily dressed and ashamed, Rachel showed up at school and did her best to try to fit in. Her efforts were met, however, with the harsh teasing of her peers. Called a "nerd" and a "weirdo," Rachel began to withdraw more and more. Failing grades replaced her once excellent ones, and her high intelligence proved to be no match for her plummeting self-esteem. The more left out she felt the more desperately she tried to fit in, and the harder she tried the more she felt the rejection of children who only wanted to associate with those they considered "cool" or popular. Rachel simply did not fit their job description.

To avoid going to school, Rachel often pretended to be sick, overslept, and arranged to have nothing clean to wear. Her mother met direct attempts to miss school with lectures on "the importance of a good education." While this is a value most people endorse, Rachel lacked an orientation toward the future that made having a high school diploma—or education in general—seem important to her; she was trying to survive on a day-to-day basis. Moreover, Rachel's associations to the concepts of lessons and learning were tinged with cruel memories of her experiences with the day-care "teacher."

Rachel would make up stories about herself in order to make herself interesting, and therefore likable, to her peers. But instead of becoming more popular, she became known as a liar. When Rachel did not turn in her homework assignments, her frustrated teachers sometimes regarded her lack of compliance as evidence of resistance or oppositional behavior and administered various negative consequences, which only heightened Rachel's dislike for and distrust of both school and authority figures.

Rachel became more and more convinced that she had somehow caused not only her sexual abuse but also all of her difficulties at home and at school. She continuously thought about things she felt she should have said or done that might have changed her situation, and she made up magic words to use as a way to stay safe.

Deciding that one way to stay safe was to shut out other people, Rachel became a loner. This way, she felt, she was in control. Others were not rejecting her, she was rejecting them. She tried to act tough and as if she did not care that she was left out of her peers' social activities. (She was, for example, the only child left in line after all the other children were chosen for teams when games were played at school.) Sometimes well-meaning teachers would try to help Rachel. However, Rachel's distrust of authority and her conviction that adults were unable to have any true positive impact on her life only made her perceive their helpful attempts as a nuisance and an embarrassment. At first Rachel felt hurt by these well-meaning efforts; then she gradually became angry.

Isolated, rejected, and alone, Rachel contemplated suicide for the first time when she was 11 years old. She was unable to think of any other way to stop the pain in her life. She wanted things to "just quit hurting." Rachel spent hours, days, and months thinking of painless and "messless" ways to end it all. She thought of hanging herself but ultimately ruled this out because she did not want an innocent passerby to find her and be upset by her "mess." She was uncertain as to what type of pill and how many she would need for a "successful" overdose. She feared she would take only enough to paralyze herself or turn herself into a helpless vegetable, an idea she could not tolerate.

Because she could not think of a good plan, Rachel decided to stop thinking about suicide for the time being. Instead, she began to drink more and more and to use chemicals on a near-daily basis. Her drug use served a couple of key needs: It helped ease her pain and gave her a sense of identity (in the world of hallucinogenic drug users, her weirdness became "cool" and her unusual style was considered arty). Rachel had at last found a home and acceptance with peers—other youth who distrusted authority; who did not like teachers, rules, or school; and for whom being unique was the norm.

Rachel's use of chemicals only added to her ever-increasing school problems. The once accommodating, people-pleasing, and compliant Rachel was now developing an "attitude problem." She became argumentative with authority figures and refused to do her "stupid homework." Because her short-term memory was affected by her chemical use, she was unable to retain the new information necessary for success on school achievement tests. Rachel was now flunking seventh grade. A knowledgeable school official who believed that Rachel had emotional problems and perhaps a learning disability arranged for special placement. This transfer to a classroom for children with emotional problems only added to Rachel's anger at the school for not understanding her. Her peers now teased her for "being in the class for geeks," and she skipped classes more and more. She also increased her use of chemicals.

Rachel then made the first real friend in her life: a drug-using peer named Betty. The two felt spiritually connected, became inseparable companions, and began to skip school together. Both girls were bright and sensitive and had been sexually abused by adults (Betty's alcoholic father was raping and molesting her). Rachel was thrilled when Betty invited her to spend the night at her house. The second time Rachel slept at Betty's house, Betty's father raped both girls at knife point and in the same bed. Rachel froze, unable to scream, fight, or summon help, reacting as many survivors do in such a situation. Betty's father continued to abuse Rachel nearly every time she spent the night at her friend's house.

Why did Rachel keep returning to that house? There are many reasons. Rachel had learned to "go away" when bad things were happening to her. An expert in both mental and emotional dissociation, she used her dissociation "skills" to cope with the situation. (Rachel disconnected not only from her own feelings but from others who might have helped her.) Moreover, Rachel felt loved by Betty. Giving up her body to Betty's drunken father for a few minutes seemed to her a small price to pay for the love and support she received from Betty. She also felt that she was helping and supporting her friend by sharing her abuse. Moreover, Rachel expected adult males to be unsafe; sexual abuse was "normal" for her. She really did not know that she had a right to say no, that she owned her own body and her own sexuality. And telling her mother did not seem like an option to her.

Rachel and Betty increased their use of chemicals. Under the influence of drugs and alcohol they could build a joint pretend world, one that was much more appealing than the real one. Chemicals numbed the pain and also supported the grandiosity of their adolescent worldview and the antisocial stance of their "fuck them all" thinking pattern. Their anger, too, fueled their feelings of strength and power.

Rachel reached sexual maturity at an early age and had a certain voluptuous quality attractive to men. She also looked older than her age, passing for 19 or 20 when she was just 13. She began to see the power she had over males because of their desire to have sex with her; she learned that she could make them call her, visit her, talk to her, and pay attention to her by the promise, spoken or implied, of a sexual favor. Being high also permitted her to be promiscuous without feeling the underlying terror that sexual activity had for her. Both she and Betty felt popular for the first time in their lives. The attention Rachel got from males gave her a sense of identity. Early in treatment she referred to herself as a "sexual goddess." She learned that young men would say or do almost anything in order to have sex with her. Seductive clothing brought her much attention and many "friendly" overtures.

Our first impression of Rachel when she came to our office was that she was 3 going on 30. Sitting in the lobby dressed in that skimpy blouse and tight miniskirt, her long legs clad in those black fishnet stockings, she was clearly responsible for the hormonal surge a young man waiting in the lobby for a counseling appointment was evidently having just by looking at her. Yet when we introduced ourselves to her and she cast her eyes downward as she spoke to us, we had the impression that we were meeting a very young child.

Rachel seemed willing to answer all our questions and attempted to please us by guessing when she was unsure of an answer. She was quite open about her drug and alcohol use. She had minimal insight into her multiple problems but readily agreed to contract for abstinence with absolutely no overt resistance or hesitation. Her immediate agreement to an abstinence contract led us to conclude that Rachel either did not truly grasp the concept of abstinence or had no intention of following through with treatment. The latter proved to be true. Over the years, Rachel's mother had taken her to several therapists, but Rachel never went to more than three or four counseling sessions. Either her authority issues would trigger a rebellion or her idealization of the counselor as the one adult who could finally help her and whom she could trust would be followed by devaluation in the wake of what Rachel considered a "stupid" or untrustworthy act on the part of the counselor.

The initial treatment plan for Rachel included an abstinence contract, psychological testing, and dual diagnosis recovery counseling with Katie (Evans) on a one-to-one basis. A longer-term objective was for Rachel to participate, when ready, in a group for teenage girl survivors in recovery. A short stint in the group made it clear that she was unable to tolerate anything more intense than a structured group assembled for the purpose of educating members about alcohol and drug use. A group other than one that felt like a class triggered Rachel's sense of danger and led to her avoidance of groups. She expressed her intolerance for group therapy both directly, by complaining about not liking the group, and indirectly, by failing to show up for group because she "missed the bus." Even when she was well into her recovery, Rachel had difficulty with groups. Her sense of distrust and paranoia made the group situation very stressful for her.

Mike (Sullivan) began family counseling with Rachel and her mother. Managing crises and basic safety were the initial goals of the family therapy. Rachel's mother complained of Rachel's noncompliance with her rules, and both mother and daughter reported serious clashes at home that sometimes ended with blows or objects being thrown. Rachel would bring years of anger and resentment toward her mother into these sessions. Often, the escalating emotions in these volatile family sessions were so intense that it was necessary for Mike to first send Rachel out of the room in order to contain them and to then provide supportive counseling to her overwhelmed mother or vice versa. Mike worked with

Rachel's mother to help her formulate and implement consistent rules and consequences at home and avoid responses that escalated tensions. He also supported Rachel's mother in her efforts to build a support network for herself and to help her daughter use the self-care skills Rachel was learning in her individual therapy to manage flashbacks and other symptoms. Overall, Rachel's mother proved to be a fairly open-minded and flexible parent. Her criticisms of Rachel were minimal, and she was emotionally supportive of her; she believed and validated her daughter's accounts of sexual abuse, paid for her therapy, and encouraged her to stay in treatment.

Rachel's own therapy continually focused on the core issue of safety. Rachel had never before known a place where people only wanted to help her stay safe. Although she attended her one-to-one appointments religiously, it was confusing to her that Katie was only interested in helping her. One day after about a month of treatment Rachel came to a therapy session and vented a great deal of anger at Katie. She tried to portray herself as "bad," expressed hostility, and then became critical of Katie's attempts to give her support when this occurred. Katie remained calm and continued to try to reinforce the importance to her client of learning to get and stay safe. She complimented Rachel on her assertive expression of emotions and calmly pointed out to her those statements that felt more "aggressive than assertive." She also tried to explain how they were caught in the same idealization–devaluation cycle Rachel had experienced with other therapists. In response to Katie's refusal to get angry with her and send her away, a consequence she feared and anticipated, Rachel appeared to deepen her trust of her therapist. She found in Katie a person it was safe to trust. Katie presented herself to Rachel as a knowledgeable mentor, not a substitute parent or friend. While withholding details, Katie did share with Rachel the fact that she too was recovering, and she offered her client suggestions based on her own experience of staying clean and sober. While transference was clearly a key part of the therapeutic alliance, Katie's lack of cool neutrality and her avoidance of the blank-slate approach common to some traditional therapy schools created an atmosphere of safety for Rachel. Such an atmosphere was an important part of the therapy, for it was in this context that Rachel's relapses were challenged—in a supportive way—with Katie often reminding her, "There are no mistakes, only lessons."

Another early therapeutic objective was helping Rachel stay safe from further abuse. The teenager's style of dress was a source of constant male attention. Mistaken for a prostitute, Rachel was frequently propositioned and harassed. Katie diplomatically identified Rachel's style of dress as "very flashy and quite original but not very safe." Gradually,

Rachel was able to tone down her style of dress to the point where she was no longer harassed on a daily basis just by walking down the street.

Katie also knew that Rachel needed to learn some ways to manage her intense mood swings, especially her acute anxiety and depression. Lacking a consistent source of nurturing in her past, Rachel needed to build her own internal nurturing voice.

Katie began "parts work" with Rachel. This work began with attempts to help her see that there was a part of her that was a wounded little girl. Most survivors are very attentive caregivers—of others, not themselves—and Rachel was no exception. The goal was to help teach Rachel how to give some of this good nurturing to the hurt part of herself. Katie, for example, went for walks with the little girl part of her client and took her out for an ice-cream cone.

Rachel's sobriety was built on the premise that drugs and alcohol are not safe. Katie would ask, "Would you tell a crying 4-year-old to go get drunk or stoned when she is sad?" Rachel would reply vehemently, "No!" Then Rachel and Katie would make a list of things one could say to a hurt child to make her feel taken care of and help her feel safe. Rachel responded to this self-nurturing exercise with a ravenous thirst that equaled in intensity her need for this type of unconditional love.

Once Rachel felt safe, she began to learn more about her diseases of addiction and of posttraumatic stress disorder (PTSD). Katie would read to Rachel the diagnostic criteria from the DSM-III-R for PTSD and substance dependence. Then she and Rachel would discuss how these issues applied to her. As they reviewed each symptom (e.g., hypervigilance), Katie applauded Rachel's strength and praised her gifts as a survivor, often reframing many of her attributes as special and unique strengths or has having both helpful and not so helpful aspects. Rachel's hypersensitivity, for example, was characterized as also an indication of her "intuitive nature," and her poetry, which Katie encouraged her to write and which was often violent and depressing, was acclaimed for its "depth and passion."

Rachel began to transform her identity from being a victim to being a survivor. No longer was she a passive reactor to the abusers in her life. No longer did she sit back and helplessly complain of the pain inflicted by others. With Katie's help, Rachel was able to get her personal power back. From that moment on she no longer feared violation. Her body, mind, and spirit were now her own, to do with as she pleased and to share with whomever she chose.

Katie continued to help Rachel increase her sense of safety by encouraging her to be assertive and to stand up for herself. She also worked with her on setting boundaries. Katie defined internal boundaries as "screens on our windows" that help us learn to filter out the unkind and cruel comments and actions of others. She explained that when someone says, "You're mean," this is not necessarily a reflection of your true self but only an indication of what that person thinks at that moment. And he or she could be wrong! This gave Rachel a new power. Always afraid that others could see her "true" self, she now could begin to own her own power and develop her own identity. Rachel also worked on external boundaries. Telling someone no became an option. She no longer had to be sexual with every male around her just because he asked. Rachel also found that it was more helpful to her to be assertive with her mother instead of passive aggressive or aggressive, a discovery that facilitated progress in their family therapy sessions. Articulate and more self-assured, Rachel could now ask directly for what she wanted and needed, and, to her surprise, people often responded. In her sessions with Katie she would marvel at how well these skills worked.

Katie also worked with Rachel to help her better manage flooding with feelings of anxiety and depression. Slow breathing exercises, relaxation training, and journal keeping became part of Rachel's "feeling management tool kit." Rachel was then able to listen to audiotapes about being a survivor without feeling fearful and overwhelmed, thus gaining further support in her attempt to reframe herself as a survivor instead of a victim. One day after about a year of therapy Katie asked Rachel what it meant to be a survivor. Rachel replied, "Survivors have many talents and skills that un-survivors don't have. We have overcome something and are stronger for it!" Rachel was at the threshold of being able to do her integration work.

It was on her first sobriety birthday (and a few days before Halloween) that Rachel began to experience her first flashbacks of what appeared to be even more extensive abuse. In later chapters we describe the strategies we used to help her work through and further integrate her old and new memories.

The Impact and Process of Abuse

Sodomy

A touch becomes too much,
Unwanted feelings come to pass.
An ugly sensation,
Sickness and dirt.
So many showers that never do any good.
Emotions and scars,
from many years of pain.
Only when your mind can become healthy,
and clean is when the pain will finally be no more.

—SHANE, age 17

Our focus in this chapter is the impact and process of childhood abuse. We can use our knowledge of the impact and process of abuse to assess our clients, make prognostic statements, educate our clients, and provide therapeutic experiences that are more likely to be effective.

THE IMPACT OF ABUSE

We define abuse as the experience of highly stressful events inflicted by another person that is beyond the individual's capacity to cope and that impairs the individual's sense of well-being. Abused persons' effectiveness in living and the quality of their relationships are also impaired. This definition is consistent with current thinking and research in this area (1, 2).

The individual who has experienced childhood abuse very often experiences a number of personal symptoms and problems in living, and

31

these take many forms. Abuse survivors very often have distressing and disabling levels of fear, anxiety, depression, and anger, which often become chronic (3, 4). Survivors can experience episodes of psychotic-like symptoms and severe dissociative disorders, including dissociative identity disorder (DID; formerly multiple personality disorder) (5, 6, 7). Substance abuse or dependency is a frequent coexisting disorder (8, 9). Survivors can exhibit high rates of self-destructive behaviors, including sexual acting out, a tendency toward revictimization in relationships and self-mutilation (9, 10). They very often have difficulty trusting others and sustaining intimate relationships (11, 12). In fact, difficulty in interpersonal relationships best distinguishes between clients seeking therapy who have a history of abuse and those with no such history, at least when the abuse involved is incest (13).

We have identified 10 core issues that we see over and over again in our treatment of survivors. Not all of these issues present in acute form or are unique to survivors, but in our experience survivors tend to have some difficulties in most or all of these areas. The ten symptoms to which clinicians must be sensitive in their work with survivors are as follows:

1. Frequent use of denial or dissociation to deal with problems
2. Strong need to be in control
3. Tendency to be overly sensitive and to take things too personally
4. Difficulty trusting others
5. Distorted sense of responsibility, being either overly responsible or irresponsible
6. Trouble being appropriately assertive and dealing with anger
7. Unusual thinking and behavior, sometimes to the point of appearing psychotic
8. Tendency to reenact or repeat self-defeating behavior
9. Sexual and somatic problems
10. Alienation from self and others

Although individuals with a history of childhood abuse often end up suffering from a number of symptoms and problems, these disturbances take a variety of forms, and no one diagnostic picture or framework appears to characterize the survivor experience (1). This holds true even when writers have limited the domain of abuse under consideration to sexual abuse (3).

Posttraumatic stress disorder (PTSD) is the diagnosis that is typically used for those who are affected by abuse in a serious and long-term way. The fourth edition of the American Psychiatric Association's *Diagnostic and Statistical Manual of Mental Disorders* (DSM-IV), used by all treatment professionals in this country, contains the official set of mental health diagnoses and the criteria for making these diagnoses (14). The DSM-IV describes the cause, symptoms, and onset of PTSD as follows:

1. Exposure to a traumatic event in which the person experienced events that involved actual or threatened death or serious injury or a threat to the physical integrity of self or others *and* the person's response involved intense fear, helplessness or horror. Children may express this through disorganized or agitated behavior.

2. The person reexperiences the event in one or more ways in an ongoing manner, including the following: recurrent and intrusive memories, images, thoughts and so forth; distressing dreams; flashback-type experiences; and strong mental, emotional, behavioral, and physiological reactions to cues that resemble or symbolize an aspect of the traumatic event.

3. The person persistently avoids stimuli associated with the event and also experiences a numbing of general responsiveness. This includes efforts to avoid thoughts, feelings or conversations as well as activities, places or people connected to the trauma. The person may have amnesia for important aspects of the trauma. The person may also show increased interest/participation in significant activities; feelings of detachment or estrangement from others; emotional numbing or a restricted range of feelings; and a sense of a foreshortened future.

4. There are enduring symptoms of increased arousal/anxiety including the following: difficulty falling or staying asleep, irritability or outbursts of anger, difficulty concentrating, hypervigilence, and an exaggerated startle response.

PTSD-type symptoms may occur immediately after the event. In this case, the diagnosis is Acute Stress Disorder unless the symptoms last more than 4 weeks. If PTSD symptoms last less than 3 months, the disorder is considered acute and, if more than 3 months, chronic. The DSM-IV also allows for a delayed onset designation for symptoms that evidence at least 6 months after the trauma. In cases of delayed onset the traumatized individual may have appeared at the time of the event to have coped well enough, and does not apparently demonstrate any obvious effects from the trauma. However, the individual may have used denial or repression to manage the trauma and may have failed to integrate the experience. Typically, some sort of trigger event, such as the loss of a love relationship or high levels of outside stress, sets off the acute symptoms of PTSD at a later time.

While the PTSD diagnosis clearly captures many of the obvious symptoms and problems associated with serious abuse, many survivors do not evidence classic signs of PTSD and do not technically qualify for this diagnosis. Our own clinical experience and the experience of many of our colleagues suggest that 40% to 60% of survivors demonstrate classic symptoms of PTSD at the time of seeking treatment (15). On the other hand, we have seen individuals in our practice who appear to have few, if any, apparent symptoms of posttraumatic stress disorder from the childhood abuse they experienced. They are, however, likely to show symptoms of major depression and/or an anxiety disorder other than PTSD. Some survivors seek treatment for distress stemming from current life stressors and qualify for an adjustment disorder diagnosis. Research studies have also discovered symptom-free survivors (3).

The mixed picture found among survivors has a number of clinical and theoretical implications. *Clinicians need to rule out childhood trauma with each client regardless of the presenting issues.* This includes clinical presentations for addiction and is especially important when the clinical picture includes chronic interpersonal difficulties.

Clinicians also need to be prepared to give clients multiple diagnoses. Within the DSM-IV framework, clients qualify for more than one diagnosis if they meet the criteria. Typically, the first diagnosis is the one describing the problem for which the client has sought treatment. Given the variety of problems survivors experience, assigning both an Axis I diagnosis, such as alcohol dependence or posttraumatic stress disorder, and a coexisting Axis II personality disorder is often appropriate.

Finally, the heterogeneity of the impact of abuse found among survivors suggests that simply focusing on abuse as a unitary event is simplistic. Clearly, it must be the case that multiple factors influence the outcome of abuse. Viewing abuse and trauma as a process and not an event is likely to result in a more sophisticated understanding of survivor treatment needs.

One final note is appropriate: We do not believe that all clients who have substance dependence problems or other emotional difficulties are survivors of abuse. We also do not believe that trauma alone always accounts for all the difficulties addicted survivors experience. However, childhood trauma plays a central role in the difficulties of many of the clients we treat, whether they are substance abusers or not, and treatment is much more likely to be effective if this is taken into account.

ABUSE AS A PROCESS, NOT AN EVENT

Mental health professionals have just begun to recognize the need to see abuse as a process and not as just an event, and their writing and research now reflect this more inclusive view. They have criticized the PTSD view of abuse for failing to account for the ongoing, multifaceted nature of incest and for failing to place abuse in a developmental perspective (3, 16); have pointed out the importance of recognizing what did *not* happen in addition to what did happen; and have made distinctions between one-time and ongoing trauma in terms of the symptoms experienced (17, 18). Finally, research has demonstrated that family characteristics predict the likelihood of abuse; that these characteristics often account for differences in outcome among survivors as convincingly as, or better than, aspects of the abuse itself; and that the presence or absence of support from others is very much a key variable for understanding the impact of abuse (19).

Specific Variables

A natural first step in elaborating the process of childhood abuse is to look at the parameters of the abuse itself. The most thoroughly investigated type of abuse is sexual abuse. Not surprisingly, the more severe the sexual abuse, the more severe the impact. The effects of sexual abuse appear to be most severe when (1) incidents are frequent; (2) the inappropriate sexual activity occurs over a long period of time; (3) the sexual activities are wide-ranging and extensive (e.g., fondling versus intercourse); (4) there is more than one perpetrator; (5) the sexual abuse involves physical violation and force; (6) the abuser is older; and (7) the relationship of the child or adolescent to the perpetrator is close, with sexual abuse by a family member, especially a parent, being particularly damaging (20, 21, 22, 23). Experiencing both sexual and physical abuse is more traumatic than experiencing either type of abuse alone (24, 25).

Unfortunately, the available literature is not as detailed for other kinds of traumatic abuse and basically consists of identifying a certain kind of experience as damaging and then labeling it as abusive. Physical abuse is certainly traumatic. Individuals who have experienced it in childhood appear to demonstrate long-term difficulties and appear to be somewhat more likely to develop acting-out defenses associated with conduct disorder in youth or antisocial personality disorder in adults. They are also somewhat more likely to develop substance use disorders than those who experienced sexual abuse (8, 26, 27). In our own clinical experience we have certainly noted a correlation between physical abuse and a clinical picture associated with serious acting out. This is in contrast to the greater likelihood we have found to exist among survivors of sexual abuse of either "acting in" (such as with dissociation) or presenting a mixed picture. Interestingly, there are some indications that an acting-out pattern *in childhood and adolescence* increases the chances of better adjustment in adulthood, suggesting that physical abuse may somehow be less damaging than sexual abuse (28). Psychological abuse, such as severe criticism, also appears to cause significant psychological difficulties (26). A negative home atmosphere, where the child experiences high levels of parental conflict, has also been shown to have deleterious effects (1).

Terr, on the basis of her extensive clinical work with young survivors of many kinds of trauma, has proposed that there are important differences in the symptom picture found in children that depend on whether they have experienced a one-time trauma such as a kidnapping or an ongoing trauma such as incest (18). According to her scheme, children who have undergone a trauma, no matter what the type, usually show the following four characteristics for long periods of their life: (1) repeatedly perceived visual, tactile, kinesthetic, or olfactory memories of the traumatic event; (2) repetitive reenactments of aspects of the trauma in play, relationships, and even in works of art; (3) trauma-specific fears that are particular rather than general in nature (e.g., fear of sex rather than anxiety about relationships); and (4) changed attitudes about people, life, and the future, with the basic thrust being a sense of danger and untrustworthiness. Within this general framework, Terr also distinguishes between Type I and Type II traumas.

Type I traumas result from single unanticipated events. Survivors of such traumas have a symptom cluster that includes the following: (1) full, clear, and detailed memories of what happened; (2) preoccupation with possible "omens" (e.g., the child constantly reviews what happened in an attempt to find warning signals that could help him or her avoid a recurrence of the event); and (3) misperceptions, including visual hallucinations and peculiar time distortions (e.g., the impression of being "visited" by a family member unexpectedly killed in a car accident).

We have treated many clients suffering from this type of trauma. One adolescent girl presented with PTSD-type symptoms and at first glance seemed like a survivor of childhood abuse. Careful questioning, however, revealed no history of abuse and a history, until recently, of good functioning. Several months prior to the intake interview, she had experienced a very traumatic event. She had broken up with her boyfriend of many months during an argument, he had sped off into the night on his motorcycle, and had died in a crash. This young lady felt responsible for the death, and her schoolmates reinforced this feeling by telling her that her boyfriend would not have died if she had not been such a "bitch." She developed a continuous high level of anxiety, began to have flashbacks of the night of the accident, began experimenting with drugs, and became oppositional at home and at school. She had rapid mood swings, quickly went through several sets of new friends, and dropped out of school. This Type I trauma survivor, however, quickly recovered. She made and kept a contract to abstain from drugs and alcohol, took antidepressants for several months, processed the event in therapy, and, with encouragement, shared her feelings with family members and old friends who were supportive, not blaming.

Terr's Type II trauma involves exposure to extreme external events that is long-standing and/or repetitive. The Type II symptom cluster includes the following: (1) denial and psychic numbing; (2) self-hypnosis, depersonalization, and dissociation; and (3) rage, turned outward toward others or inward toward the self. This, of course, coincides with symptoms of PTSD and is the classic picture we associate with serious childhood abuse.

Abuse by Omission

The literature exploring issues germane to the topic of abuse by omission is based less on research findings than on theoretical elaborations of clinical observations. Object relations theories are the predominant paradigm currently used to frame these observations (29, 30, 31). This paradigm has several postulates, including the following: Humans form their general sense of self, of others, and of the connection between the two in the crucible of the relationship with the primary caretaker, most often the mother. The child goes through various stages of development that involve such things as differentiating self from others and creating internal images of self and others that integrate the good as well as the bad qualities. Primary caretakers must provide "optimal frustration" of the child's needs during each stage of development for balanced development to occur. Too much or too little gratification of these needs causes difficulties.

Joselyn has summarized this literature, identifying eight important aspects of human relatedness, the caretaking processes influencing their development, and the negative consequences for the individual of inappropriate caretaking (32). Table 3.1 summarizes her condensation of this material.

Careful examination of this table gives us hints about those "missing experiences" that constitute abuse. Some of these experiences, when "supplied" in too great a quantity, fall under the rubric of "abuse by commission." But more important for our purposes here is consideration of those experiences that might constitute abuse by omission. Failures in containing, predictable responsiveness, validation, and so on, result in an inadequate sense of self, deficits in self-regulation, and problems relating to others (16).

The classic example of abuse by omission is the failure to validate the child's experience of sexual abuse if and when the child tells an authority figure who should support and validate him or her. This double dose of abuse is very much associated with an increased risk of long-term

TABLE 3.1. Aspects of Human Relatedness, Caretaking Need, and Negative Consequences of Imbalanced Caretaking

Aspect	Need	Negative consequence (too little versus too much)
Holding	Containing Physical support Stimulation barrier	Sense of falling versus sense of suffocating
Attachment	Predictable responsiveness	Aloneness versus clinging
Passionate experience	Safe touch Play Union Expression of sexuality	Inhibition versus obsessive love
Validation	Mirroring Empathy Regard	Rejection versus transparency
Idealization and identification	Role models worthy of appreciation	Purposelessness versus slavish devotion
Mutuality	Affective attunement	Loneliness versus merging
Embeddedness	Balance of self versus society	Alienation versus conformity
Caretaking	Balanced parental caretaking (neither neglectful or "smothering"	Indifference versus compulsive caregiving

negative outcomes (16, 33). Telling children they imagined the molestation or dreamed about it, calling them liars, or telling them they deserved the abuse is extremely damaging. When any such reaction occurs, children not only undergo abuse of the active kind but also abuse of the abandoning sort. Their caretaking situation, among other things, fails to provide adequate protection (holding) and gives them a basis for concluding that they are alone in this world and that no one will be there for them (attachment, validation, mutuality).

The literature on attachment probably constitutes the most thoroughly researched and developed body of knowledge regarding specific caretaking ingredients and the consequent adjustment (19). Attachment refers to the nature of the relationship between caretaker and child as well as to the resultant personality style demonstrated by the child later in life. Investigators observing the behavior of young children in a laboratory setting during brief separations from and reunions with the mother have identified four styles of children's responses when the mother returns. These four styles of attachment have been labeled the secure, the avoidant/dismissive, the preoccupied/resistant, and the fearful/disorganized, with each of the last three being an insecure style. Researchers have correlated these attachment styles with parental caretaking styles and with the child's level of functioning over the course of several years. Studies have also looked at adult functioning in terms of attachment style and have correlated these observations with retrospective accounts of parents' caretaking styles. Not surprisingly, insecure attachment predominates in populations of children who have experienced abuse, and the particular symptoms abused children exhibit appear to be mediated by their attachment experiences. Table 3.2 summarizes the links found between parental caretaking style, attachment or personality style, and various personality features.

TABLE 3.2. Attachment Style and Associated Parental Caretaking Style and Consequent Personality Characteristics

Attachment style	Caretaking style	Consequent personality characteristics
Secure	Supportive Responsive Predictable Attuned to all needs	Socially skilled, empathetic, resilient, comfortable with a wide range of emotions, self-confident, trusting, comfortable with intimacy, able to reflect coherently on the past, positive view of self and others
Avoidant/ dismissing	Insensitive Unemotional Unavailable Not attuned to child's need or comfort	Emotionally insulated, hostile or antisocial, attention-seeking, lacking in empathy, lonely, uncomfortable with intimacy, unable to recall childhood, positive view of self but negative view of others, compulsive sexuality, compulsively self-reliant, covert fears
Preoccupied /resistant	Inconsistent, "parentifies" the child, sometimes attuned to need	Needy, tense, impulsive, passive, helpless, dependent, jealous, negative view of self but positive view of others, target for victimization, desperate love style, compulsive caretaking, anxious and depressed, negative self-esteem
Fearful/ disorganized	Chaotic, fear-inducing, disoriented, randomly attuned to need	Disorganized, undirected fear and distress, socially inhibited, negative view of self and others, dissociative, unstable and intense affect, poor impulse control, hot and cold relationships

The literature on attachment contributes greatly to our under-standing of abusive processes. The descriptions of various attachments styles coincide well with observations from clinical experience. Profes-sionals can easily recognize clients they have treated and can perceive similarities between these attachment styles and some commonly encoun-tered personality disorders (14). The avoidant style seems to correspond closely to narcissistic personality disorder or, in more extreme cases, to antisocial personality disorder; the preoccupied style appears to accord with so-called codependent-type personality disorders; and the fearful style seems amazingly similar to borderline personality disorder.

These descriptions of attachment, or personality style also allow us to conceptualize in more detail the forms of abuse that are less obvious and traumatic than those associated with severe PTSD-type symptoms but that nonetheless leave their mark on our clients, a mark that often determines their presenting complaint when they enter therapy. Knowing which set of personality traits goes with which childhood caretaking experience gives us the ability to quickly ask the right questions and zero in on the pertinent issues. Because they have found someone who seems knowledgeable and appears to understand them well, clients typically feel not only supported and validated but hopeful about their treatment.

Information about significant aspects of the nature of the abuse has several implications for the assessment and treatment of survivors. Infor-mation on the parameters of the abuse itself (e.g., how long the abuse lasted, who the perpetrator was, the type of abuse) gives a good indication of the extent and nature of the damage the client has probably sustained and therefore of the likely extent and emphasis of the treatment needed. The clinician must be alert to the importance of abuse other than sexual or physical abuse, such as severe emotional abuse or exposure to so-called secondary abuse (such as domestic violence between parents), which is less immediately obvious and therefore susceptible to minimization. The clinician must also be alert to what at first glance looks like a classic PTSD-type syndrome but may differ enough in its exact symptom struc-ture, depending on whether the trauma was a one-time occurrence or ongoing in nature, to have implications for prognosis and the pacing of treatment. Of crucial importance is the role of abuse by omission, which is more easily overlooked than abuse by commission because it is "not there." Understanding both what did happen and what did not happen is also important because they probably existed together and their sequelae interact in a synergistic fashion. Finally, understanding that normality consists of caretakers providing a balance of necessary rearing ingredients gives the survivor a vision of what should have been and of what needs to be, a vision that can help both client and therapist set the goals of therapy, and provide the necessary corrective experiences.

Individual Differences

A growing body of literature looks at so-called person variables that appear to interact with abuse, produce differences in outcome, and have implications for treatment. For example, knowing that "fighting back" appears to be a more successful strategy than "placating" has immediate, clear-cut therapeutic implications (34).

Temperament, or the behavioral expression of genetic and constitutional factors, also appears to have some relationship to the process of abuse. Infants and children with more "difficult" temperaments (e.g., those who are distractible or who have a low threshold to stimulation) appear to have more difficulty handling stress and are more likely to elicit parental irritability, criticism, and hostility (35). Somewhat surprisingly, intellectual ability has no reliable relationship to outcome, with some studies showing that high ability helps, others showing that it makes no difference, and still others showing that it makes things worse (1). Gender, on the other hand, does appear to make some difference, although the results are not clear-cut. While males appear somewhat more likely than females to respond to experiences of sexual abuse and other forms of abuse with acting-out symptoms such as anger and fighting—cultural values undoubtedly play some role in this difference—for the most part males and females report similar problems associated with a history of sexual abuse (1, 3).

Human beings go through stages of development from birth to death. While these stages have some social and cultural components, especially in the adult years, constitutional and genetic influences are paramount. Persons must accomplish certain developmental tasks at each stage of development if they are to build the foundation for later stages and if they are to evolve into their full potential. Abuse disrupts the smooth progression of development in several ways (36), including (1) intensification, aggravation, and fixation of the current stage; (2) regression to previous stages and/or reactivation of previously unresolved developmental issues; and (3) pseudo maturity and premature acceleration into advanced stages of development. Knowing the age/stage of development at which the abuse started and the ages/stages during which the abuse continued is invaluable in understanding many of the survivor's core issues and the dynamics likely to be present in therapy.

Cole and Putnam (16) present a review of the literature on stages of development and the likely developmental impact of incest. They argue that incest has uniquely negative effects in the general domains of self-definition and integration; self-regulation of feeling, thinking, and behavior; and a sense of security and trust in relationships. They also argue that the exact nature of these disruptions depends on the particular developmental stage at which they occurred. We present a summary of their overview of the developmental issues and tasks associated with different ages in Table 3.3 to serve as a general guide and reference to help our readers integrate a developmental perspective into their assessment and treatment of survivors.

Obviously, the earlier the abuse, the more profound the damage, both because the distortions are more basic and because the foundation for later stages is so shaky. The profound damage from early abuse manifests itself clinically in a variety of ways: Some survivors seem perpetually stuck in childhood despite the trappings of being older, such as being married or having children. They evidence black-and-white thinking when under pressure, and in a group therapy situation may exhibit resentment toward a new group member (as if the latter were taking attention away from them). Survivors of serious and early abuse sometimes regress to infantile states (e.g., hiding in a closet after making a mistake or crawling around on the floor and using baby talk when in a dissociated state); some survivors

TABLE 3.3. Developmental Stages and Issues

Stage/age	Developmental issues and tasks
Infancy/toddler (birth–2 years)	Discovering a world of objects and people Establishing secure family relationships Establishing a basic sense of self Developing autonomous awareness Acquiring an initial sense of right and wrong
Preschool years (ages 2–5)	Integrating self with social restrictions Elaborating sense of self in concrete terms Making use of denial and dissociation Making egocentric attributions Using black-and-white thinking
Childhood (ages 5–13)	Elaborating sense of self in abstract terms Developing shame and pride Developing friendships Making use of rationalizing, blaming Inhibiting self for the sake of social relations
Adolescence (ages 13–18)	Integrating emerging sexuality Developing intimacy Increasing use of abstract thought Articulating an integrated identity Exploring boundaries of self and others
Early to middle adulthood (ages 18–40)	Integrating roles of worker, spouse, parent, etc., into identity Regulating self to take care of others and fulfill responsibilities Reflecting on self and paths taken or chosen or still available

suddenly lose the ability to solve problems in a coordinated way when faced with stress. Adult survivors can experience a kind of second adolescence when their survivor issues begin to emerge and they start to question adult commitments such as marriage.

Adding a developmental perspective to our understanding of a survivor client can be very helpful clinically. If, for example, the client at times sounds and acts like a 7-year-old, there is an excellent chance that the abuse started at that age. Pinpointing developmental deficiencies can help us tailor our "talk" in treatment sessions; for example, a client in a "5-year-old state" needs many concrete examples and demonstrations; much modeling; and simple, direct limits, not elaborate interpretations. It can also help alert us to skills clients are likely to need particular assistance in learning and to issues they may need guidance in resolving. We can avoid assuming that clients, no matter how mentally healthy they look at the start, have truly acquired such basics as the ability to plan for the future or the notion that when someone is mad at them, it does not necessarily mean that the relationship is over. Finally, we can appreciate transference phenomenon better when we understand that at times we will become the parent for a client and that he or she may age regress during the session because of a reactivation of these developmentally-based issues during sessions.

A survivor's sense of control over abusive events at the time they occurred appears to be a key factor moderating the impact of these events, both in the past and in their current lives. Studies have consistently shown that it is not so much the "objective" stress associated with a noxious event that determines its impact but, rather, the person's subjective sense of control over stressors that modulates their effects (37, 38). Interestingly, these same studies show that persons can maintain a sense of "controllability" not only if they have the means to actively decrease the frequency or intensity of the stressor but even if they merely have information that allows them to predict when a stressful event will occur. The classic studies (involving both animals and humans) on this phenomenon used electric shocks administered on a schedule of some sort. We can easily understand that the person who can press a button to ward off some of the shocks feels more in control of the situation and therefore less stressed than when no such device is available. Less intuitively obvious, however, is the established fact that when persons are able to see a light warning of impending shock and are thus able to predict the occurrence of the stress, they also experience less stress than when no such warning device exists. In other words, individuals can cope with stress not only by attempting to master the stress but also by just attempting to predict the pattern of painful events.

The longitudinal study showed that adult survivors who used different strategies as children had different outcomes later in life. Are some coping strategies more helpful than others? Abused children who evidenced fatalistic attitudes were found to have poorer long-term outcomes than abused children who maintained a belief that there was hope for the future. Higher-functioning survivors were also found to have a better self-image even as children; interestingly, they often maintained a sense of hope through fantasy, imagining themselves surmounting their current situations and having a brighter future. Moreover, these more "successful" survivors had behavioral patterns that were belligerent, demanding, and provocative, and that turned their aggressiveness outward. The less functional survivors were more self-destructive and had used either yielding behavior (characterized by isolation, defeatism, and passivity) or placating behavior (characterized by people pleasing, obedience, and attention to the needs of others). Readers should note, however, that even the more "successful" adults had difficulty expressing emotions and establishing intimate relationships (28). It also appears that individuals with an internal, as opposed to an external, locus of control weather stress better (1). Whereas persons with an internal locus of control have a strong faith in their ability to control their world, those with an external locus of control believe that there is little they can do to influence their world. Research has found that adult female survivors of childhood sexual abuse had poorer current functioning if they had an attributional style for negative events that was internal ("It's all my fault"), stable ("It will always be this way"), and global ("It's this way for everything") as compared to those who had opposite beliefs about the causes and reasons for negative events (33). Finally, the lack of any consistent coping strategy—as is typically true for the fearful/disorganized child—is associated with the poorest outcome of all (39). Finally, many survivors blame themselves for the trauma; this is known as survivor guilt. The need to maintain a sense of control probably accounts for at least some of this self-blame and represents a last-ditch attempt to assert control by seeing themselves as the cause.

Certain experiences also appear to help compensate for the damage inflicted by the abuse. Survivors who did well in school or sports seem to do better, probably because they had "data" that contradicted negative messages at home and that supported a more positive self-image (1, 34). Survivors who had responsibility for taking care of others as children seemed more insulated than survivors who did not (34). Undoubtedly, this caretaking behavior served a protective function by giving meaning and purpose to the abuse.

Survivors, no matter how strong their subjective feelings of having been a victim, were not passive receptacles of abuse but in some fashion defended themselves as best they could. Furthermore, they had a strong incentive to develop strategies, in both their thinking and actions, for "understanding" and "doing something" about their experience of abuse.

To the extent that these strategies "worked," survivors are likely, for better or worse, to carry these styles of coping into their current life. However, some strategies appear to be more helpful than others. Assessing survivors' coping skills and attributional styles is clearly important, and assisting them to understand and evaluate these styles and to adopt potentially more productive ones is a key task of treatment. Part of our efforts as therapists can focus on encouraging survivors to learn to "take charge, get mad, and fight back" in ways that are not destructive to self or others. We can improve our clients' abilities to assert themselves, to solve problems, to ask for help, and to contain and dissipate unpleasant feelings and destructive impulses. We can help them modify destructive attributional biases by working with them to achieve success in their daily lives, to rethink assumptions about what they truly can and cannot control, to reframe their theories of why they were abused, and to recognize the implications of these theories for their sense of themselves and of their power in the world. We can even ask them to develop and use their imaginations to provide more helpful and hopeful "stories" for themselves, about both the past and the present.

Family and Social Factors

The family and the "extended family" of relatives, neighbors, teachers, and so forth, provide the prime context for the child's experience of the world. Childhood abuse occurs in this context. Not surprisingly, clinical experience and a growing body of evidence indicates the importance of this context for understanding the process of abuse and its ultimate impact. Parental conflict, family isolation, poor cohesion in the family, and excessive paternal dominance, for example, have all been found to be as important as, or even more important than, the actual abusive events in accounting for survivors' outcomes (19). An absolutely critical issue is the nature of the survivor's relationship with the nonabusive parent (who is, more often than not, the mother). Children who experience abuse but who have a relationship with a warm, competent, and supportive caretaker survive better than those who do not have such a relationship (1, 16). As discussed earlier (but worth repeating), an absolutely critical factor is the nonabusive parent's reaction to the abuse upon discovery or disclosure (16, 33). If the caretaker supports the child, validates the child's reality, and takes steps to protect him or her, the child is likely to do better.

Another critical variable contributing to differences in outcome among survivors is the quality of the family's social support before and after disclosure of the abuse. At-risk children who cope better with trauma appear to use a network of informal relationships with friends, neighbors, and others to obtain support, and at-risk parents who have support appear less likely to engage in abusive caretaking (1). Of particular importance is the availability to the abused child over time of a supportive adult (not necessarily one of the parents) who treats the child as special and with whom the child feels safe (34). We have often noted the importance of such relationships (and of their absence) among our own clients, and we refer to this as the "fairy godperson" effect. Whether this person is a relative, neighbor, teacher, coach, or member of the clergy, contact with such an individual provides a partial antidote to the toxicity of the abuse the child experiences. We have found that those of our clients who had such a fairy godperson (who, e.g., spent summers with a beloved grandparent) or who were able to make extensive use of a church youth group, a sports team, or other group of peers almost invariably coped better with their abusive experience and respond more quickly to therapy.

In general and across a wide range of psychiatric disorders, access to current social support also appears to lower the risk of developing psychological symptoms and of exhibiting interpersonal difficulties (40). Survivors of abuse are no exception (33). Survivors who have people in their current lives who can offer them emotional and material support have, of course, not only survived better than those who lack this advantage but also are better able to cope with current difficulties.

The research on family and social factors has shaped our clinical practice in many ways. We ask our clients the following key questions as part of our assessment process: What was it like in your family growing up? What sort of relationship did you have with your mother when you were younger? With your father? With your brothers and sisters? Have you ever told anyone about what happened to you? What was their response? When you were growing up, was there anyone who thought you were wonderful and who made you feel special and loved? How are your current relationships with your parents, spouse, siblings, significant other? If you need help, is there someone you can call to get some support? The answers to these questions and information gleaned from the client's own report about current resources for and impediments to recovery yield important information for prognosis.

The findings on social and family factors also have implications for treatment. One obvious implication is that we therapists must strive to be the supportive, validating person so many survivors never had in their lives. We must help our clients review their abusive experiences, place them in a broader social context, and rewrite their life script in a way that uses the point of view not of the isolated, egocentric, self-blaming child but of the more objective, connected-with-others adult. Above all, we must help our clients build and use social support systems in their lives. This is a high priority and a crucial therapeutic ingredient. Not only do these systems assist the survivor's own healing for the long term, but they also help take the pressure off the therapist to provide all the support, thus decreasing the chances of a skewed therapy relationship and of therapist burnout.

Big-Picture Models

Multifactor models of abuse as a process are currently few and far between in the literature. A few investigators have used statistical procedures such as path analysis (a way of numerically correlating factors to demonstrate the sequence and importance of different variables with regard to outcomes) to explore this issue, but these efforts are rudimentary to date (41).

Attachment Model

Alexander (19) has applied the insights of attachment theory (discussed earlier) to describe and understand the dynamics of the sexually abusive family. She argues that there is intergenerational transmission of insecure attachment, that distorted attachments are a breeding ground for sexual abuse, and that viewing abusive families in terms of attachments is consistent with the available literature on the dynamics of families associated with abuse.

Families characterized by rejecting/avoidant attachments appear to have fathers who view other family members as being their property and as responsible for meeting their needs and who are likely to deny the impact of abuse on the child; mothers who are unavailable physically or emotionally because of the demands of such things as work, illness, or depression and who are less likely to notice or to follow up on suspicions of abuse; stepparents who do not take on the role of protector; and children who are at increased risk for sibling incest and less primed to seek out help when abused.

Families characterized by preoccupied/resistant dynamics appear to have parents who feel that children should meet their needs, just as they met their own parents' needs (whether these needs are for sexual gratification or emotional nurture), or who are more involved with taking care of their own parents than their children, or who, in the case of the nonabusive parent, are unable to oppose the abuse; the children in such families appear to be more vulnerable to manipulation to meet the needs of others who are older, both inside and outside the family.

Families characterized by fearful/disorganized attachment appear to have parents who were seriously abused or neglected themselves or who, because of the extensive use of dissociation, serious substance abuse problems, or both, are unaware of their abusive behavior or that of others or unable to respond effectively; the children in such families have no models of any effective coping strategy and have no hope of finding any ally at all other than the abuser. Thus, any pattern of distorted parental attachment appears to provide a fertile breeding ground for the abuse of children.

Examining the roles of the family cast of characters within this framework is a fruitful source of therapeutic strategies and tactics for working with survivors. One of the things that this procedure does is remind us that we must provide a therapy relationship that promotes "secure attachment" for our clients. Thus, for therapy to be successful we must provide structure and reliability for fearful/disorganized clients, encourage a certain level of dependence on the part of avoidant/dismissing clients, and encourage rejecting/preoccupied clients to take care of themselves. Balanced and predictable responsiveness on our part also establishes a healthy therapeutic alliance.

Another thing the attachment model does is encourage us to assist clients to broaden their view of who is to blame for the abuse and to redistribute responsibility in a more realistic and healthy fashion. We worked with one male client, for example, who presented with problems with anger and intimacy. He was very open about the sexual abuse he had experienced from age 5 to age 13 at the hands of his stepfather but tended to minimize the contribution of his mother. One of the triggers for his anger revolved around incompetence in others. During our exploration of this issue we asked the client a series of questions about his relationship with his mother, his answers to which suggested an ongoing pattern of neglect on her part. A key breakthrough occurred when the client recalled cutting himself badly at the age of 4 and feeling, despite "the pool of red blood" on the bathroom floor, reluctant to "bother" his mother for help. When asked why a 4-year-old would not feel comfortable asking his mother for help in an emergency, the client experienced an "a-ha" reaction that resulted in the recovery of a torrent of memories of other incidents with his mother, all of which conveyed the message "Don't bother me" or "You're on your own." Not only did this realization help the client begin to understand why he might have an "incompetence" button for his anger, but it also helped him understand why he submitted to the abuse all those years, a revelation that lightened his load of shame.

The Two-Factor Model

Another model that we have developed and used over the years is the "two factor" model of abuse. The first factor is the trauma factor, which refers to all the things that *did* happen, such as sexual or physical abuse, domestic violence, and so forth. The second factor is the abandonment factor, which refers to all the things that did not happen, such as protection and validation. Either one alone, especially if intense, can produce difficulties. Both together multiply harmful effects in an interactive manner. The child who is sexually abused without force for a short period of time by someone outside the family and who, when he or she tells the secret of the abuse, receives the full support of a well-functioning family is likely to be much less damaged than the child who is exposed to a more toxic set of circumstances. Readers can imagine the less benign situation and its impact, an impact that is likely to result in the classic posttraumatic stress disorder syndrome and the more severe personality disorders, such as borderline or narcissistic personality disorders.

We implicitly use this model to formulate our assessment and exploration questions with our clients and later use it explicitly to help our clients understand and organize their experience. We help our clients understand that both what did happen and what did not happen are important. We explain that it is difficult but nevertheless important to recognize and acknowledge abuse by omission. We encourage clients to gain control of their experience by identifying both their trauma and their abandonment triggers. We explain that trauma triggers are likely to produce intense reactions characterized by anxiety or anger and by a narrowing of activity and attention. Trauma triggers are also more likely to be highly specific. We clarify for our clients that abandonment triggers are likely to be more general and pervasive and to be characterized by depression, resentment, and shame. Our clients almost universally respond well to this framework.

The Mind Control Model

We have also drawn from the literature on brainwashing and mind control to develop another model that we have found very useful for helping us and our clients get the "big picture" of the process of their abuse (42). Survivors so often beat themselves up with the question of why they submitted to the abuse and why a part of them perhaps even enjoyed it that it is immensely helpful to reframe their experience through a comparison with that of, for example, "strong, committed American fighter pilots in the Korean war." To achieve this end, we review and explore with our clients in a checklist fashion the following elements of brainwashing:

1. *Obtain substantial power and control over the person's time and location.* In a very real sense, parents and other authority figures have great power and control over children by virtue of custom and law and by the innate powerlessness of children and their consequent dependence on adults.

We can legitimately view children under adverse conditions as hostages and prisoners of war.

2. *Cut off other sources of support and validation.* Whether by making threats to kill children or their loved ones, by telling them that no one would believe them, by relying on their own sense of shame, or by counting on the children to follow family rules about "not talking," abusers function as "programmers" who ensure that children are even more dependent on them for their safety, health, and view of reality. It is consistent with this picture that families where abuse occurs are notorious for being socially isolated (22).

3. *Further increase the person's sense of powerlessness.* Abusive parents can do this in several ways. For example, they can assume a mantle of authority and have others obey them by staging demonstrations of their power, such as beating the child or the other parent, destroying household furnishings, or pulling the phone cord out of the wall, or by appealing to the Bible to support their claims to their rights as a parent. Another way is by forcing compliance in the child in small matters, such as requiring permission to go to the bathroom. Abusive parents also commonly increase their children's sense of helplessness by mounting a consistent attack on their sense of self-esteem, for example, calling them sluts or bitches or telling them they will never amount to anything.

4. *Manipulate rewards and punishments to inhibit resistant behavior and to promote submission.* Abusive parents may threaten to send their children away to an orphanage if they are "bad" and may buy presents for them when they are "good."

5. *Shape compliance by getting the person to take small steps toward the desired "controllable" state.* For example, the abuse may start with a request for a kiss, proceed to backrubs, and escalate to genital contact. Or it may start with a brief spanking and then escalate to severe beatings over time if the child is not more compliant. Clinicians use the term "grooming" to describe this shaping procedure. Offenders are adept at identifying needy children and insinuating themselves into a position of power by gratifying the child's wishes, giving presents, and gradually becoming more and more of a key figure in the child's life.

6. *Maintain a system of logic that explains away all contradictory facts and always frames the person who is questioning the relationship as the problem.* Offenders are deft at rationalizing their behavior and blaming others. They are also skilled at making distinctions that are artificial but sound impressive. For example: "It's important that you learn about sex from someone who loves you," or "Our family is special and so are you," or "What's the matter? Can't you take it like a man?" Particularly pernicious is when the offender can point to previous seemingly voluntary behavior

on the child's part and then use that to convince the child that he or she "wanted it" or will be in big trouble if the secret gets out or is "just like me."

7. *Encourage disorientation, confusion, and trance states.* Abusers can bring about these conditions in a number of ways. One means of doing this is to interfere with the child's physiology, for example, by administering drugs; disrupting sleep; pairing pain with pleasure; maintaining ongoing high levels of stress through aggressive attacks, either physical or psychological; and inducing sensory deprivation by keeping the child locked up in a bare room. Another method of doing this is to encourage dissociation by suggesting to children that they pretend they are somewhere else (e.g., at Disney World), by vividly describing to them past or future abuse experiences, or by exposing them to chanting, rhythmic music, or dancing (as occurs in ritualistic abuse). A common means of inducing confusion is through "good guy/bad guy" strategies, where the abuser is awful one minute and wonderful the next or where the other parent actively enables the abuse but is especially nice to the child the next day. The double-bind paradigm is a classic statement of conditions conducive to inducing confusion and trance states (43). An individual is in a double bind when an authority figure commands belief and/or compliance simultaneously with respect to two contradictory messages and the individual is not free to leave the situation or even to comment on the existence of the double bind. A child receiving the messages of "I love you" and "I will abuse you" faces such a double bind and is likely to become frozen with fear and experience increased confusion and suggestibility.

This mind control model of abuse is invaluable. It pinpoints for us important questions to ask about the context of our clients' abuse. Even when clients cannot remember specific incidents of abuse, it alerts us to the likelihood of such abuse having occurred when they describe a home that had or still has a "brainwashing" atmosphere. In general terms, the model suggests that therapeutic objectives need to include helping our survivors establish equitable power and control relationships and contacts with validating others; enhance their self-esteem and their ability to spot seduction and the "con"; and, as described in more detail in the next section, learn to identify and dissolve dissociation and trance states. When we work with our survivor clients to identify how they were brainwashed (when they are ready to deal with this material), they generally gasp upon recognizing the elements of brainwashing in their past; they then experience a strong sense of relief as they let go of shame and blame for their abuse.

Small-Picture Paradigms

We now return to a focus on paradigms of the internal responses and processes that result in psychiatric symptoms in the person exposed to abusive conditions. Recent years have witnessed the elaboration of more sophisticated frameworks for understanding the impact of trauma. We have found three of these paradigms particularly useful for understanding and helping our survivor clients.

Biphasic Paradigm of PTSD

The first paradigm is a biphasic model of posttraumatic stress disorder that combines theory and research on conditioned fear responses, state-dependent learning, and the brain biochemistry associated with these phenomena and with various psychiatric disorders (44, 45). According to this formulation, high stress that is ongoing ultimately produces not only a chronic state of *physiological hyperarousal* but also an imbalance and disequilibrium between approach and avoidance mind–body systems that are normally "in phase" but now are "out of phase" and operate as two systems. Chronic hyperarousal in the autonomic nervous system leads to the following symptoms: (1) exaggerated startle response, (2) affective hyperarousal, (3) frenetic overactivity, (4) sleep disturbance, (5) hypervigilance and scanning, (6) sensation seeking, and (7) pronounced autonomic activity (e.g., rapid heart beat) associated with the trauma. This permanent state of high alert takes some time to establish, but if relief does not occur in the early hours and days of the trauma, it tends to become established in the nervous system. Moreover, this chronic hyperarousal is associated with increased sensitivity and responsiveness not only to stressors related to the original trauma but also to other stressors that occur later on.

Trauma also decouples the usually coordinated and balanced excitatory and inhibitory physiological/neurochemical response systems and leads to out-of-kilter and overly intense swings between the two systems. The sympathetic-adrenal-medulla system associated with catecholamine-based neurochemistry constitutes the excitatory system. The pituitary-adrenal-cortical system associated with cholinergic-based neurochemistry constitutes the inhibitory system. Table 3.4 summarizes the psychological/behavioral correlates and trauma-induced problems of these two systems as outlined by Wilson (36).

Neutral aspects of one situation become capable of eliciting fear when associated with painful aspects of another situation through classical conditioning in the conditioned fear response paradigm. For example,

TABLE 3.4. Psychological/Behavioral Correlates and Trauma-Induced Out-of-Phase Problems of the Body's Excitatory and Inhibitory Neurological/Physiological Systems

Excitatory System	Inhibitory System
Right hemisphere	Left hemisphere
Undercontrol	Overcontrol
Reenactment	Protective
Visual memory	Verbal/auditory memory
Increased arousal, irritability, anger	Depression, loss of interest in meaningful activities
Fight–flight response	Blocked awareness, responsiveness
Intrusive imagery	Denial
Disturbing emotion	Emotional detachment
Affective flooding	Withdrawal, estrangement
Hypervigilance, lability	Numbing
Sensation of recurrence	Inability to remember
Overgeneralization of associations	Selective inattention
Flashbacks, dissociation	Amnesia, impaired concentration and constricted cognition
Intensification by exposure to trauma stimuli; anniversary reactions	Developmental arrest, foreshortened future

sounding a tone prior to administering an electric shock to an animal or human soon results in the tone alone producing anxiety and fear even in the absence of the electric shock. Numerous research studies suggest that fear responses from conditioned stimuli are long-lasting and never really disappear. However, if organisms have new and repeated experiences that indicate that a stimulus no longer "means" pain, their fear responses gradually decrease. This is known as extinction and forms the basis for therapies that involve desensitization through repeated but now safe exposure to a formerly painful stimulus (46). However, extinction can produce only mixed results. What seems to occur in extinction is not the elimination of the association but the learning of a new one that suppresses the fear response, and this can limit not only the generalizability of the newly acquired fearlessness but its durability as well. The disappearance of the fear connection is limited to specific situations and easily returns with the slightest reexperiencing of pain (47). Moreover, avoidance (if at all possible) of the feared situation is the normative response; thus, there are few natural opportunities for extinction to take place and avoidance becomes firmly established as a coping mechanism.

We find that this model helps us make sense of our survivor clients' symptoms, problems, and treatment needs. For example, survivors generally seem overly reactive to a wide variety of stressors and have more difficulty handling life's upsets in general. This seems to be related to chronic hyperarousal and increased sensitivity to any kind of stress. The return of PTSD symptoms when tugged after many years of lying dormant reflects the permanent nature of conditioned fear responses and the relatively fragile and limited effect of any new safety and extinction experiences provided by life. This same phenomenon may also account for the slow gains that those with PTSD experience in treatment and suggests that it may be necessary to think of PTSD as a chronic condition potentially requiring lifelong management. Facing one's fears is easier said than done and completely goes against the natural avoid-at-all-costs defense that clients have developed.

Many of our clients who present with depression paradoxically respond with increased symptoms of anxiety when they take a so-called activating antidepressant medication such as Prozac. Instead, they sometimes appear to do better on less activating antidepressants. Listening to music is a right-hemisphere function, and many of our clients use music to manage high levels of arousal. In fact, we sometimes prescribe music to help clients who are struggling with flashbacks and flooding. We sometimes encourage clients who are flooding to temporarily engage in "healthy" compulsive behavior such as exercising or housecleaning if this is what they have done in the past to manage intense disruptive emotions. We also prescribe hot baths, saunas, and (if tolerable) massages to help soothe and give at least a moments peace to our chronically uptight clients. The rationale for using imagery and art with survivors to access and process material in right-hemisphere channels suddenly becomes clearer. Many of our clients use high-risk, high-intensity activities such as motorcycle riding at high speeds or self-mutilation in order to feel something or to refocus themselves away from the internal pain and flooding to external and more manageable pain. We attempt to help our clients develop safer ways to manage their pain by encouraging them to channel their need for excitement and relief into sports such as skiing or by teaching them relaxation techniques.

Thinking of PTSD as a conditioned emotional response having two phases or components points to the relevance of various cognitive–behavioral techniques for treating these phases. For example, therapists help clients attempt to eliminate their problematic avoidance responses by encouraging them to desist from responding in these ways (response prevention), to use new ways to cope (skills building), and to face their fears (exposure) to help them desensitize to feared situations (46, 47). These fears can, of course, refer to frightening situations that are outside the individual (such as telling the secret or confronting the perpetrator) as well as to those that are inside (such as recalling memories of the abuse).

Conceptualizing PTSD as a learned response that is state dependent and that requires extinction in a wide variety of situations points to the need to encourage wide-ranging healing experiences that involve the re-creation (in at least some small fashion and in a safe way) of the original mind–body state in which the "abuse learning" took place in order for new learning to establish itself (48).

State-dependent learning is a well-researched phenomenon that shows that what is learned and remembered depends on the psychophysiological state of the individual at the time of the experience. The classic example is the student who takes methamphetamines to cram for finals, takes the exam, crashes, and later can barely remember taking the exam much less what he or she studied. Yet if the student takes speed again, he or she suddenly remembers in much greater detail the material studied. It appears that treatment for PTSD must include some sort of "real-time" relearning in a variety of situations to be effective. Merely chatting about issues in the office is not likely to transfer to the outside and to result in genuine and deep changes. This explains why so many survivor clients forget what they discuss in sessions and have difficulty transferring what they learn. Sending home an audiotape of part or all of a session and using written reminders as behavioral tactics are remedies for this problem. The trance busting technique described later on also address this issue.

Finally, medications to address the biological components of PTSD appear to be an important tool in our treatment kit, particularly with the increased understanding of the biochemistry of PTSD. Some authors, for example, have suggested that neuroleptics designed to treat psychotic-type conditions are likely to be effective for serious PTSD (45). Unfortunately (and as discussed in more detail in Chapter 6), no one class of medications has achieved the status of being the medication of choice for treating PTSD symptoms, and neuroleptics also have serious side effects that have to be taken into account when considering their use.

The Parts Paradigm

A second paradigm that has greatly influenced our thinking about helping survivors heal is the "parts" paradigm (49). This paradigm encompasses ideas and observations about dissociative phenomena. Dissociation refers to the ability of the mind–body to erect barriers between an individual's awareness and his or her past and current experience. Thus, it can be thought of as a coping skill that humans can employ to help themselves deal with anxiety-inducing experiences. Abusive experiences are by definition strongly anxiety producing, and high levels of dissociation are likely to be a result of abuse, especially if ongoing.

While dissociation can help persons survive abuse, the disruption of normally integrated systems of experience (disruption such as the loss of awareness of thoughts and feelings through repression or through amnesia-based identity disorders) indicates that the solution can become part of the problem. A classic example of this is what we call "codependent confusion," or the scattered, disorganized and blank thinking that many survivors show in the face of conflict and disagreement.

Originally identified by the early psychoanalysts as the basis of hysteria and other subconscious "complexes," the concept of dissociation has begun to appear again, with writers now using it to account for the wide range of responses to abuse. The recent upsurge of interest in DID has accelerated the use of the concept of dissociation (50).

Braun is the writer who has most thoroughly developed the concept of dissociation to understand and explain a wide range of psychopathology, including that caused by abuse (51). He proposes a continuum of awareness that ranges from normal, to suppression, to denial, to repression, and on to partial and then full dissociation. He further proposes that awareness has four components summarized by the acronym BASK. The B stands for behavior or what we do, the A for affect or what we feel, the S for sensation or what we perceive in our bodies, and the K for knowledge or what we think and remember. Integrated and congruent "BASKing" represents mental health and optimal functioning within this model. Trance-inducing occurrences (including abuse) produce a disconnection between some or all components of our BASK experience. Hypnosis used to promote anesthesia for control of surgical or chronic pain is an example of benign dissociation in the S modality. Problematic dissociation occurs in cases of psychogenic fugue, where memory, or the K component of a person's identity, is lost in response to a serious stressor. Severe cases of abuse can result in the ultimate dissociative phenomenon, the development of DID, where the individual manifests completely organized BASK subsystems ("personalities") that have no awareness of or control over each other. Braun also specifies that dissociation is a form of state-dependent learning.

Braun's ideas, together with notions of our own, have proven immensely valuable in our work for understanding and treating our survivor clients. Reenactments in this framework represent a triggering of dissociated and state-dependent BASK complexes. The triggered complex can be entire and whole as in DID, or it can be partial and fragmentary as when a survivor suddenly and overwhelmingly floods with tears at feedback that objectively seems benign and constructive but subjectively feels massively critical. Survivors can continue to experience somatic flashbacks of the abuse, such as the reappearance of raised welts on their skin where they were tied or beaten, the sound of the abuser's footsteps coming into their room at night, or the feeling of the abuser's hand over their mouth. We have even witnessed "cross-triggering," where feelings of being trapped in a bad job situation prompt memories of the abuse with associated feelings of being "trapped" by the abuser.

We use the BASK model of triggering to make interpretations and to reframe our clients' experiences, a process that at first astounds them and then comforts them as the mysterious becomes comprehensible. We can continue to monitor their progress in therapy by noting which parts are still being dissociated. We also teach our clients the BASK model so that they can begin to identify their own trance states. We might, for example, ask a client what she is *feeling* as she discusses an issue with us in a coldly intellectual manner. Or we might observe that a client constantly stiffens his back and lets out a nervous giggle when he talks about how often he got into trouble and how often his stepfather had to punish him; asking more questions about these punishments might reveal that the stepfather would have the client bend over with his pants down and hold on to his ankles while he beat him mercilessly with a leather strap for minor infractions. Or we might witness a client suddenly dissociate or space out and curl up in a ball in the chair when beginning to discuss her sexual abuse; realizing that the abuse was probably profound and at an early age and that the client cannot tolerate work in this area at this time, we would bring her back to the here and now and institute other measures to help her feel safe.

Survivors' treatment is incomplete if any BASK component remains unintegrated. Unfortunately, many survivors, even those with years of therapy, still trigger and flood and have pockets of their own past or present experience that are not integrated. They can talk at length about their abuse, they can tell people why they are not to blame, and perhaps they are generally somewhat more assertive and less anxious. However, these same survivors might still produce an angry tirade at the slightest provocation or lapse into a profound, long-lasting depression that is above and beyond the usual when a romantic relationship ends. Survivors who have achieved some progress in treatment often recover more quickly following the floods after triggering better than they did before, but they still flood. And survivors whose treatment is incomplete and who have unintegrated parts often evidence affective and somatic numbing that alternates with ongoing reenactments of aspects of their abuse.

We have come to regard the ultimate goal of treatment with survivors as one of integrating parts of themselves that are habitually dissociated. Although much of the writing about recovery from trauma refers to a peeling-away process to get at the underlying core conflict or unresolved trauma, we find it more fruitful to think in terms of helping survivors put back together the parts of their experience and lives that fragmented, split, and disconnected under the impact of the abuse. Our work involves assisting survivors to internally integrate their BASK components from both past and present. But it also involves helping them externally integrate with others. Abuse disrupts and disconnects victims from others, whether it is abuse of the traumatic kind at the hands of supposedly safe adults or abuse of the abandoning kind from the failure of supposedly nurturing adults to protect and nourish. In fact, until the survivor connects with others in safe and supportive ways, internal integration is not likely to occur.

We introduce the notion of parts to our clients once treatment is under way. Speaking to clients about "that part of you that wants to hurt people" or "that part of you that wants to drink" is a way of giving information, feedback, and interpretations that is less likely to trigger their defensiveness, whether in the form of denial or full-blown dissociation. It also lays the groundwork for future interventions.

In later stages of treatment we use a general tripartite model to help our survivor clients label, explore, develop, and, finally, integrate these parts of themselves. The three parts of our schema have certain functions with respect to the client's actions, feelings, thinking, and sensations associated with the abuse. That is, the function of the "wounded part" is to hold the pain of the abuse, both the trauma and the abandonment; the function of the "protective" part is to hold all the defenses the individual has evolved to stay safe and to avoid further pain; and the function of the "nurturing" part is to hold all the ways he or she has developed to support, validate, and care for the self. We first try to increase the functional capacity of these parts by, for example, adding assertion skills to the protector part or by having the client read affirmations to strengthen the nurturing part. We later work with the client to create a map—or clear picture of—the function, triggers, feelings, behaviors, and beliefs of these parts as they operate currently, and we also try to help the client understand the original "learning environment" that influenced these parts. Finally, we focus on integrating clients' new skills and understanding into their appropriate parts and then fusing the parts into a more coherent whole. This framework suffices for most clients, but in the case of clients suffering from DID the parts are typically more numerous and differentiated and require modifications in the sequencing of these interventions. (Later chapters describe these strategies and tactics in more detail.)

The Trance Paradigm

The final paradigm that we have found useful is one that views the major symptom of abuse as the occurrence of problematic trance states and the goal of treatment as a "de-trancing" of the client. This paradigm uses the concept of state-dependent learning (a construct common to the biphasic and parts paradigms as well) and the concept of dissociation (which also underlies the parts paradigm).

According to the trance paradigm, trance and hypnotic phenomena are everyday occurrences, although there are individual differences in "tranceability." Most people have experienced a trance, which is characterized by a narrowing and intensifying of attention, when, for example, they arrive safely at their destination but cannot recall driving there (highway hypnosis) or become so engrossed in a book that they do not hear the phone ringing.

Furthermore, hypnotic trances seem to occur spontaneously in times of high stress; they are, in other words, state dependent. Since abuse is by definition a high-stress state, it is hypothesized that it induces trances and that symptoms of abuse therefore represent hypnotic phenomena. For example, flashbacks can be seen as time regression and as so-called positive hallucinations (seeing something not really there; negative hallucinations refer to not seeing something that is there). Obsessive worry involves positive hallucinations of negative outcomes and represents a projection forward in time. A great deal of research on hypnosis and state-dependent learning is available to support these general hypotheses and their application to survivor issues (48, 52). Even research in the cognitive–behavioral tradition indicates that certain affective states distort the individual's perception and memory. Depressed individuals, for example, are more likely than nondepressed individuals to remember negative descriptions of themselves (53).

A key and crucial implication of this paradigm is that the task for therapists is to help survivors "detrance." In the old view, the therapist uses hypnosis to put clients into a trance and help them uncover the repressed trauma and work it through. In the new view, the therapist's job is to recognize that clients are already in a trance and to help them get out of their "abuse trance" (54).

The trance paradigm has enormously enriched our understanding and treatment of survivors. We are much more sensitive to the internal workings of our clients in our sessions, being more observant of such things as changes in breathing, shifts in posture, and spaced-out looks when we assess for possible survivor issues and treat survivors for abuse-related conditions. Our clients enthusiastically respond to our reframing their problems in trance terms (we introduce this viewpoint by saying something like "It's as if you are in a trance") and then educating them about trances and about how normal such a response is to abuse experiences. The notion of a trance fits the client's subjective sense of being somewhere else and of being in the grip of a process that defies rational control. The trance reframe also is exciting, mysterious, and intriguing for most of our clients and engages them more firmly in the therapy process. While we have had formal training in hypnosis and strongly recommend this to other therapists, just recognizing when survivor clients are in a trance and using such simple techniques as asking them to breathe, maintain eye contact, and notice what is going on with them as it happens require no specialized training and go a long way toward helping clients come into the here and now.

THE PROCESS OF ABUSE AND THE CONTINUUM OF OUTCOMES

We now return to our original questions about the abuse process with an enhanced understanding of the factors that form the tapestry of abuse and influence the pattern of outcomes that survivors experience. Abuse takes many forms and differs in kind and severity. Globally speaking, abuse includes both trauma and abandonment and the interaction of these two experiences constitutes abuse. Survivors-to-be bring to their experience of abuse certain adaptive abilities and skills, and these, along with a particular life situation and the presence of significant others, further modulate the impact of the abuse. Abuse represents a disconnection between a child's needs for protection and nurturing and the gratification of these needs by the family and society. This disconnection reverberates throughout survivors' experience, dissociating them both "outside" (i.e., from others) and "inside" (i.e., preventing them from being balanced and whole in their mind and body and creating a sense of shame) and can become acute when triggered.

We think of abuse outcomes as falling along a continuum of severity on which a survivor can receive any diagnosis from being the child of an alcoholic (COA) to having a DID. Figure 3.1 depicts such a continuum.

COAs experience a profound sense of abandonment during childhood because of parental preoccupation with substance use. While parental substance dependence is associated with a high probability of physical and sexual abuse as well, abuse of the abandoning kind is a key theme for COAs and leads to a number of serious problems for them in adulthood (17, 55). In our counseling of COAs we have found that many do not know how to really take care of themselves physically or emotionally and that it is important to prompt them toward better self-care by encouraging them to eat well and maintain proper levels of activity and by helping them learn to manage unpleasant feelings such as anger, depression, fear, and stress. Often COAs take excellent care of others but do not consistently take care of themselves; as children they very often took care of their parents and learned to survive this way. It is important for therapists to help these clients integrate and direct their caretaking to include themselves as well.

Clients can have COA-type issues when their background includes not only a parent who was chemically dependent but also one who was unavailable for other reasons, such as chronic physical or mental illness, severe workaholism or other preoccupation, or premature death. Black-and-white thinking, fear of abandonment, hypersensitivity, and difficulty setting limits often characterize these clients.

Individuals with an identity disorder typically have experienced not only family failure to care for their needs but also some kind of physical abuse as well. Often angry and frustrated as children, these persons enter adolescence acting out their anger through such delinquent activities as school truancy, running away from home, and drug and alcohol use. These teens are at high risk for gang affiliation and often drop out of school. Their anger at the world in general and authority figures in particular leads to countless conflicts with school officials, police, parents, and the therapists who try to help them. We use the term *identity disorder* rather than such diagnoses as oppositional defiant disorder or even conduct disorder (although such diagnoses are commonly applied to these adolescents) to underscore our belief that it is the abuse-based internal and external disconnections in the experiences of these individuals that cause their difficulties.

Persons suffering from borderline personality disorder have usually suffered both serious abandonment and sexual abuse at an early age (24, 27). Individuals with this disorder are extremely volatile and have major difficulty with their emotions, relationships, and their sense of identity. Under stress their thinking is infantile and can even appear psychotic. They often engage in very dangerous behaviors and are quite often suicidal. Chaos characterizes both their internal and external worlds. Clinicians often talk about the need to provide "holding" environments during a crisis for persons with borderline personality disorder because

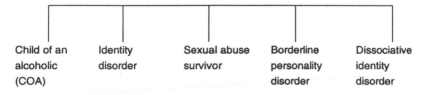

| Child of an alcoholic (COA) | Identity disorder | Sexual abuse survivor | Borderline personality disorder | Dissociative identity disorder |

FIGURE 3.1 Continuum of outcomes of abuse.

they have so little ability to organize and modulate their feelings, impulses, and responses to the world. The need for such an environment reflects the very early failure of the family to provide even basic protection and nurturing during the childhood of such persons.

Persons suffering from DID have usually experienced not only severe abandonment but trauma of the most vicious kind (50). Torture and other forms of horrific abuse are common. Persons with this disorder survived by dissociating so completely that they created new personalities with different functions and attitudes and even different physiological responses. We have seen clients with DID in the hospital whose personalities had different basal blood pressures and medication allergies and differed with respect to their need for reading glasses.

Viewing survivors on a continuum, instead of as collections of diverse symptoms and problems, helps us to ferret out common themes and treatment needs. Thinking in terms of a continuum helps to account for a commonly observed clinical phenomenon as well, namely, the tendency of clinicians to sometimes overestimate the baseline pathology of survivors. Many such clients are very volatile and resistant to treatment, and clinicians often have strong negative feelings toward them. Because survivors typically enter treatment in a crisis, we tend to see them at their worst. It is not uncommon for clinicians to abruptly and mistakenly label a client as a "severe borderline," and therefore as very difficult to treat, when in fact in more stable times the client would be recognized as a COA with strong codependent features, a more hopeful prognosis. We have more than once had to remind both ourselves and clinicians we are supervising to go slow and to be patient in such situations. Rediagnosing a client as a "survivor of abuse in a crisis" instead of a "bad, untreatable borderline" assists us in maintaining a therapeutic attitude. Conversely, keeping in mind that even COAs, like their MPD brethren, are likely to have dissociative symptoms helps us to take even more seriously the pain of these relatively less damaged clients. We have worked with many COA clients who told us that other clinicians viewed them as just fine after a cursory assessment that failed to look beyond their seemingly healthy presentation and take into account subtle but important dissociative signs such as their relentless, exhausting workaholism. Until we learned differently, we sometimes made the same underestimation ourselves. We have also learned not to prematurely diagnose with a more serious disorder those adolescent female COAs who cut on themselves or engage in other forms of self mutilation (often taken as a classic sign of borderline personality disorder) after breaking up with their boyfriend.

The continuum notion also helps us account for other clinical observations. For example, our clients refuse to fall into neat diagnostic categories. Not only do COAs dissociate and show "personality fragments" resembling DID personalities, but borderlines often show a range of strengths and functional capabilities. The diagnostic rules of the DSM-IV acknowledge these possibilities by allowing for multiple diagnoses for a given client (14). Persons suffering from DID have often received borderline personality diagnoses and when integrated often continue to evidence signs of difficulties further down the continuum. Finally, we see among all survivors the same kinds of problems, although differing in extent and intensity, problems such as black-and-white thinking, triggered and dissociated behavior, and avoidance behaviors. This has encouraged us to believe that a common treatment model is possible for all survivors.

Seeing survivors on a continuum permits us to consolidate the insights and wisdom of the literature on a variety of different problems and client populations. The more tools we have, the more likely we are to be helpful to our survivor clients in helping them to put together what their abuse broke apart; and the further up the continuum a person falls, the more likely it is that he or she will need dual-diagnosis treatment.

Later chapters explore treatment issues in more detail. In our review of the abuse process in this chapter we have indicated that the provision of conditions for secure attachment, protection, and nurturing in therapy sessions, the building of social supports, the teaching of coping skills, and work on desensitizing and detrancing clients will be fundamental to helping them overcome shame, fear, and a sense of abandonment, and to integrate their experiences, and achieve wholeness.

REFERENCES

1. Luthar, S. S., & Zigler, E. (1991). Vulnerability and competence: A review of research on resilience in childhood. *American Journal of Orthopsychiatry, 61*(1), 6–22.
2. Lazarus, R. S. (1980). The stress and chronic pain paradigm. In C. Eisdorfer, D. Cohen, & A. Kleinnian (Eds.), *Conceptual models for psychotherapy*, (pp. 173–209). New York: Spectrum.
3. Finkelhor, D. (1990). Early and long-term effects of child sexual abuse: An update. *Professional Psychology: Research and Practice, 21*(5), 325–330.
4. Perry, J. C. (1985). Depression in borderline personality disorder: Lifetime prevalence at interview and longitudinal course symptoms. *American Journal of Psychiatry, 142*(1), 15–21.
5. Chopra, H. D., & Beatson, J. C. (1986). Psychotic symptoms in borderline personality disorder. *American Journal of Psychiatry, 145*(12), 1605–1606.
6. Coons, P. M., & Milstein, V. (1986). Psychosexual disturbances in multiple personality disorders: Characteristics, etiology, and treatment. *Journal of Clinical Psychiatry, 47*, 106–110.

7. Ellenson, G. S. (1986). Disturbance of perception in adult female incest survivors: Social casework. *Journal of Contemporary Social Work, 67,* 149–159.
8. Brown, G. R., & Anderson, B. (1991). Psychiatric morbidity in adult inpatients with childhood histories of sexual and physical abuse. *American Journal of Psychiatry, 148*(1), 55–61.
9. Gelinas, D. J. (1983). The persisting negative effects of incest. *Psychiatry, 46,* 312–332.
10. Shapiro, S. (1987). Self-Mutilation and self-blame in incest survivors. *American Journal of Psychotherapy, 41,* 46–54.
11. Lowery, M. (1987). Adult survivors of childhood incest. *Journal of Psychological Nursing, 25,* 27–31.
12. Briere, J., & Runitz, M. (1987). Post-sexual abuse trauma: Data and implications for clinical practice. *Journal of Interpersonal Violence, 2*(4), 367–379.
13. Conte, J. R., & Shuerman, J. R. (1987). The effects of sexual abuse on children: A multidimensional view. *Journal of Interpersonal Violence, 2,* 380–390.
14. American Psychiatric Association (1994). *Diagnostic and statistical manual of mental disorders* (4th ed.). Washington, DC: Author.
15. Famularo, R., Kinscherff, R., & Fenton, R. (1991). Post-traumatic stress disorder among children clinically diagnosed as borderline personality disorder. *Journal of Nervous and Mental Disease, 179*(7), 428–431.
16. Cole, P. M., & Putnam, F. W. (1992). Effect of incest on self and social functioning: A developmental psychopathology perspective. *Journal of Consulting and Clinical Psychology, 60*(2), 174–184.
17. Cermak, T. (1986). *Diagnosing and treating codependents.* Minneapolis, MN: Johnson Institute.
18. Terr, L. C. (1991). Childhood traumas: An outline and overview. *American Journal of Psychiatry, 148*(1), 10–20.
19. Alexander, P. C. (1992). Application of attachment theory to the study of sexual abuse. *Journal of Consulting and Clinical Psychology, 61*(2), 185–195.
20. Hartman, M., Finn, S. E., & Lean, G. N. (1987). Sexual abuse experiences in a clinical population: Comparison of familial and nonfamilial abuse. *Psychotherapy, 24*(2), 154–159.
21. Herman, J., Russel, D., & Trocki, K. (1986). Long-term effects of incestuous abuse in childhood. *American Journal of Psychiatry, 143,* 1283–1296.
22. Harter, S., Alexander, P. C., & Neimeyer, R. A. (1988). Long-term effects of incestuous child abuse in college woman: Social adjustment, social cognition and family characteristics. *Journal of Consulting and Clinical Psychology, 51*(1), 5–8.
23. Briere, J., & Runitz, M. (1988). Symptomatology associated with childhood sexual abuse: Victimization in a nonclinical adult sample. *Child Abuse and Neglect, 12,* 51–59.
24. Bryer, J. B., Bernadette, A. N., Miller, J. B., et al. (1987). Childhood sexual and physical abuse as factors in adult psychiatric illness. *American Journal of Psychiatry, 144,* 1426–1430.
25. Brown, G. R., & Anderson, B. (1991). Psychiatric morbidity in adult inpa-

tients with childhood histories of sexual and physical abuse. *American Journal of Psychiatry, 148,* 55–61.

26. Sanders, B., & Giolas, M. H. (1991). Dissociation and childhood trauma in psychologically disturbed adolescents. *American Journal of Psychiatry, 148,* 50–54.

27. Zanarini, M. C., & Gunderson, J. B. (1987). Childhood abuse common in borderline personality. *Clinical Psychiatry News, 6,* 1.

28. Zimrin, H. (1986). A profile of survival. *Child Abuse and Neglect, 10,* 339–349.

29. Mahler, M. S., Pine, F., & Bergman, A. (1975). *The psychological birth of the infant.* New York: Basic Books.

30. Masterson, J. F. (1976). *Psychotherapy of the borderline adult.* New York: Brunner/Mazel.

31. Hartocollis, P. (Ed.). (1977). *Borderline personality disorders: The concept, the syndrome, the patient.* Madison, CT: International Universities Press.

32. Joselyn, R. E. (1992). *The space between us: Exploring the dimensions of human relationships* (1st ed.). San Francisco: Jossey-Bass.

33. Gold, E. R. (1986). Long-term effects of sexual victimization in childhood: An attributional approach. *Journal of Consulting and Clinical Psychology, 54*(4), 471–475.

34. Zimrin, H. (1986). A profile of survival. *Child Abuse and Neglect, 10,* 339–349.

35. Rutter, M. (1979). Protective factors in children's responses to stress and disadvantage. In M. W. Kent & J. E. Rolf (Eds.), *Primary prevention of psychopathology: Vol. 3. Social competence in children* (pp. 49–74). Hanover, NH: University Press in New England.

36. Wilson, J. P. (1989). *Trauma, transformation and healing: An integrative approach to theory, research and post-traumatic therapy.* New York: Brunner/Mazel.

37. Gazzaniga, M. S. (1992). *Nature's mind: The biological roots of thinking, emotions, sexuality, language and intelligence.* New York: Basic Books, Harper Collins.

38. Seligman, M. E. P. (1975). *Helplessness.* New York: W. H. Freeman.

39. Conte, J. R., & Schuerman, J. R. (1987). Factors associated with an increased impact of child sexual abuse. *Child Abuse and Neglect, 11,* 201–211.

40. Brown, G. W., & Harris, T. O. (1978). *Social origins of depression: A study of psychiatric disorders in women.* London: Tavistock.

41. Harter, S., Alexander, P. C., & Neimeyer, R. A. (1988). Long-term effects of incestuous child abuse in college woman: Social adjustment, social cognition, and family characteristics. *Journal of Consulting and Clinical Psychology, 56,* 5–8.

42. Singer, M. T., & Ofshe, R. (1990). Thought reform programs and the production of psychiatric casualties. *Psychiatric Annals, 20*(4), 188–193.

43. Bateson, G. (1972). *Steps to an ecology of the mind.* New York: Ballantine Books.

44. Wilson, J. P. (1989). *Trauma, transformation and healing: An integrative approach to theory, research and post-traumatic therapy.* New York: Brunner/Mazel.

45. Charney, D. S., Deutch, A. Y., Krystal, J. H., et al. (1993). Psychobiologic mechanisms of posttraumatic stress disorder. *Archives of General Psychiatry, 50,* 294–305.

46. Foa, E. B., Kozak, M. J., Steketee, G. S., et al. (1992). Treatment of depressive and obsessive-compulsive symptoms in OCD by imipramine and behavior therapy. *British Journal of Clinical Psychology, 31*(3), 279–292.
47. Fairbank, J. A., & Nicholson, R. A. (1987). Theoretical and empirical issues in the treatment of post-traumatic stress disorder in Vietnam veterans. *Journal of Clinical Psychology, 43*(1), 44–55.
48. Rossi, E. (1986). *The psychobiology of mind-body healing.* New York: Norton.
49. Kimmel, S. (1992). Personal communication.
50. Ross, C. (1990). Twelve cognitive errors about multiple personality disorder. *American Journal of Psychotherapy, 44*(3), 348–355.
51. Braun, B. G. (1988). The BASK model of dissociation. *Dissociation, 1*(1), 4–23.
52. Spiegel, D., & Cardeña, E. (1990). Dissociative mechanisms in post-traumatic stress disorder. In M. E. Wolf & A. D. Mosnaim (Eds.), *Post-traumatic stress disorder: Etiology, phenomonology and treatment.* Washington, DC: American Psychiatric Press.
53. Prieto, S. L., Cole, D. A., & Tageson, C. W. (1992). Depressive self-schemas in clinic and non-clinic children. *Cognitive Therapy and Research, 16*(5), 521–534.
54. Wolinsky, S. (1991). *Trances people live: Healing approaches in quantum psychology.* Norfolk, CT: Bramble Books.
55. Brennan, K. A., Shaver, P. R., & Tobey, A. E. (1991). Attachment styles, gender, and parental problem drinking. *Journal of Social and Personal Relationships, 8*, 451–466.

Addiction and Survivors

Forgotten

If she could only remember,
If she could only say,
Maybe death would seem farther away.
—AUBRY, age 17

Our goal in this chapter is to discuss in more detail drug and alcohol use, abuse, and addiction as well as related assessment and treatment concerns. The discussion covers these issues in general terms and in regard to addicted survivors.

ALCOHOL AND DRUG USE DISORDERS

Alcohol and drug *use* is the benign use of a potentially addictive substance either in social situations or under medical supervision. Alcohol and drug use may or may not lead to abuse or addiction but can be a warning sign of future chemical use problems. This is especially true for individuals with mental or emotional difficulties, who are at higher risk for developing problems with chemicals that alter mood.

Alcohol and drug *misuse* is the use of drugs outside medical supervision or inconsistent with medical advice. Substance misuse may or may not involve abuse or addiction. Drug misuse is not necessarily a sign of a substance use disorder but may be a warning of future substance use problems. It indicates the tendency of an individual to self-prescribe or overindulge, a tendency suggesting a life-style that could evolve into the misuse of drugs.

Substance abuse is, according to the DSM-IV (1), a maladaptive, recurrent pattern of substance use leading to significant impairment or distress within a 12-month period as indicated by: (1) a failure to fulfill major role responsibilities at work, school, or home; (2) use in situations which is physically hazardous (e.g., when driving); (3) legal problems; and (4) social and interpersonal problems.

Thus, alcohol and drug abuse is defined as the use of a chemical to the extent that it seriously interferes, or very well might, with the health or the occupational and social functioning of an individual. Individuals may, for example, suffer from colitis due to heavy drinking; they may have work problems, such Monday morning absences owing to hangovers or difficulty working as a team member or getting along with coworkers; and they may experience increased marital conflict.

Alcohol and drug *dependence* is a chronic, progressive, and often fatal illness that includes the following elements: (1) compulsion to use or reuse a drug, (2) loss of control over the drug, and (3) continued use despite adverse consequence.

DSM-IV (1) describes seven criteria, with the diagnosis of substance dependence requiring the presence of three or more of these at the same time in a 12-month period to make the diagnosis. These criteria include: (1) tolerance, with either a need for increased amounts of the substance to achieve the same effect or a diminished effect from the same amounts; (2) withdrawal symptoms that vary depending on the substance; (3) the person takes larger amounts of substance or uses over a longer time period than intended; (4) persistent desire or unsuccessful efforts to cut down or control substance use; (5) the person spends a great deal of time in obtaining, using, or recovering from use; (6) substance use leads to giving up important social, occupational, or recreational activities; and (7) the person continues the substance use despite knowledge of having persistent or recurrent physical or psychological problems that are likely to have been caused or made worse by the use of the substance. The DSM-IV allows specification of course as well, allowing, for example, designations of early full (no criteria of dependence present) or early partial remission (at least one of the criteria present intermittently or continuously) in the first 12 months and sustained full or sustained partial remission after the first 12 months when the individual has evidenced none of the criteria for dependence for a full month. This takes into account the reality that relapses are very common for many individuals in recovery from substance dependence (2).

PSYCHOLOGICAL AND PHYSICAL ADDICTION

The term *substance dependence* refers not only to the negative consequences associated with the substance use but also to the compulsive use of these chemicals. The American Society of Addiction Medicine describes drug dependence as having two possible components: (1) psychological dependence and (2) physiological dependence. The former refers to the need of drug users to reach a certain drug effect, which can be quite subjective, in order to feel that they can function normally. Even if their body has not developed tolerance or any sort of dependence on a chemical, persons who develop a psychological dependence on drugs or alcohol believe they cannot function without their drug of choice—although they may substitute another chemical when their drug of choice is not available. Individuals who psychologically crave alcohol or drugs begin to believe that they must use chemicals; consequently, they devote a great deal of time and energy to ensure a continuation of this use. Panicky and frantic efforts to obtain the chemical are signs of psychological withdrawal. Psychological addiction is so powerful that there are even people who are mentally dependent on taking a single aspirin at bedtime; if they run out of aspirin or for some other reason are unable to take the aspirin, they are unable to sleep. Examples of the mental obsession involved in psychological addiction include such preoccupations as planning the day around drinking or using, ensuring an adequate supply by anticipating and then avoiding situations that may lead to the necessity of sharing the substance with others or by hiding a little extra, and thinking about drinking or using when at work or during other activities.

Another aspect of addiction is the physiological dependence on chemicals. Physical dependence refers to tissue dependence on the drug and is evident in a tolerance for it and in the presence of withdrawal symptoms when the drug is no longer ingested. If persons continue to ingest a mood-altering substance over a long period of time, they eventually develop a metabolic tolerance for it and their body will need the drug to feel normal and to prevent withdrawal symptoms (3). That is, with exposure to a chemical over time the body can develop the capacity to more quickly and efficiently neutralize the chemical and compensate for its effects. Moreover, this tolerance extends across all substances of the same chemical class, a phenomenon known as "cross tolerance." In other words, the establishment of biologic tolerance to one drug means that there is also tolerance to others of the same drug class. Alcohol, for example, is "cross-tolerant" with other depressant-type drugs.

Abruptly removing a chemical from a person who is physiologically dependent on it will cause withdrawal symptoms, which vary from drug to drug but often include symptoms such as confusion, anxiety, insomnia, and nausea (4). In general, withdrawal symptoms are the opposite of the usual effects of the drug: Depressant withdrawal causes anxiety whereas amphetamine withdrawal causes mental and physical fatigue (3).

Tolerance and withdrawal set up a vicious cycle. As chemically dependent persons develop a tolerance for the chemical, they have to take more of it in order to get high, but they soon develop a tolerance for the increased dose, which leads to the need for even more of the chemical. Soon addicts, whose body now requires the drug to function normally, are using chemicals to avoid the withdrawal symptoms. This is referred to as relief drinking or using. Desperation has now replaced "recreation."

SYMPTOMS OF THE DISEASE OF ADDICTION

Blackouts

An important sign of chemical dependency is the occurrence of blackouts, which are periods of time during which the alcoholic or addict, despite remaining fully awake, appearing to an observer to be alert, and being capable of walking and talking, cannot recall any of his or her behavior. Some individuals suffer blackouts that last only a few minutes, others have blackouts that last for hours, and still others (some binge drinkers) have blackouts in which they lose days or even weeks. There are alcoholics who tell stories of getting on an airplane to visit a sister in California and waking up 2 weeks later in England with no clue as to how they got there, their last memory being one of ordering a drink on the plane.

Life Problems

Other symptoms of chemical dependency include drug-related life problems. Being late to work, calling in sick on Mondays and Fridays, and recurrent conflicts with coworkers are all work-related symptoms of drug addiction. Family problems include extramarital affairs, increased fighting among family members, the diverting of family income to support the chemical use, and a breakdown of communication between family members (5). Social symptoms related to chemical dependency include a turning away from long-term friends in favor of new drinking buddies, borrowing money from friends and failing to repay them, making caustic and unkind comments to others while under the influence of chemicals, social isolation, and avoidance of previously enjoyed activities.

Addicted persons often have legal difficulties. Alcoholics may get arrested for drunk driving, lose their driver's license, or even cause an accident when driving under the influence. Addicts desperate for money to buy drugs may resort to stealing, dealing, or even prostitution to support a growing and expensive drug habit.

Control and Loss of Control

Loss of control, perhaps the key feature of the disease of addiction, refers to the loss of ability of the addict to effectively control his or her use of chemicals (3,6). Drinking or using more than intended, drinking or using more often than planned, unsuccessful attempts to cut down or quit, and loss of control of behavior when drinking or using (such as promiscuity or excessive spending)—all are examples of loss of control, a phenomenon that distinguishes substance abuse from addiction.

In the earlier stages of the disease of addiction, loss of control happens sporadically; in the middle stages it happens more frequently; and in the late stages of the disease the addict is out of control almost immediately. This is, of course, why there has not been much success in teaching alcoholics to control their drinking. It would be much like trying to teach a diabetic who is supposed to limit his or her intake of sugar how not to react after indulging in an excessive amount of sugar. A disease process is not under the control of the person who suffers from the disease. We cannot control illness any more than we can chose who our ancestors were.

Some alcoholics have brief success trying to control their alcohol use. Others force periods of abstinence in attempts to prove to themselves and others that they do not have a problem with alcohol. The Big Book of AA suggests the following test to determine if a person has lost control of his or her drinking (7). If a person can drink two drinks each evening—no more, no less—for a month without feeling any strain or frustration, he or she is not an alcoholic. If, however, this test is frustrating or difficult or if the person fails it altogether, then he or she is considered to have lost control over alcohol use. Chemically dependent people can often stop their use of substances for a while. It is moderating or limiting their use that is the problem. Once the chemical is ingested, it takes control of the alcoholic's will and behavior and the alcoholic loses control.

Most addicts and alcoholics have issues with power and control that encompass more than their use of substances. They try to manipulate circumstances and the people around them in order to continue their substance abuse. Their attempts to keep things under control by such acts as lying, scheduling long lunches, and forging checks indicate their increasing desperation to control what is out of control. Confronting alcoholics and addicts about their control issues is a key part of treatment.

One sign that someone is beginning to have issues of control around their chemical use is the existence of "rules" for using, such as only drinking beer and not "hard" stuff, only using on weekends, and only drinking when with others. The stricter and more numerous these rules, the more likely it is that the individual is into an addictive process. And, of course, going on to break these rules is a sure sign of loss of control.

Denial

Denial is a term often used when discussing the chemically dependent person and is a common characteristic of addiction. Denial is distorted thinking and refers to addicts' lack of insight into their substance use problem and its effects on themselves and others. *The disease of addiction is a disease of denial.* This is extremely important for professionals to remember. It is not realistic to think that addicted persons are going to have much insight during the assessment interview into the extent of their problems with chemicals; in fact, the presence of denial is often the best clue about the severity of an interviewee's chemical use problem. Denial, or defensiveness about drinking and using, indicates a need to protect the all-important relationship with chemicals, and its presence suggests that a problem exits. Counselors need to be skilled at identifying denial and its distorted thinking patterns to effectively assess and treat addicted individuals. This distorted thinking includes minimizing the amounts of the substance used, justifying the use, rationalizing its consequences, and lying to oneself or others about the use. Clients seeking an assessment because their spouse thinks they have a drinking problem might say, for example, "I only drink one glass of wine a night." However, the savvy drug and alcohol counselor will ask how big the glass is and may find that it is a very large goblet. A college student may attempt to justify the use of amphetamines or cocaine by saying, "I have to lose weight, and besides I could never get all my studying done without it." Both are examples of denial.

All people use some denial at certain times or with certain issues. It is part of everyone's psychological defense structure. However, extensive use of denial for important issues inevitably leads to negative consequences. If someone minimizes the fact that he or she is overeating and not exercising, for example, the consequence will be weight gain. If someone ignores a limited budget and spends money constantly, bankruptcy may be the result. Denial, moreover, can be insidious. Often, the person in denial is the last person to figure out what is really going on. Many of our clients express what appears to be genuine surprise when they finally recognize their addiction. Unfortunately, it often takes a significant or substantial crisis before a person dependent on chemicals (or anyone in denial about anything important) surrenders to the reality of the situation.

Denial can be very frustrating both for the addict's therapist and for the significant others in his or her life. We find it helpful to remember that most addicts and alcoholics are not personality disordered and are not deliberately and maliciously trying to mislead us. Their use of drugs and alcohol puts them in a values conflict. If one of a person's values is honesty in marriage and yet that person drinks each time his or her spouse is not around, then it will be necessary for the person to either change the drinking or change the way he or she views it. The change that is made is the latter, and this "decision" constitutes the beginning of denial. Recovery requires "rigorous honesty," according to the Big Book of AA, this being the antidote for the denial and the dishonesty of the disease of addiction (7, 8, 9).

Yokelson and Samenow have developed the concept of "thinking errors" to describe denial and the associated distorted thinking found among individuals with antisocial behaviors (11, 17). We have adopted their work for use with alcoholics and addicts and with persons who have one of the acting-out personality disorders. The list of thinking errors in the next paragraph contains examples of denial in the form of easily recognized statements that clients in denial are likely to make, either out loud or to themselves. We have found that keeping this list in mind during assessment interviews and treatment sessions helps us to spot denial quickly. Anyone who uses many of these thinking errors in general and particularly in response to questions about substance use is likely to have an active substance use problem. The notion of thinking errors and these examples give us a language to use when we give feedback to clients about their denial process. We also share this list with clients to help them identify and conquer their own denial.

The following is a list of the various kinds of distorted thinking patterns that are present in denial:

Excuse making: "I drink because my wife nags me."

Blaming: "They made me relapse!"

Justifying: "I deserved to get stoned; I had thirty days clean!"

Redefining: "I'm not an addict; you just like to pick on people!"

Superoptimism: "I can stay sober on my own!"

Lying by omission: "I forgot to tell you all of the story."

Overt lying: "I never drink alcohol."

Assent: "If you think I have a problem, well maybe I do."

"I'm unique": "The rules in the treatment program shouldn't apply to me."

Ingratiating: "You are such a smart counselor that I'm sure you will be able to help me get out of jail early."

Fragmented personality: "Well I did rob a guy on the way to my AA meeting, but I gave some of the money to AA." (A true example!)

Minimizing: "I only had one drink. Does that count as a relapse?"

Vagueness: "Oh, you know, I just have a couple of drinks now and then."

Power play: "I'm rescinding my release of information, and if you report my relapse to the court, I will sue you for breach of confidentiality."

Victim playing: "People are always dumping on me!"

Grandiosity: "What is the deal with these AA dudes going to meetings for years? I got it after one meeting: Don't drink!"

Intellectualizing: "When was the last time your laboratory had its equipment checked? I know my urine drug screen had to be clean because I am clean!"

ASSESSMENT TOOLS

There are a number of standardized assessment tools for determining whether a person has a drug or alcohol problem, including some very simple ones (11). The CAGE is an acronym for the basic ideas within four simple questions that explore whether a person has a problem with alcohol (12). Those ideas and the questions in which they are embedded are as follows:

*C*ut down: Have you ever tried to *cut down* your use of chemicals?
*A*nnoyed: Has anyone ever *annoyed* you by criticizing your drinking?
*G*uilty: Have you ever felt *guilty* about your behavior when drinking?
*E*ye opener: Have you ever used alcohol *in the morning* in order to reduce the effects of a hangover?

There are several other brief screening interview tools for rapid assessment of alcoholism that are also acronyms. They are the FATALDT, HALT, and BUMP (13). FATALDT stands for the following elements:

*F*amily history of alcoholism
*A*lcoholic's Anonymous attendance
*T*houghts of having alcoholism
*A*ttempts or thoughts of suicide
*L*egal problems
*D*riving while intoxicated
*T*ranquilizer or disulfiram use

The HALT asks about the following:

Do you usually drink to get *high* (*H*)?
Do you sometimes drink *alone* (*A*)?

Do you find that you are *looking* (L) forward to drinking or using?
Do you have a *tolerance* (T) to alcohol?

The BUMP asks about the following:

Have you ever had *blackouts* (B) from drinking?
Have you ever used alcohol in an *unplanned* (U) way?
Do you drink in the *mornings* (M)?
Do you ever *protect* (P) your supply?

An important principle to keep in mind when asking clients questions about their chemical use and evaluating whether they have a problem is that the cardinal indicator of alcoholism and addiction is negative consequences of use. The novice evaluator often focuses on how much and how often. While this information is helpful, it is more helpful to determine what happens when the individual does drink or use. One individual we evaluated, for example, only drank two or three times a year, a report confirmed by family members. However, he always drank to the point of intoxication, would go into a blackout, and would always end up wrecking furniture and starting fights with family members, often even assaulting them. Yet he clung firmly to the belief that he did not have a problem because he only drank a few times a year.

Unless they are in a "surrender" state, most clients give distorted information, ranging from minimizing to outright lying, in interviews because of their reliance on denial. Experienced counselors know that the substance use history clients give later in treatment is very different from the one they give at the intake interview (14). Relying only on interview information is almost always likely to yield a less than accurate picture.

We have already discussed using the material on thinking errors to spot denial. As a rough guideline, the more evident the thinking errors, the more likely clients are to be in trouble with chemicals. Other assessment procedures besides standardized assessment tools and intake interviews are also helpful. We always try to obtain collateral data whenever possible. While family members may also be in denial, more often than not they can provide a less distorted view of the client's chemical use patterns and the consequences of that use. A client's refusal to allow us to contact anyone is a serious sign that something is amiss. Occasionally, the reasons for this are legitimate, but generally a refusal is a reflection of client denial and control issues in action. Random urinalyses while not perfect, help clients remain honest. Because most of the adolescents we treat come to our clinic at someone else's insistence, we routinely have them take a urine test. We treat a refusal as indicating that the test will come back positive for a substance of abuse. Adults who are under some sort of work or legal mandate also have urinalyses done, and we request a urinalysis from any client whose behavior indicates a possible relapse, a request that often, especially with clients who are survivors, must be made with a great deal of tact. We try, whenever possible, to encourage clients to regard the urinalysis not as an attempt to catch or humiliate them but as a useful tool in promoting rigorous honesty and combating the denial that the part of them that holds the disease constantly promotes. Finally, after evaluating several psychological tests, we are increasingly using the Substance Abuse Subtle Screening Inventory (SASSI) as part of our assessment package (15). Easy to complete and quickly scored, the SASSI has both a section of obvious questions about alcohol and drug use and a section of subtle questions whose purpose is hard for interviewees to recognize and that detect chemical dependence even when they are in strong denial. There are forms and norms for both adults and adolescents, and the available research and our own experience indicate very good accuracy for the results (16).

STAGES OF ADDICTION

Addiction is a progressive disease. Things get worse over time with continued use of substances. The Jellnick progression chart (of which Table 4.1 is an adaptation) shows the progression of the disease of addiction from early to middle, and then late stages. These three stages are widely used to determine where a person is in the progression of his or her disease. Table 4.1 correlates specific symptoms with progressive stages of the disease (6).

Early Stage

In the early stages of the disease the addict/alcoholic may occasionally lose control. He or she may begin to avoid some activities where alcohol is not served and may occasionally experience a blackout. An occasional conflict with spouse or friend may occur that is related to the drug or alcohol use. There is only minimal social or occupational impairment in the early stage, but there is a growing preoccupation with the importance of the chemical. Persons in the early stage may begin to feel defensive about their substance use, although they have not yet experienced many negative consequences of it.

Middle Stage

In the middle stage of the disease the addicted person develops increased metabolic tolerance. In this stage conflicts with family members and

TABLE 4.1. Progression of Addiction

Early stage

Sneaks drinks/drugs
Preoccupied with alcohol/drugs
Avoids reference to alcohol/drug use
Increased tolerance
Relief drinking/using
Drinks or uses before and after social drinking/using functions
Memory blackouts

Middle stage

Beginning of loss of control
Is dishonest about substance use
Tries periods of forced abstinence
Hides or protects supply
Commits thinking errors about chemical use
Feels guilty about drug/alcohol use
Quits or loses job
Drinks/uses alone
Neglects physical health and nutrition

Late stage

Experiences tremors or shakes
Early morning drug/alcohol use
Binge use
Loses tolerance for substance
Unable to work
Loses friends and family

friends are more common; legal problems, such as drunk driving tickets, may have occurred; and blackouts may become more frequent (3). The addict/alcoholic is now experiencing more frequent loss of control over the drug/alcohol use. In the middle stage of addiction withdrawal symptoms, such as hangovers, shakiness, and nervousness, may appear in milder forms with cessation of use.

Late Stage

Tolerance may change at the late, or chronic, stage. It may no longer take large amounts of the chemical to achieve euphoric effects but only small amounts. By the time this drop in tolerance occurs, the user has suffered serious medical problems, such as damage to the liver and pancreas. The liver can no longer metabolize and clear the body of the drug. Other medical problems, such as heart disease and cancer, can be a result of long-term use. Impairment of mental processes may also occur, including damage to memory functions, as in a condition known as "wet brain," or Korsakoff's psychosis, which is characterized by profound short-term memory loss.

In this late and chronic stage of the disease of addiction the addict or alcoholic has already lost his or her job, family, and friends and may have already been unsuccessfully treated for the addiction. Frequent failed attempts at sobriety are common at this stage. Sufferers at this stage of the disease often have a hopeless attitude about their ability to improve their life's situation, and almost all their activities now involve the obtaining and using of the addictive substance or substances if they are polysubstance dependent. Many addicts and alcoholics die in this stage from a medically related illness or as a victim of violent crime (2).

THE RECOVERY PROCESS

Recovery is the general and inclusive term used to describe the process of healing for the chemically dependent person. Recovery involves not only abstinence from mind-altering chemicals but also taking steps to repair the damage caused by the disease of addiction. Recovery is a process, not an event. The individual will never be "recovered" but can stay "recovering" if he or she continues to work a program that supports recovery concepts. Recovery from a life-threatening disease deserves and demands commitment and must be a priority! Treating the disease of addiction as secondary to anything else will lead to resumption of the chemical use and further progression of the disease. The priority given to the treatment of addiction in a survivor of abuse must equal that given to the treatment of PTSD or any other survivor syndrome. Recovering survivors need to respect the power of the disease of addiction as being not only a threat to their sobriety but also to their recovery from their childhood abuse. Treatment professionals, especially those with a background primarily in mental health and not in drug and alcohol treatment, must also come to respect the power of the disease of addiction and recognize the need to give it attention at least equal to that paid to any other survivor syndrome. The most common source of treatment failure we have seen in our own practice and in supervising others is the "mental health relapse" of therapists in their implementation of treatment, that is, the inclination of therapists to focus on the psychiatric disorder, either from the onset or gradually over time. Almost inevitably, clients then relapse not only in their substance dependence but, because of the synergistic effect, in their survivor syndrome.

In the paragraphs that follow we discuss the essential elements of an effective recovery program both for clients with the single diagnosis of substance dependence and for addicted survivors (6).

Abstinence

An addict's commitment to eliminating all addictive substances from his or her life is key to building a strong foundation in recovery; trying to control or simply cut back the use of chemicals is not the solution to a problem with chemicals. Some addicts try to quit one drug but still continue to use another (very often the new drug is alcohol). In our experience this is *not* an effective strategy. Those employing this strategy of "partial abstinence" usually either return to using their drug of choice or. There is also a state, referred to as a "dry drunk" syndrome, in which individuals stop using mood-altering chemicals but never work a program of recovery. In our experience these individuals are often angry, depressed, rigid, and controlling and continue to have life problems despite no chemical use. These "personality traits," which are not a cause but a consequence of addiction, continue to interfere with all therapeutic interventions and with the attainment of a quality recovery.

Education

Teaching recovering addicts and alcoholics about their disease is an important part of recovery. By understanding the signs and symptoms of their disease they can give up their sense of themselves as a "bad person trying to get good" and replace this with a view of themselves as "a sick person trying to get well." Understanding the biological basis of addiction, identifying their own signs and symptoms of the disease, discussing the relapse process and applying this information to their own situation—all such steps should be part of the education process for clients (2). It is also important that clients have information regarding the stages of addiction, the progression of their disease, and the medical effects that abuse of their chemical has on the human mind and body. Information about the effects of addiction on family members helps recovering persons increase their sense of responsibility and empathy toward their own family members (5).

A good education for recovery includes information on a 12-step recovery program and on how to "work the steps" (7, 8, 9). This can be done initially through group discussions. However, requiring clients to go to 12-step meetings outside of group help to anchor their recovery and to assist them in building new relationships with sober individuals is essential. Discussing such topics as the role played by various members in alcoholic families and the phenomenon of enabling (see Chapter 9) allows the alcoholic to understand the need for the whole family to be in recovery if sobriety is to be maintained. Newly recovering addicts/alcoholics can also begin to apply the information they are receiving about the influence of and interdependence within families to a new understanding of the impact of growing up in their family of origin.

Involving other family members in the recovery process is also important. For example, some family members have difficulty with the frequent absences of the newly recovering person who attends many 12-step meetings. They may complain about and even sabotage the attempts of the recovering person to reach out and develop a support group of abstinent persons, and they may feel left out of the recovering person's life because of all the new 12-step jargon and all the events that revolve around the recovery group. Participation in a group of their own (e.g., Al-Anon) offers family members an opportunity to work through their own feelings and issues around the disease of addiction and the effects it has had on their family.

Sober Support

Support comes in many forms. Active participation in such 12-step groups as AA, Narcotics Anonymous (NA), and Cocaine Anonymous (CA) promotes abstinence for the recovering alcoholic/addict, both short- and long-term. Active participation in 12-step programs might include a goal in the early weeks of recovery of attending 90 meetings in 90 days. We recommend no less than three meetings a week to provide adequate 12-step support in the early days of recovery.

Another form of support for the recovering person is the presence of a sponsor, or someone who is further along in the recovery process and who thus serves as a mentor. He or she acts as a guide to working the steps and understanding the philosophy and principles behind a 12-step self-help program. A sponsor should be someone who has at least a year of continuing abstinence and who is the same sex as the newly recovering addict/alcoholic. Sponsorship with members of the opposite sex have the potential of confusing support with sexual or romantic issues and thereby complicating the relationship. The term "13th stepping" refers to the development of a romantic or sexual relationship between a newcomer to a 12-step program and an established member. Such a relationship is strongly discouraged. A newcomer can choose a sponsor by attending meetings and finding someone there who seems to have quality abstinence and who appears to be a person with whom he or she can form a relationship.

Participation in 12-step groups can help newly recovering individuals develop a circle of sober friends. Such groups often sponsor dances, potluck dinners, and other activities around which friendships can develop. For newly recovering persons to continue to associate with their old addicted friends at the local tavern, even if they have a soft drink or coffee while their friends drink, is a precarious recovery at best.

A "home group" is the group whose meetings the newcomer chooses to attend regularly. Choosing a home group instead of drifting from meeting to meeting helps the newcomer meet new friends and develop a sense of belonging. Most cities have what is called an "intergroup office" for 12-step meetings, and the phone number for such an intergroup office is in the phone book. By calling any such office one can get a schedule of when and where 12-step meetings occur. Some of these meetings are "open" meetings, which means that even people who are not addicts can attend. A "closed" meeting, on the other hand, refers to one that is only open to people who are trying to become abstinent. Many newcomers are confused by the notion of a closed meeting, thinking that attendance is by invitation only. This is not the case! It is an oft-repeated principle of 12-step programs that "all newcomers are wanted and needed for the program to work."

Structure

Having a great deal of unstructured time on their hands is not helpful to persons in early recovery. Making a daily schedule of work and sober activities assures that newly recovering persons will fill their time with helpful instead of hurtful practices (17, 18). Most recovering addicts and alcoholics have spent a great deal of time and energy thinking about and using chemicals, and these activities become woven into the fabric of their daily lives; for example, most of an addicted person's social activities (especially in later stages of the disease) involve drinking and using. No longer playing pool at the tavern, dancing in bars, or drinking wine with friends can pose a problem for the newly sober person who has no substitutes.

A full week of work and family responsibilities followed by a weekend that is unstructured and boring is likely to lead to relapse for individuals who were weekend users. "Plan, Plan, Plan" is our motto. Most alcoholics/addicts are compulsive people anyway, and giving them the task of planning a daily schedule, especially for weekends, suits their nature and preempts hours of worry about what to do other than use chemicals. If the newly recovering person has a drinking style that includes stopping by the neighborhood bar on the way home from work, planning an alternate route or activity for that time slot is very helpful.

Structure is particularly important for addicted survivors. Structure equals safety. Making use of a daily schedule, which can be thought of as a tool for creating a healthy balance of activities in life, helps addicted survivors avoid both a return to drinking and using and the possibility of anxiety attacks and flashbacks, which can occur in the unstructured hours. However, some survivors jam-pack their schedule for the day with more projects than they can possibly accomplish; they then either become stressed trying to do the impossible or become so immobilized when they look at their lengthy "to do" list that they feel overwhelmed and go back to bed. Other survivors leave the entire day open with no real structure. The days pass, one by one, with the survivor drifting along, not going anywhere or getting anything done.

Skills

Many addicts and alcoholics lack skills to manage life problems. Perhaps they come from families where such skills were never modeled, or perhaps their learning stopped when they first began drinking or using. Often addicts and alcoholics are stuck emotionally at the age they first began drinking or using drugs, and when they are faced with the difficulties that life inevitably presents, they resort to using chemicals rather than coping in more functional ways.

Learning and practicing such skills as managing anger and depression, being assertive, and structuring one's time and taking responsibility for such things as filing a tax return are an important part of treatment. Many alcoholics, whether survivors or not, need to work early in the recovery process on how to set boundaries with themselves and others. They need to learn to say no to chemicals and to unsafe places that may jeopardize or compromise their recovery. Many alcoholics have a hard time telling friends that they are alcoholic and cannot drink. It is especially important for those who have a need to please others to learn how to set boundaries and be assertive about getting their own needs met. Saying no to the excessive demands one puts on oneself and saying yes to self-care activities are also part of boundary setting.

Working the Steps

To "work the steps" means to apply the concepts of the 12 steps of AA to all areas of life (7, 8, 9). For example, an addict's admission that he or she is powerless over the abused substance is the first part of recovery and the antidote to living with a disease that is out of control. Learning to accept one's powerlessness over other situations that are beyond one's control can help develop a life-style that is gentler and more stress free. The 12 steps are as follows:[*]

1. We admitted we were powerless over alcohol—that our lives had become unmanageable.
2. Came to believe that a Power greater than ourselves could restore us to sanity.
3. Made a decision to turn our will and our lives over to the care of God as we understood Him.
4. Made a searching and fearless moral inventory of ourselves.
5. Admitted to God, to ourselves and to another human being the exact nature of our wrongs.
6. Were entirely ready to have God remove all these defects of character.
7. Humbly asked Him to remove our shortcomings.
8. Made a list of all the persons we had harmed and became willing to make amends to them all.
9. Made direct amends to such people wherever possible, except when to do so would injure them or others.
10. Continued to take personal inventory and when we were wrong promptly admitted it.
11. Sought through prayer and meditation to improve our conscious contact with God as we understood Him, praying only for knowledge of His will for us and the ability to carry that out.
12. Having had a spiritual awakening as the result of these Steps, we tried to carry this messages to others and to practice these principles in all our affairs (7, 8, 9).

Sometimes recovering persons will do all their 12-step work under the guidance of their sponsor and within the fellowship of their 12-step group. Others have a chemical dependency counselor to assist them. We use simple written assignments based on the 12 steps, a great deal of group discussion, and individual counseling to help the chemically dependent person understand and apply the concepts embedded in the 12 steps (19, 20).

Although the 12-step program has a strong spiritual emphasis, it is not a religion. People with deep religious beliefs as well as those who lack such beliefs are comfortable in the meetings. The AA Big Book even has a chapter titled "To the Agnostic" to help such individuals understand that they are welcome and that no specific Christian, or any other, belief

[*]From Alcoholics Anonymous (1976). Copyright 1976 World Services Association of Alcoholics Anonymous. Reprinted by permission.

is required (7). The emphasis is only on having a belief in some sort of power greater than one's self. Besides a traditional God this power can be karma, nature, the universe, even the 12-step fellowship itself. The idea is to believe in something beyond one's own mere willpower. Making the home group the higher power and listening for the miracle of recovery through the sharing of other people in meetings is a very helpful start for the addicted agnostic.

The 12 steps rescue the newly recovering person from a life dominated by drinking and using by means of a comprehensive course of recovery that builds faith and hope, teaches self-appraisal and responsibility for behavior, and ultimately brings a sense of altruism to those previously lost in a world of chemicals and self-centered thinking and behavior.

Family Recovery

As we mentioned earlier, families can be profoundly affected by the drug or alcohol use of a member (6). Resentments over episodes of drunken behavior, broken promises, and the squandering of family resources on drugs or alcohol need to be addressed as part of treatment. Receiving marital or family therapy is helpful. Family members also need to be educated about the disease of addiction so that they can begin to understand that their loved one is sick, not bad. They also need to learn how the illness has affected them and what they must do to work their own recovery program. Attendance at their own 12-step meetings is very helpful for the family members' recovery.

The issue of enabling, which refers to the inadvertent support by a family member of the addicted member's unsafe or sick behavior, requires attention. Enablers, in their attempts to be helpful, protect addicted family members from the negative consequences of their behavior and sometimes make excuses for them. Enabling is any behavior that helps keep a person sick rather than promote recovery. An enabling wife who tells a complaining husband that maybe one drink will not hurt is minimizing the importance of abstinence and inadvertently encouraging relapse.

SURVIVORS AND RECOVERY FROM ADDICTION

Survivors of trauma who are also abusing substances or who are chemically dependent are more likely to succeed if they confront both their illnesses and work a dual recovery program. As we have seen in previous chapters, survivors are at especially high risk for getting into trouble with chemicals. Their severe mood swings, dissociative episodes, and suicidal experiences make any use of mood- or mind-altering chemicals problematic. Alcohol is a depressant and increases the risk of self-harm. Although hallucinogens such as marijuana or LSD can cause psychotic symptoms in any user (10), they can further escalate, even to the point of inducing a psychotic break, bizarre and unusual thinking in survivors who already have psychotic-type features. Similarly, while amphetamines increase energy and arousal in almost all users, they can cause acute panic attacks and even anxiety-based psychoses in survivors, who are already likely to be in a chronically anxious state (5, 10).

Besides the escalation of psychiatric symptoms, there are other concerns with chemical use that are unique to survivors (19, 20). The progression of alcohol and drug use to abuse and then to addiction can be very rapid for survivors. Studies show that the two reasons people most often give for using drugs or alcohol are to enjoy life more and to reduce negative feelings (2). Since survivors' intense negative feelings—including depression, fear, guilt, shame, hopelessness, helplessness, anger, and resentment—leave them frantically looking for some sort of relief to help them numb the psychological pain, it is not difficult to understand how the idea of using a chemical to relax or feel better can be so seductive for them.

Most survivors experience chronic depression, which causes them to have difficulty deriving pleasure from normal activities in life. Their longing to have some enjoyment in life and to be like other people makes chemical use a tempting solution for many survivors. Sooner or later, however, this solution turns into an additional problem the survivor must overcome.

As with singly diagnosed addicts and alcoholics, the first step in recovery for addicted survivors must be abstinence. Even if the survivor is only abusing chemicals and is not addicted, no recovery can begin as long as he or she continues to use drugs or alcohol. Therapists who believe they can effectively work through recovery issues related to the trauma and not contract for abstinence are building a program of therapy without first establishing safety—the core ingredient necessary for successful work with survivors. And since chemical use is not safe for survivors, survivor work that has not developed a firm foundation of safety is likely to be ridden with client crises and instability. Any use of mood-altering chemicals that is not specifically prescribed with survivor issues in mind is not safe. If survivor clients can keep a contract for abstinence without working an active recovery program, they may not need to follow the dual recovery program that we describe in the next several chapters. However, it has been our experience that the general elements, suitably modified, of a good recovery program (such as the social support and the teaching of skills, as discussed earlier in this chapter) are helpful for work with any survivor of trauma.

Acceptance

Client acceptance of the fact that he or she suffers from both PTSD (or a related trauma syndrome) and addiction is the second key element of a recovery program for addicted survivors. Survivors benefit greatly from understanding that they are "sick getting well" and not "bad getting good" because it helps them deal with their feelings of shame about their history of both substance abuse and other out-of-control behavior as well as about the abuse itself.

Meetings and Sponsors

All of the ingredients of working an active program for addiction are relevant for addicted survivors. However, sometimes helping them work a program requires creativity and flexibility on the part of therapists. Therapists may find that they have trouble getting survivors to attend 12-step meetings. Survivors may feel unsafe around people, especially people who are strangers, and may balk at the notion of attending meetings. We have found that having a trusted person accompany a survivor to meetings can help allay these initial fears, although some survivors may still not feel safe even under these circumstances. In these cases, we find that a professionally led, same-sex relapse prevention group can serve as an initial substitute for a 12-step group and can prepare survivors to ultimately join such a group for the long-term support they will need.

Another issue is that of choosing a safe sponsor. The importance of the need for a same-sex sponsor cannot be stated too strongly. The newly recovering survivor is a prime candidate for a predatory person. Owing to the dynamics of being a mentor, sponsors have psychological power over the people they sponsor. If a sexual or intimate relationship develops, it can mimic the dynamics of the survivor's childhood abuse relationship—leading the survivor to feel vulnerable to manipulation by a more powerful person and to reenact the abuser–victim relationship.

Even in same-sex sponsor relationships there are challenges for most survivors in finding a sponsor who is right for them. Most survivors have difficulties with, and unresolved issues toward, authority figures. Parents who failed to protect and nurture have typically left the survivor distrustful of adults with any sort of authority, benign or not. This distrust may play itself out in a sponsor relationship. Fragile survivors might choose, for example, a sponsor who is very directive and controlling. Unassertive survivors may not have the skills to stand up for their own needs in such a relationship and may feel overpowered; they may then retaliate by not going to meetings or by "firing their sponsor"—but without ever having tried to directly address these issues. Sometimes survivors choose a kind, gentle, less directive sponsor and then fail to call the sponsor out of a fear of bothering him or her. This sort of sponsor then passively waits to hear from the newcomer who may begin to feel abandoned by the sponsor, experiencing a rejection when none exists. We encourage our clients to use their newly learned skills to ask for what they need from a sponsor. If they are asking directly for things that are appropriate and still feel rejected, hurt, overly criticized, or abandoned, a change of sponsor may be in order.

We are happy to meet or talk with the sponsor of any client after getting a release of information form signed by the client. This way we and the sponsor can share the tasks of recovery and work as a team to support the client. This can prevent future problems of triangulation between client, therapist, and sponsor.

Types of Support Groups

AA is designed to help those who desire to stop drinking (7), that desire being the only requirement for participation. The survivor may attend AA meetings even when in relapse. There are many different types of AA groups (and 12-step groups in general): nonsmoking, smoking, women only, men only, gay/lesbian, dual diagnosis, and so forth. The variety of meetings offered varies from area to area and often depends on whether clients live in a rural community or in a large metropolitan area. In Portland, Oregon, for example, there are over 400 AA meetings a week. NA, like AA, has numerous groups all over the country, although in most areas NA is not quite as available as AA; the only requirement for joining is the desire to stop using drugs (8). There are fewer groups of CA, designed to meet the needs of those trying to end their addiction to cocaine, than of AA or NA in most parts of the country.

Al-Anon (Al-Anon Family Groups) is designed to meet the needs of family members of alcoholics. These groups often meet at the same time and in the same building as AA groups so that family members can go to meetings together. Alateen is for older children from families in which a member, usually a parent, has a problem with alcohol. Naranon, affiliated with NA, is very much like Al-Anon and is for family members of those having drug problems.

Adult Children of Alcoholics (ACOA) meetings are designed to meet the needs of those adults who have issues related to being a child of an alcoholic. Some ACOA groups can be identified and located through Al-Anon; others have their own meeting schedules and intergroup offices.

Adults Molested as Children (AMAC) is a self-help organization whose program is not based on the 12 steps, as are those of all the groups just mentioned. AMAC groups in different parts of the country vary in the format of their meetings and in the issues they address. The key function of AMAC is to provide a safe, therapeutic environment for recovery from childhood sexual abuse. Some AMAC groups are led by a trained therapist. We believe these groups are preferable because the volatile and often intense subject matter discussed can cause age regression and flooding in survivors and having a trained therapist in the room can help maintain safety.

We believe that 12-step groups can be an option for the survivor in any stage of recovery from PTSD and addiction and that he or she should have at least 6 months of quality sobriety and be working on integration issues prior to attending ACOA or AMAC meetings. We have seen many survivors regress and go into crisis when they prematurely begin working on their survivor issues in depth before a proper foundation for their dual recovery is achieved.

AA and NA Slogans and Stories

Members of 12-step programs repeat various slogans and stories that have developed over the years as part of the lore of recovery. These slogans and stories, which are pithy and memorable ways of reinforcing the principles of recovery, are useful in therapy sessions. They are a means of teaching new ways of thinking—for example, recognizing that it is a lot easier to live life without alcohol if one can learn to take things easier and "live life on life's terms"—in order to encourage behaviors that promote recovery. These slogans and stories are a part of the 12-step culture. Therapists benefit from being familiar with at least some of them because they can then reinforce recovery precepts in language that is familiar to clients who are members of that culture. Here are some examples of 12-step slogans:

- Live in today.
- If you don't take the first drink, you won't get drunk.
- One drink is too many, and a thousand is never enough.
- Live and let live.
- Easy does it.
- This too shall pass.
- One day at a time.
- First things first.
- Turn it over.
- Just for today.
- More will be revealed.
- You're right where you are supposed to be.

- Stinking thinking.
- Progress, not perfection.
- Let go and let God.
- Powerless over people, places, and things.
- Keep it simple.
- God works through people.
- Live in the solution, not in the problem.
- Live life on life's terms.

Survivors and the 12 Steps

We believe strongly in the usefulness of the 12 steps in treating addicted survivors. We understand, however, that some special concerns and issues arise when using the steps with this client population. We discuss specific concerns in great detail in later chapters of this book, and the appendix contains specialized 12-step work sheets for different subgroups of survivors. At this point we wish to give the reader a general understanding of the special concerns for the survivor using a 12-step program.

Step One, for example, states that "we admitted that we were powerless over alcohol/drugs and that our lives had become unmanageable." This first step deals with the individual's loss of control and the negative consequences of his or her chemical use. Survivors can have a difficult time dealing with the issue of powerlessness; they often misinterpret Step One to mean that they are being asked to admit helplessness. This threatens their sense of safety. Assisting clients to get past this concrete thinking and to understand how both chemical use and out-of-control survivor symptoms have made their lives unmanageable is the task facing counselors. A related task is to emphasize the paradox of Step One, namely, that letting go of attempts to control the uncontrollable results in regaining power. Obsessive worry is a good example to illustrate this concept: If someone is apprehensive and concerned over getting a new job or a promotion, he or she may experience some worry and stress. Fear and worry before the interview, however, will not affect the outcome in any way. The person either will or will not get the job, and worrying about it only makes life unmanageable. Or take the example of chemical dependency. Alcoholics spend a huge amount of time, money, and energy trying to manage a substance that has begun to manage them. They may find that they are trying to drink only beer or to limit themselves to two drinks, and when they have met their self-imposed limit, they may feel angry and deprived; then they either have to refrain from drinking and remain unsatisfied or lose control and admit that they cannot adhere to their commitment. Acceptance of the fact that their chemical use is out of control is therapeutic.

Step One assists addicts/alcoholics in admitting to their addiction. Steps Two and Three encourage reaching out for help—and throw survivors into a bit of a quandary as they face the issue of God. Most survivors are either angry at or afraid of God. We have heard many hurt survivors make statements like "If there is a God, why did he let these things happen to me?" Struggling with the concept of either a new, more forgiving, God or an "alternative God" (such as "a higher power") is often a productive way for survivors to deal with these issues. We have found that most survivors eventually make peace with their childhood God and that in the meantime these solutions suffice to prevent further delay in step work.

Step Four helps the recovering person begin a journey of realistic self-appraisal. Writing down and honestly acknowledging character defects, however, can be an experience of shame and depression for survivors and not the exercise in balanced and realistic self-knowledge that is intended. Most survivors are highly self-critical and can turn this fourth step into an opportunity to beat themselves up. We have found it very helpful to have clients write the word *faith* or *hope* at the top of their Step Four paper and begin by listing some of their strengths. In Step Five the client reviews the character inventory with a trusted person who helps teach him or her how to admit mistakes and learn from them. This person could be a sponsor, clergyperson, or therapist. Steps Four and Five therefore reinforce psychotherapy and counseling, and it is important for therapists not only to help survivors pick a person they can truly trust for sharing these steps but also one who will monitor the survivor's progress to make certain he or she is not being overwhelmed with shame.

Steps Six and Seven emphasize the need for further self-actualization and the importance of selflessness in this pursuit. Steps Eight and Nine afford persons a chance to clean up the wreckage of their past by taking responsibility for their part in problems and by apologizing to those who have been harmed by their behavior. Many guilty and shame-filled survivors want to rush into these steps. However, these steps should be taken only in conjunction with adequate social support and only after the previous steps have been mastered. Rushing through the steps too quickly can lead to a relapse or, at the very least, a setback in treatment. For example, we do not want to see a newly recovering survivor making amends to an abusive or abandoning parent too early in recovery (if at all), for this could invalidate his or her survivor work.

Step Ten encourages individuals to take personal inventory of themselves on an ongoing basis. Again, this reinforces the rest of treatment and vice versa. Learning to set good boundaries and speak assertively gives survivors tools to help make this step a part of their daily routine. Step Eleven assists recovering persons with the continued development of the spiritual part of themselves. This is the step that helps survivors maintain an optimistic outlook that includes hope and faith, commodities lacking in the lives of most survivors. Step Twelve brings survivors full circle. They have now developed a sense of altruism and community: They are now reaching out to other sick alcoholics and addicts in attempts to help them get clean and sober. Reaching out to other survivors also fits with the intent of Step Twelve.

PREVENTING AND MANAGING RELAPSE

Relapse refers to the recurrence of a behavior that was previously in remission (2, 18). For the chemically dependent person in recovery, a relapse is the use of a mood- or mind-altering substance. For the survivor, a relapse could be a return to an old unsafe behavior, such as self-mutilation. An "unraveling" process typically takes place prior to the actual relapse. This process often involves, for example, the gradual return of old attitudes ("stinking thinking") and a gradual decrease or even total halt in recovery activities.

We strongly believe that addicted survivors who relapse in either of their illnesses require support and encouragement, not condemnation and discharge from treatment. Such responses only reinforce old shame-based self-descriptions and usually lead to further decompensation. Simultaneously supporting recovery and not enabling the disease of addiction can indeed be a delicate balancing act for the therapist. Characterizing relapses as "unsafe" (instead of "bad") behavior, we encourage the attitude that they are not mistakes but opportunities for learning. This helps remind survivors of their core issue, namely, their need to feel and be safe. We then work with clients to identify the triggers that led to their relapse and help them devise ways to respond differently the next time. If, however, the relapses become more frequent or more intense, we then consider some other type of therapeutic intervention, such as a residential or inpatient treatment stay. We continue to work with clients as long as they demonstrate some reasonable level of honesty and willingness to continue to work on their dual recovery.

It is important for the clinician to prepare the survivor very early in treatment for the probability of a relapse—without, however, at the same time providing an excuse for a relapse to take place. We discussed earlier in the chapter the fact that negative emotions are often a common reason for drug/alcohol use. Studies have demonstrated that negative emotions are a major cause of relapse in those suffering from chemical dependence as well as in those with other psychiatric disorders (2, 18). Intense insecurity and emotional pain, coupled with poor self-esteem and limited skills, clearly make survivors likely to relapse.

Survivors also frequently show a pattern of self-sabotage: When they start to experience success, they may find it overwhelming and may react with behavior that risks disappointing and letting down their therapist and loved ones. Their sense of being "bad" and incapable of success feeds into this as well. Sometimes survivors, who usually develop extremely strong transference reactions toward their therapist, test the relationship by having one sip of wine after 6 months of sobriety and then asking the therapist if this is a relapse. A rigid, critical, or crisis averting response on the part of the clinician may damage the therapeutic alliance. However, the therapist who dismisses the relapse without much emphasis on its importance establishes a permissive attitude that may promote a future relapse. We have struggled and continue to struggle with this balancing act. We constantly remind our clients (and ourselves) that there are "no mistakes, no failures, only lessons" and that we are ahead of where we started if we have learned from our mistakes. If there are two steps forward and one step backward, then we are still getting ahead.

We often ask ourselves which response is the most helpful reaction to a relapse. Given that there are very few absolutely right or wrong responses in these sorts of clinical situations, we often are forced to give the situation our "best guess" and go with whatever response seems most therapeutic and most likely to produce a step toward recovery. At times these decisions are difficult to make. Outside supervision and help from a team staff can help the therapist walk the thin line.

Terrence Gorsky has published excellent material, outlining the most common signs of relapse, which is helpful to the higher-functioning survivor (18). Educating survivors on these signs and symptoms can help them (and their therapist) intervene prior to a relapse. We employ the thinking error material described earlier as a way to detect "stinking thinking" in our clients, that is, thinking that generally signals the beginning of a relapse. We encourage our clients to use this material to become experts at detecting their own relapse thinking.

CONCLUDING COMMENTS

Clients with a history of childhood trauma are showing progress in treatment when they transform their identity from victim to survivor. By abstaining from drug and alcohol use, survivors are learning how to better nurture and protect themselves. Hypervigilance, part of the survivor's protector part, works better if it is not clouded by substance abuse, for example. Seeing oneself as a "survivor in recovery from dual diseases" acknowledges and emphasizes success and strength and is part of the transformation from the victim identity.

In this chapter we have discussed the assessment and treatment of chemical dependence in general and with addicted survivors in particular. We hope readers find this material at least a useful review—or perhaps even a useful introduction to the entire field. In the next chapter we combine the material presented in preceding chapters and introduce an integrated model for treating addicted survivors.

REFERENCES

1. American Psychiatric Association. (1994). *Diagnostic and statistical manual of mental disorders* (4th ed., rev.). Washington, DC: Author.

2. Marlatt, G. A., & Gordon, J. K. (1985). *Relapse prevention: Maintenance strategies in the treatment of addictive behaviors*. New York: Guilford Press.

3. Milam, J. R., & Ketchum, K. (1981). *Under the influence*. New York: Bantam Books.

4. Kranzler, H. R., & Liebowitz, N. R. (1988). Anxiety and depression in substance abuse. *Medical Clinics of North America, 72*(4), 867–881.

5. Picard, F. (1989). *Family intervention: Ending the cycle of addiction and co-dependency*. Hillsboro, OR: Beyond Words Publishing.

6. Brown, S. (1985). *Treating the alcoholic: A developmental model of recovery*. New York: Wiley.

7. Alcoholics Anonymous World Services. (1976). *Alcoholics Anonymous*. New York: Author.

8. *Narcotics Anonymous*. (1982). Baltimore, MD: Carena.

9. Alcoholic Anonymous World Services. (1965). *Twelve steps and twelve traditions*. New York: Author.

10. Yokelson, S., & Samenow, S. (1976). *The criminal personality: Vol. 4. The drug abuser*. New York: Jason Aronson.

11. Blum, A. (1984). *Handbook of abusable drugs*. New York: Gardner Press.

12. Ewing, J. A. (1984). The CAGE Test for alcoholism. *Journal of the American Medical Association, 252*(14), 1905–1907.

13. (1987, Sept.). Three rapid assessment questionnaires for the detection of alcoholism. *Journal of American College Health, 36*.

14. Lowinson, J. H. (1982). Group psychotherapy with substance abusers and alcoholics. In H. I. Kaplan and B. J. Sadock (Eds.), *Comprehensive group psychotherapy* (pp. 45–64). Baltimore, MD: Williams & Wilkins.

15. Available from the SASSI Institute, P.O. Box 5069, Bloomington, IN 47407-5069.

16. Creager, C. (1989, July/August). SASSI Test breaks through denial. *Professional Counselor*, p. 65.

17. Evans, K., & Sullivan, J. M. (1991). *Preventing relapse from your dual diagnosis*. Center City, MN: Hazelden Foundation.

18. Gorskie, T., & Miller, M. (1986). *Staying sober: A guide for relapse prevention.* Independence, MO: Herald House/Independence Press.
19. Evans, K., & Sullivan, J. M. (1990). *Dual diagnosis: Counseling the mentally ill substance abuser.* New York: Guilford Press.
20. Evans, K., & Sullivan, J. M. (1990). *Step study counseling with the dual disordered client.* Center City, MN: Hazelden Foundation.

A Model for Dual Recovery and Crisis Stage Interventions

Self-Harm

A slice of skin, the sight of my own blood,
Relief at last from the pain.
The emptiness inside will swallow me.
Pain relieves the numbness, I know that I am alive.
I pray for the freedom of death.

—LORIE, age 22

In this chapter we explore issues that arise in blending mental health and chemical dependence treatment approaches for addicted survivors. We present in some detail our views on controversial issues and then provide a general overview of a five-stage systematic model for treating survivors of childhood abuse who are also chemically dependent. We focus at great length in this chapter on the first, or crisis, stage and leave examination of the other four stages for later chapters.

KEY ISSUES IN BLENDING APPROACHES

We argued in Chapter 1 for the importance of an integrated model for treating the addicted survivor. Such an approach provides for the simultaneous treatment of the coexisting disorders that these clients present. It also provides comprehensive treatment that identifies common themes and condenses interventions in a coordinated fashion that effectively addresses the synergism in these disorders.

The survivor and addiction recovery approaches discussed in the last two chapters share a large number of common treatment elements. However, there are some areas of conflict that arise and that require working through if a successful marriage is to take place. Table 5.1 compares details of these two models to help the reader identify areas of agreement and disagreement.

A glance at Table 5.1 reveals that the two models have a great many features in common. They share similar or highly compatible etiological influences, courses, symptoms, problems, treatment goals, concerns, and interventions. Both syndromes have a chronic course. Helping clients deal with cues that might trigger a relapse is an important feature of treatment with either disorder, as is the notion of recovery as an ongoing process. In both disorders it is crucial for the therapist to deal with the client's denial, at whatever depth and intensity is appropriate, and to promote self-acceptance, a major objective of treatment. Having a significant "helping other," whether therapist or sponsor, is necessary for the client to experience validation and learn how to reach out to others for support. Encouraging clients with a traumatic history to reframe their sense of self from being a victim to being a survivor has its parallel in helping chemically dependent persons come to see themselves not as bad, weak, and without willpower but as sick and suffering from the disease of addiction.

The 12 steps represent a psychotherapeutic paradigm with parallels to other schools of therapy (1). For example, followers of the strategic school of therapy believe that the client's solution to the perceived problem actually maintains the problem, and they encourage the client to do the opposite to paradoxically achieve a resolution. In a similar way, Step One of the 12-step program encourages alcoholics to give up trying to control their substance use and to achieve control, paradoxically, through surrender. Clients' experience in telling their story—which involves discussing what it was like before recovery, what happened that broke their denial and forced a change, and what it is like now in recovery—whether it occurs in a 12-step meeting or in a therapy session, serves to simultaneously increase their sense of ownership of their problem and decrease feelings of shame. In addition it offers them the sense of a new beginning. Teaching the client in counseling to engage in more positive thinking or self-talk (e.g., "I've gotten through worse than this, and I will get through this, too," or "All a mistake means is that I need to change my approach, not that I am a mistake") is basically the same as encouraging the client to use recovery slogans heard in AA meetings and from sponsors (e.g., "This too will pass" or "Progress, not perfection"). The client's newly developing recovery voice uses these slogans to override the old defeatist/victim voice.

TABLE 5.1. Comparison of PTSD and Substance Addiction

Survivor treatment	Addiction treatment

Etiological factors

Some genetic influence	Genetic influence
Life experiences very important	Life experiences important
Neurophysiological component	Neurophysiological component
Usually family-of-origin issues	Usually family-of-origin issues

Courses

Variable onset	Variable onset
Variable course	Progressive
Fatal: suicide	Fatal: death
Chronic disorder	Chronic disease
Triggers and relapse	Triggers and relapse
Ongoing recovery	Ongoing recovery

Symptoms

Substance use as self-medication	Substance use as the prime cause of all presenting problems
Denial/dissociation	Denial
Depression, anxiety, anger	Depression, anxiety, anger
Stigma/shame	Stigma/shame
Powerlessness versus control	Powerlessness versus control
Distorted victim thinking	Distorted addict thinking
Disrupted relationships	Disrupted relationships
Impaired role functioning	Impaired role functioning
Demoralization	Despair
Existential issues	Spiritual issues

Treatment goals

Early treatment goal: stability	Early treatment goal: abstinence
Empowerment	Surrender
Control distortions	Control distortions
Accept survivor reframe	Accept alcoholic label
Insight/awareness	Self-acceptance
Behavior change	Concrete action

Interventions

Support groups	12-step groups
Psychotherapy	Step work
Wellness	Self-care
Practice new skills	Practice new skills
Education	Education
Use of psychotropic medication	No mood-altering substances
Positive self-talk	Eliminate "stinking thinking"
Therapist and "helpers"	Counselor and sponsor
Individual/group therapy	Individual/group counseling
Family work	Family work
Continuum of care	Continuum of care

Working the first three steps of a 12-step program is the same process as being willing to reach out and engage in a therapeutic relationship. The faith required in the first three steps is parallel to the initial transference relationship with the therapist in that in both cases there is the hope that someone can finally help with all the pain. The "moral inventory" in Step Four is similar to the self-observation and self-examination that insight therapies encourage clients to undertake. Steps Five through Ten teach the recovering person to identify negative and positive personal characteristics that both assist recovery and have the potential to impede it. These steps encourage the open expression of thoughts and feelings and the breaking of old secretive or otherwise unhelpful patterns, much as psychotherapy does. Steps Eleven and Twelve encourage recovering persons to listen to their intuitive part, let go of old narcissistic wounds, and reach out to help others through altruism. Meditation, yoga, and self-defense classes all offer the survivor a sense of empowerment, hope, and faith. A therapist's suggestion that a survivor work in some capacity to help others overcome the effects of trauma (e.g., working as a rape prevention advocate) mirrors the goals of Step Twelve.

Professionals in both areas are likely to recommend physical exercise to their clients to help them manage stress better and to promote a sense of well-being and are likely to help clients make a decision between inpatient, or residential, treatment and outpatient work. And, of course, working with family issues, both current ones and those from the past, is common to clients in either area.

Several areas of potential conflict between the mental health and chemical dependence treatment approaches for addicted survivors exist, however, and need resolution before any nuptials can take place. These are discussed in the following paragraphs.

Chemical Abuse versus Dependency

The first area of conflict between the two approaches revolves around the issue of whether most survivors are just self-medicating their pain and merely abusing drugs or whether they are truly chemically dependent. The literature on PTSD and survivor issues tends to show a persistent bias toward the self-medication/abuse stance although the DSM-IV takes a more neutral stance than previous editions (2, 3). Our policy is to avoid black-and-white thinking in this area. We believe that any significant level of substance use poses risks for survivors and that abstinence must therefore be a goal of treatment for these clients. Survivors are at risk for developing problems with addictive substances. Survivors are also at risk in this area because they typically enter treatment feeling acutely stressed and are likely to experience periodic recurrences of this throughout treatment. The decision to turn to chemicals as a means of managing emotion leaves survivors with the belief that chemicals and only chemicals can relieve the pain and make them feel better. This is psychological dependence. Since survivors are often at higher risk of addiction due to genetic predisposition, the progression of the disease of addiction may already have begun in the chemical-using survivor. If clients use substances to manage the unpleasant emotions that are stirred up in therapy, the old way of dealing with difficult issues through avoidance is likely to be reinforced and new ways of coping are not likely to take root. Chemical users have the attitude that instant gratification takes too long. "Why spend 1 hour walking or 30 minutes meditating," they might think, "when it takes 20 seconds to consume a shot of whisky?" As discussed in earlier chapters, chemicals that are mood altering typically increase the degree of depression, anxiety, and anger with high and/or sustained levels of use. Furthermore, the mood that is altered is very likely to be, at least in part, a consequence of the chemical use in the first place, and a brain affected by chemicals has reduced impulse control. This further increases the probability that some sort of unsafe acting out, such as a suicide attempt or aggression toward others, might occur.

Our policy is that any chemical use by survivors is very likely to be a problem. Regardless of the outcome of our careful assessment of substance use patterns in the past and present, we obtain an abstinence agreement from all our survivor clients and reserve the right to monitor their compliance with this agreement. Strong resistance to an abstinence contract is an indication that there may be problems in this area. If a client is unable to "just say no" and violates this abstinence agreement, it is highly likely that there is a coexisting addiction problem. We are very careful to explain to clients the rationale for the abstinence agreement. We present the agreement in terms of their need for safety and stress the fact that a brain affected by drugs or alcohol cannot be trusted to make therapeutically wise and safe decisions and the chemicals will interfere with achieving longed-for outcomes in treatment.

We explain to our survivor clients that the need for honesty about violations of the abstinence agreement is not a matter of our "catching" them but a reflection of our care and concern for their well-being. We also discuss how important honesty is as a part of the developing mutual trust between client and therapist. Survivors' trust and shame issues make it important for us to pay careful attention to how we present this "no-use safety" contract. This sort of joining is important even with survivors who are angry and acting out, because they will balk at treatment unless they feel it is in their best interests. We also explain that the abstinence agreement covers all classes of mood-altering substances. While some exceptions are made for the use of nicotine and caffeine, we still discuss how even these substances are potential impediments to the recovery process.

Medication for Coexisting Mood and Thought Disorders

Traditional drug and alcohol counseling has a strong bias against the use of any psychotropic medication. Addicted survivors, however, are very likely to have coexisting and quite disabling mood or thought disorders. We respect the power of the physiological components of the severe melancholic depressions, the "I'm going to die" panic attacks, and the psychotic-like aspects of the acute dissociative states that survivors can experience. Failure to address the biochemical aspects of these psychiatric symptoms significantly reduces the probability of successfully treating the addicted survivor. Indeed, survivors who are immobilized by a severe endogenous depression, barely able to get out of bed, and preoccupied with suicide as the only solution now that the use of drugs and alcohol is no longer an option, are not likely to respond very well to exhortations to go to their 12-step meetings or to call a friend and talk. We support the use of prescribed, nonaddictive medications after a careful evaluation suggests that they are indicated.

Drug-Affected Thinking versus Coexisting Psychiatric Disorder

The material in Chapter 3 of this book suggests that survivors are likely to evidence a number of different psychiatric disorders and that achieving a differential diagnosis can be a challenge. Moreover, survivors who are abusing or dependent on chemicals can have symptoms that mimic those of a host of psychiatric conditions, ranging from substance-induced psychoses to major depressions and generalized anxiety states, but that are related to the effects of the chemical use. (Such symptoms are especially likely to occur in alcoholics and addicts just prior to their entering treatment and in the first several weeks and months of abstinence.) Consequently, addicted survivors often prove to be a major diagnostic challenge.

In some ways, the question of functional rather than differential diagnosis is the more important one, at least at the very beginning of treatment: If clients are confused, suicidally depressed, or unable to carry out activities of daily living, the treatment plan must take these issues into account no matter what the diagnosis. This might mean, for example, referring clients to more intensive levels of care (such as residential or inpatient treatment), instituting a suicide watch, or ensuring that instructors in classes on substance abuse use simple materials, repeat key ideas several times, and use visual and auditory aids to make their points. In other ways, however, the issue of differential diagnosis remains an important one. Achieving a differential diagnosis does have important implications for prognosis, the prescribing of medication, and, of course, for treatment planning.

Certainly all clients seeking treatment, whether for chemical dependence, other psychiatric difficulties, or both, require a comprehensive assessment at intake to identify all relevant issues and possible diagnoses. We evaluate any client seeking treatment for substance dependence who has a history of childhood trauma or signs and symptoms of such trauma for coexisting psychiatric disorders. These include PTSD, major depressive disorder, somatoform disorder, the dissociative disorders, other anxiety disorders, and psychoses. The intake evaluation should include questions assessing potential psychiatric disorders and, when available, psychological testing.

We have found that using a combination of some standard mental states questions and questions targeting substance dependence issues (as described in Chapter 4) provides a good overview of the alcohol/drug use pattern as it interrelates with any coexisting psychiatric disorder. The Dual Diagnosis Assessment Tool in the appendix outlines the questions we ask to help us evaluate our clients, particularly dual diagnosis clients. This tool is an interview guide; we do not use it as a test that produces scores. Chapter 7 discusses specific data that we utilize to make differential diagnoses among various clusters of addicted survivors.

We use several decision rules, based on our own clinical experience, to establish whether someone abusing or dependent on chemicals has a coexisting psychiatric disorder. These rules are based on answers to the following questions (presented in order of importance): (1) Did the client have symptoms of the psychiatric disorder prior to extensive involvement with chemicals? (2) Do the psychiatric symptoms continue or worsen during a 4-week or longer period of abstinence? (The answer to this question can be obtained either by history or by current observation.) (3) Do the client's responses to interview questions, his or her observed behaviors, or the results of psychological testing indicate that the symptoms and problems are substantially more intense than those typically seen in cases of substance abuse or dependence? (4) Does the family history, genetic or otherwise, indicate possible familial transmission of a coexisting disorder? (5) Is there a history of positive response to psychotropic medication or other specific psychiatric treatment? (6) Is there a history of multiple chemical dependency treatment failures, and has the client tried to work a 12-step program of recovery? The greater the number of these questions that can be answered in the affirmative for clients with chemical use problems, the more likely it is that they have a coexisting psychiatric disorder. Readers interested in further information about the rationale and specifics of our decision rules are referred to our book *Dual Diagnosis: Counseling the Mentally Ill Substance Abuser* (4).

Labeling as a Therapeutic Tool

A standard objective in the treatment of clients with trauma issues or substance dependence problems is to strongly encourage them to apply the labels "survivor" or "alcoholic" or "addict" to themselves (e.g., when they introduce themselves to members of a support group, as in "I am a survivor of abuse," or "Hi, I'm Joe, and I am an alcoholic"). Some professionals have expressed strong concerns to us about the possible negative effects on clients of adopting such labels. They argue that this encourages clients to think of themselves (and encourages others to think of them) as being only their disorder or their disease and thus increases their exposure to the negative effects of the stigma still associated with these labels. Or they argue that this promotes the formation of a negative self-identity, one that overemphasizes limitations and ignores strengths.

Our view is that these labels can be liberating. We certainly do not want to reduce clients to one-dimensional caricatures or to strengthen what is almost certainly an already negative sense of self. Note that it is not labeling that is the real issue. People say "I am a Democrat," or "I am a nurse," or even "I am a diabetic," without any implication that their identity is limited to only these things. In addition, labeling is a universal human activity and will occur no matter what anyone wants. Finally, our clients have already labeled themselves or have been labeled by others, in one form or another, as bad, shameful, or weak. The issue is the stigma and stereotyping attached to certain labels; very few people want to call themselves or their loved ones "victims" or "drunks." The task is either to change the negative connotations of these labels or to adopt labels with a more positive but still realistic tone. This approach would help not only to dilute discrimination but also to reduce denial.

Spiritual Growth versus Agnostic Belief Systems

It is true that the 12-step approach explicitly incorporates spiritual notions into its recovery program for substance dependence. In fact, the spiritual aspect of the steps is seen as a major element necessary for successful recovery. Phrases such as "power greater than ourselves" and "Let go and let God" are often heard at 12-step meetings. Proponents of the 12-step approach hold that it is crucial for the success of a treatment program for people to have a sense of hope and faith that one day at a time things will get better even though they may be difficult, painful, and frightening today. We also believe that faith and hope are important, particularly for addicted survivors.

We are careful, however, to avoid promoting a specific doctrine. We work with our clients to help them understand that 12-step groups do not attempt to convert anyone to a specific set of beliefs or to any specific religion. We explain that members of such groups take seriously the phrase "God as we understood Him" in Step Three of the 12 steps and that each person's concept of a higher power is his or her personal interpretation. We emphasize that these concepts vary and include nature, the universe, other conceptions of a supreme being besides the traditional notion of God, and even AA itself. We make clear to our clients that the goal is to help them understand that they are not alone, that there is help, and that things will improve. Finally, we explain to clients that their strategy of attempting to protect and nurture themselves and manage their drinking/using on their own through willpower has not worked and that a spiritual program will help them develop a realistic view of the limitations of willpower and the strength of turning to "safe others" for assistance.

As our clients progress in their recovery, we view certain activities in therapy and their actions outside the office as having this sort of spiritual component. We also make use of our clients' growing spirituality. Calling someone for help when one is flooding and suicidal, for example, is Step Two in action. Relaxation training that combines deep breathing with exercises in which clients are encouraged to imagine being in a safe place is more effective if clients can associate their sense of a higher power with that safe place. During a relaxation exercise we might, for example, say to a client, "Sense the peace that your higher power gives you," or "Imagine a symbol of your higher power that sends out healing rays of light." Learning to "turn it over" in Step Three (i.e., to turn over one's will and life to the care of God or a higher power) can be a wonderful anodyne to anxiety, and embracing Step 6 (i.e., being "ready to have God remove all these defects of character") can be a wonderful antidote to the shame that clients typically experience.

The Paradox of Powerlessness

One of the goals of treating survivors is to help them empower themselves, since feelings of having been helpless and powerless at the hands of unsafe others constitute a core aspect of their experience; moreover, a pervasive sense of the possibility of losing control at any moment is a key dynamic of many PTSD-type syndromes.

Yet one of the goals of treating alcoholics/addicts is to assist them to admit their powerlessness over their chemical use; losing control of their chemical use is a cardinal aspect of substance dependence, and frantic efforts to maintain the desired effects of the chemical are a central feature of addiction. A person's attempt to control chemical use by making up and then trying to follow rules about when and how often it is permissible or safe to use the chemical is an indication that he or she is trying to manage an addiction that is increasingly out of control. As we discussed in Chapter 4, the loss of control over use of the chemical is the key feature of addiction. Many addicts and alcoholics become psychologically rigid in their attempts to control the uncontrollable; they then begin to generalize this controlling coping style to many areas of living. Is asking substance-dependent survivors to surrender to the reality of their addiction and the failure of their best efforts to be in charge of their chemical use and its effects on their lives countertherapeutic? Is this, in fact, revictimizing them? Or are we feeding the grandiosity of their denial by asking them to gain control of their lives and develop a sense of mastery while ignoring a core dynamic of their addiction?

The two apparently different positions of survivors and alcoholics/addicts with respect to power can be resolved through reframing some concepts that are more paradoxical than oppositional. We help clients make a distinction between those things that can be controlled and those that cannot. We help them to develop a realistic appreciation of the strengths and limits of the power of willpower and to understand the paradoxical freedom of letting go of attempts to control the uncontrollable. We address these control issues with our substance-dependent survivors both by respecting the sensitive nature of these issues and by making use of a combination of the first three steps of the AA program and other survivor therapy strategies. We explore with our clients how their efforts to control their addiction and their PTSD have not been "helpful" and encourage them to accept the fact that their well-intentioned but misguided efforts have made their life unmanageable.

Now on to the marriage.

THE DUAL RECOVERY MODEL

The cornerstone and organizing principle of our dual recovery model is the concept of safety. Recall our review in Chapter 3, where we made the point that safety (including both protection and nurturing) was the missing experience for survivors. Chemical abuse or addiction is also unsafe, a fact that provides a link for addressing both the issue of abuse and the issue of substance dependence under the same rubric. Thus, we need not argue with addicted survivors over the semantics of whether or not they are really addicts; we can help them come to view their substance use behavior simply as "not safe." We encourage these clients to "keep safe" by contracting for no self-harm *and* for abstinence from mood-altering chemicals. In both individual and group sessions we encourage our clients to discuss how they can stay safe, and we help them develop "safety skills," that is, skills for self-protection and self-nurturing. We work with clients to develop safe (i.e., sober) social support, arrange for safe abreactions, and so forth. "Safety first" is our motto.

We include several sets of therapeutic interventions in our model that are designed to help our clients achieve a sense of safety. As discussed in greater detail in the following sections, we emphasize developing and utilizing social support, which ideally involves a combination of a therapist who has expertise in the treatment both of addiction and survivor issues, a 12-step group supporting sobriety, group therapy, friends, and even "rediscovered" and safe relatives. We assist our clients to more competently protect and nurture themselves by helping them learn and practice such skills as problem solving; boundary setting; and mastering such 12-step concepts as "Let go and let God," "First things first," "One day at time," and "Turning it over." We help them transform their identity from drunk victim to recovering survivor by encouraging them to share their story with others in recovery and to work Steps Four through Nine of the 12-step program. We help clients mitigate ("burn off") strong emotions associated with the past and integrate all aspects of themselves, past and present.

More specifically, our model organizes recovery for survivors who are chemically dependent into five stages, namely, the crisis stage and the stages of skills building, education, integration, and maintenance. Each stage has its own set of clinical indicators, therapy goals, and treatment interventions. Table 5.2 outlines this model.

In each of these stages clients need to accomplish certain recovery tasks before they can be successful in achieving the goals and objectives of the next stage. Our clinical experience suggests that prematurely going to the next stage is futile. At best, this results in little or no progress; at worst, it precipitates a relapse to earlier stages. For example, having clients talk about explicit details of their abuse in the first 3 months of recovery in an attempt to help them work through these issues will most likely be extremely overwhelming for them and may lead to a relapse. They may comply superficially but remain dissociated the whole time, or they may flood and experience urges to use chemicals or hurt themselves in other ways.

Even with properly timed and clinically appropriate interventions, substance-dependent survivors progressing in their recovery typically revisit each of these stages many times in response to a variety of triggers and issues. Each time clients return to an earlier stage, however, the clinical work is at a more advanced level and the progress is more profound. The hoped-for result is an upward spiral of healing. The

TABLE 5.2. Five-Stage Model of Dual Recovery for Substance-Dependent Survivors

Stage	Goal	Indicators	Intervention
Crisis	To maintain immediate safety and health	Chemical use; strong urges to use; need for detox; suicidal/homicidal ideation; potential for self/other harm; chaotic/disorganized thinking or behavior; intense flooding and flashbacks; poor self-care (e.g., not sleeping or eating); denial	Abstinence/safety contracts; intensive out-patient treatment or hospitalization; fail-safe plan involving safe persons (e.g., therapist, friend, relative) and safe people and places; simple alternatives to old, unsafe behaviors; develop joint treatment plan; daily/weekly schedule; medication; meeting basic health needs; strong support for sobriety through counseling and self-help groups; help in working Step One
Building skills	To promote self-protection and nurturing	Immediate safety and health obtained; some commitment to recovery; some follow through on treatment plan; trouble using social support, problem solving, managing feelings, setting boundaries	Help in setting boundaries; instruction in self-defense and assertion techniques, in how to manage negative feelings (e.g., time-outs, breathing), in self-monitoring and self-care practices (e.g., exercise), and in how to use affirmations; social support; help in working Steps Two and Three

TABLE 5.2. (continued)

Stage	Goal	Indicators	Intervention
Education	To transform sense of self from victim/ "drunk" to recovering survivor alcoholic	Increased ability to protect/nurture self; limited intellectual understanding of own issues; feelings of shame	Recovery materials and workbooks; increasing depth of involvement with support groups; encouragement to client to tell own story, name personal triggers and parts of self, including (trance and parts mapping); help in working Steps Four to Nine
Integration	To enable client to stay in the here and now and to resolve problems of the past	Firm "recovering" identity; unresolved grief; continued susceptibility to triggering and trancing	Trigger/desensitization/exposure therapy; fusion/trance work; healing ceremonies; grief work; help in continuing to work Steps Four to Nine
Maintainance	To maintain recovery and prevent relapse	Full engagement in the here and now; congruent "BASKing"	Help in working Steps Ten through Twelve; encouragement for service work

survivor who is 30 days into recovery and experiences urges to use chemicals in response to increased flooding typically is in an acute crisis and requires very firm guidance and support. Those who are a year into recovery and experience flooding are more likely to announce that they are in a relapse mode, to talk about how they called their sponsor, to increase their attendance at meetings, and to start writing in their journal again. In both cases the crisis stage is involved, but clients differ in their ability to manage the crisis.

We apply the stage model of recovery not only to guide the broad course of treatment over time but also to orchestrate the pacing and timing of interventions in individual sessions. For example, if we notice while working with survivors in the education stage that they appear to be flooding or dissociating as they tell us their story, we might call this "minicrisis" to their attention, encourage them to use their skills to assert themselves with us and say no to continuing with this issue in the session, and advise them to use deep breathing to regroup. We might then go back to explore the trigger, and the client's response to it, and its role in his or her life; as part of our return to the education stage and in keeping with our function in that stage, we might give the trigger a name and discuss ways to manage the flooding.

THE CRISIS STAGE

The goal of treatment for clients in the crisis stage is to maintain their immediate safety and health. The general strategy for this stage is to explicitly assess for high-risk behaviors and, as the very first task of treatment and recovery, to provide the structure necessary to manage these behaviors .

Most often, clients enter treatment in the crisis stage. They may be flooding with strong negative feelings, experiencing intense and frightening flashbacks, or having suicidal or homicidal ideation. Or they may have recently overdosed, either in a suicide attempt or in an extensive binge. Or their spouse may have threatened to leave unless things change. Perhaps the state is planning to remove their children because of neglect or a judge has mandated treatment for assault charges. Perhaps they are massively out of control of their lives or feel they just cannot cope with their daily existence. Perhaps a family- or work-sponsored "intervention," in which family and friends lovingly but firmly confronted the client with the stressful impact of his or her actions, has engendered a "therapeutic crisis" (5). Some people present without an immediately obvious crisis, or, rather, they present with an impending crisis. These clients have typically attained a period of recovery, either through attendance at meetings of a self-help group or through formal treatment (or both). However, they evidence signs of being in what is called "relapse mode" (6), or a state in which people are at high risk for a return to chemical use or the reemergence of abuse-based symptoms and problems. Signs of being in a relapse mode include a decrease in attendance at support group meetings or therapy sessions, a reduction in other self-care activities, and a return of denial. Such clients are very angry and blaming, restless and dissatisfied, and often have feelings of helplessness and hopelessness. Sometimes these clients present with a flare-up of their survivor issues that leaves them feeling overwhelmed; having decided previously that drinking or using is not an option, they, believing there is no other way to escape the pain, are strongly considering suicide. Many kinds of events can trigger this relapse-mode thinking, but generally they involve some upsurge of strong distressing and disabling feelings.

A past history of being able to truly abstain from chemical use for at least several weeks, as with harmful behavior in general, is a good indicator that a person can again control the behavior. Carefully exploring whether clients were truly abstinent is important. Many people quit one chemical but switch to or increase their use of another. We often see survivors who have switched chemicals because they have rationalized that some are "okay"; thus, they may go from "bad" chemicals like cocaine to "better" chemicals like cannabis or alcohol. Other indicators increasing our confidence that a client is likely to maintain abstinence include a clear and firm willingness to admit to problems with chemicals and to commit to abstinence; an absence of significant withdrawal symptoms; evidence of high functioning in other life areas; a belief on the client's part that he or she can maintain abstinence; and the availability of social support in the client's life.

TREATMENT TACTICS

We use a number of tactics for treating clients in the crisis stage. The primary theme that most of these tactics share is the use of external structure to "hold and contain" clients whose own ego strength is unequal to the task at this time. Structure involves establishing kind but firm limits, providing copious quantities of information and support, and supplying predictable and clear policies, procedures, and rules for how treatment works and what clients need to do to keep safe.

We always make contracts for safety, making a verbal or written agreement with clients that they will stay safe. Clients agree to abstain from mood-altering substances except as prescribed by a physician who is knowledgeable not only about addiction in general but also about this particular client's addiction (an important qualification for prescription drug addicts). They agree to "abstain" from suicide, self-mutilation, contact with a dangerous person (if possible), and/or harming others. Clients also agree to not run or move away from the general vicinity. The first is important in the case of an adolescent who is oppositional; the second is important in dealing with an adult who has a history of exposure to abuse. Survivors contemplating a "geographic cure" to deal with their issues need to understand that they will carry their problems with them. Clients also agree to see a physician if necessary and to follow any prescribed medical treatment.

We ask clients to commit to attending therapy sessions and scheduled meetings of a support group. We ask them to agree to be truthful as a matter of honor and because this is the only means to our assisting them in their attempts to get and stay safe. We stress that we are not attempting to "catch" them at doing something "bad" but to help them—and perhaps those they come into contact with—stay safe. We clarify that while it is very important to abstain in the interest of safety from all harmful behavior (such as using drugs and alcohol or self-mutilation, and so forth), honesty is even more important. We explain that it is not our policy to simply discharge from treatment anyone who relapses into unsafe behavior. Instead, we make it clear to clients that we will work with them to help them find and learn new ways to stay safe or to find a treatment setting that meets their needs if relapses continue.

This latter point of discussion is important for two reasons. Some of our clients come to us from previous treatment with therapists or programs that discharge clients who relapse. Most of these clients believe that they are bad and that we will abandon them if we discover this. We develop an initial "fail-safe" plan as part of the contract (to be discussed in more detail shortly). We work with clients to outline what they might do if they feel they cannot keep their agreement. Generally, this involves contacting some safe person to ask for support but can also include other actions, such as leaving an unsafe situation. We explain our on-call system for handling emergency phone calls, and as part of our presentation of this initial safety plan we explore with clients what might constitute an emergency.

We generally trust that most of our clients will honor their contracts and be truthful about them, and this has been our experience. We have found, however, that it is usually the addiction that is most likely to go unreported and that if a client's recovery is not progressing, the chances are high that he or she is continuing to use mood-altering chemicals.

Sometimes we determine that a client will need residential or inpatient treatment for detoxification or to manage an acute crisis. Health care cost containment efforts make referral to such settings no longer a first-resort option for many people, and the average length of stay is now shorter, with the emphasis being on detoxification and immediate stabilization of the psychiatric crisis. However, we generally find that our substance-dependent survivors' symptoms and problems are sufficiently acute, intense, and numerous (because of their dual diseases) that they usually qualify for at least short-term residential/inpatient stays when they are unable to get safe on an outpatient basis. We also find, more often than not, that the survivors we see are willing to consider such a stay when we present it as a matter of safety. It also helps to articulate to a client clear goals for the hospitalization, for example, complete detoxification and psychiatric stabilization. We have also found that some sort of residential/inpatient stay is almost always necessary for clients with serious PTSD symptoms and more advanced chemical dependency in order to establish a recovering identity.

We make extensive use of fail-safe planning early in treatment. We explore with clients their past reaction patterns in order to identify high-probability triggers for unsafe behavior (including substance use) and suggest alternative safe responses. We make use of what we call "fail-safe cards," which are index cards on which clients describe their triggers for relapse and list one to three options for managing the trigger other than drinking or using drugs or engaging in other unsafe behavior. The following is an example of a dual-recovery fail-safe card:

Trigger: Feeling lonely and alone
Old response: Drinking or self-harm
New response: (1) Call my sponsor, (2) go to a 12-step meeting,
    (3) go for a walk.

The information on these cards should be clear, brief, and specific. A client's past history often provides clues for identifying triggers. Simply asking clients what their risky situations are likely to be is also a good source of information about triggers. "Fail-safe-ing," as we call it, can also be a useful group exercise for a survivors' group. We make sure that we do fail-safe cards with clients very early in treatment, not at some later time during a "relapse prevention" exercise.

Safe People, Places, and Things

The early identification or creation of safe persons and places is important even when a client's living situation is not immediately and obviously unsafe. Clients, nonetheless, may continue to feel unsafe for a variety of reasons: They may be living with individuals who are highly critical or demeaning or who trigger them. Or clients may be flooding and may feel so overwhelmed that they feel internally unsafe. With a little encouragement, some clients can pinpoint a least one person they can rely on for support, whether emotional or material; we sometimes have to help clients reevaluate their thinking about the safe person, since they often fear that the person will blame them for having such problems and will find them to be a burden. Occasionally, we have to challenge a client's notion that a particular person is really safe (e.g., when the person is a drinking buddy). In the beginning some clients have only their relationship with us, and we have to work with that. As quickly as the tolerance of clients allows, we work with them to get some social support in the form of group therapy, especially if they have resistance to attending a

12-step program. We do spend time orienting clients to the process of 12-step meetings, and we encourage them to try five to ten meetings before deciding whether the program is for them.

Safe places can, of course, include the therapy office or clinic, the 12-step meeting location, and other recovery environments such as the 12-step (Alano) club. (An Alano club is a nonprofit club dedicated to recovery where many 12-step meetings are held. They also often have pool tables and the atmosphere of a drop-in center.) Our clients have also used a local coffee shop (serving no alcohol), a local church, and a local public garden as their safe places. We also encourage our clients to establish a safe place in their home, which may be their bedroom or even just a special chair. We once worked with an alcohol-dependent man with a horrific history of physical and sexual abuse who kept empty whiskey bottles and numerous books on sexual abuse in his bedroom. A committed Christian and nature lover, he found that he could literally rest easier after he cleared his bedroom of these items and made sure that he had a Bible and plants there instead. Having a peaceful sanctuary is immensely beneficial for most people but especially so for those who must work through both addiction and trauma issues.

We have learned through hard-won experience to be careful in our phrasing of questions about safe persons and places. In the past we would ask questions such as "What might be a place that you would feel safe in?" and many clients would reply, "Nowhere!" We now ask clients where or with whom they might feel *safer*. This phrasing helps clients, who are usually stuck in either/or thinking, to begin to see options where none seemed to exist.

Sometimes we use visualization techniques to assist our clients in their creation of a safe place they can go to in their mind. This technique is a tool they can always have with them, a tool that enables them to enter this safe place in their mind whenever they feel upset or unsafe.

Learning the Symptoms of the Dual Disease

We discuss with our clients the diagnosis of both the chemical dependence and the PTSD-type syndrome. Having a label to explain their difficulties can validate survivors to themselves as being people who have real issues and not as complainers who are just trying to get attention or people who are uniquely "bad." This is especially true for the survivor who has been diagnosed as having borderline personality disorder. In the mental health community this diagnosis is often synonymous with "bothersome person-ality" in the minds of many overly taxed therapists. By explaining to survivors that they are suffers of PTSD and that they are having a normal response to what was an abnormal situation, we can help them finally forgive themselves for being sick and begin the recovery process.

We discuss our treatment plan with clients very early in treatment. We do this partly to fine-tune our assessment and partly to address the issue of denial. We literally read to clients the diagnostic criteria from the DSM-IV and explore with them the ways they meet these criteria. We use this as an opportunity to give clients basic information about the causes and remedies of their dual disorder, paying particular attention to challenging their beliefs that they are bad, weak, or shameful with a discussion of such things as the genetic basis for chemical dependence and the tendency of offenders to rely on victims' blaming themselves. This is also an opportunity to develop some instant positive transference; if the survivor feels that someone finally knows what is wrong with him or her, this translates into a strong therapeutic foundation to build from.

Clients who express strong disbelief in having either PTSD or addiction or who consistently dispute our conclusions clearly need more work on acceptance. We might then suggest that they wait and see what they think as we work together; we also suggest that they wait for the results of the psychological testing for another opinion. Most clients experience some ambivalence after receiving a dual diagnosis. They simultaneously feel overwhelmed, as their denial breaks down further, and a tremendous sense of relief that their problems have a name and a solution. Knowing that others with a similar diagnosis are in recovery and that there is a specific and concrete way to deal with survivor and dependency issues allows clients to hold on to something. We show our clients the outline reproduced here as Table 5.2 and provide them with a published self-help pamphlet we wrote for them to take home and read (7). Many clients find the authoritative look of this pamphlet and the information it contains on symptoms of PTSD, addiction, and dual recovery very comforting. In addition, knowing the official terminology for their symptoms—"Okay, I'm experiencing flooding" or "What's happening to me now is called preoccupation with use"—is therapeutic for clients. It begins to give them psychological distance from their symptoms and helps them become less reactive. Information and self-awareness also help to establish a sense of hope.

Taking Care of the Physical Self

Early in therapy we ask our clients if they are receiving treatment for any medical problems and if they are getting sufficient sleep and adequate nutrition and are otherwise taking care of their basic health needs. We talk about the need for eating balanced meals several times a day; the benefits of taking vitamins, if this is approved by their physician; and the importance of adequate sleep and rest. We assess their compliance in taking medications, both psychiatric and medical (such as insulin). If there is a problem in this area, we address it in our sessions.

We encourage clients to set up an appointment with their physician for a physical if they report feeling sick or have symptoms suggesting an acute or serious medical condition. One issue we address with clients, especially those with a history of multiple or high-risk sexual contacts, is the need for HIV screening and for safe sex. When doing so, we keep in mind the sensitive nature of sexual issues for most of our clients and proceed carefully with this sort of discussion.

Structure Equals Safety

Another tool that we use is a daily/weekly schedule to help clients who are disorganized and who are having trouble going about the activities of daily living. We help such clients fill out planning sheets during the therapy session itself. We ask them to indicate the blocks of time already committed to work and other responsibilities, including their appointments for treatment, and make sure they leave time for such activities as eating, sleeping, and taking medication. By working on such a schedule with our clients, we are able to pinpoint problems they are having in carrying out their activities of daily living and help them find solutions. We are especially alert to large blocks of uncommitted time, because these are often times of high risk for using chemicals, obsessing about suicide, or experiencing flooding and flashbacks. We encourage our clients in the crisis stage to fill in these gaps in their schedule to decrease the chances of these things occurring. Incidentally, one positive by-product of helping our clients construct a schedule for themselves is that we often gain a much better understanding of our clients' world.

Psychotropic Medication

A thorough evaluation using the diagnostic guidelines mentioned earlier in this chapter may indicate the need for nonaddictive psychotropic medication. The literature on pharmacological aid for PTSD yields several conclusions (8): (1) Most studies on PTSD have used Vietnam veterans as subjects; (2) there is no single general medication specifically used to treat PTSD, meaning that professionals instead prescribe a variety of medications to treat the symptoms associated with PTSD; (3) antidepressants are the most studied psychotropic medication for treatment of PTSD and appear to have the most promise, although there are case reports or open trial studies supporting the usefulness of neuroleptics, lithium, carbamazepine, beta-blockers (such as clonidine), and the minor tranquilizers with PTSD; (4) antidepressants appear to help only with intrusive symptoms and hyperarousal and not with avoidance symptoms (such as numbing) or with problems such as anger and social withdrawal; and (5) PTSD is so highly correlated with ("comorbid with") personality disorders, chemical abuse and dependence, and major depressive and anxiety disorders that treatment must take these coexisting disorders into account. One controlled study of hospitalized patients with the diagnosis of borderline personality disorder demonstrated that low doses of a neuroleptic were more effective than therapeutically equivalent doses of an antidepressant (9). We will discuss the issue of specific medications for specific groups of chemically dependent survivors in later chapters.

Taking a Step for Safety

Step One of the 12-step recovery program has the goal of decreasing clients' denial and convincing them that trying to solve their problems "their way," through willpower, has not worked. Corollary goals of Step One are to help clients accept the true nature of their situation and to prepare them to try a different solution. Step One provides a general guideline for orchestrating sessions in the crisis stage, especially as the crisis begins to resolve. Although we do look at control issues, we emphasize unmanageability of drug and alcohol use and translate this into our safety framework. We use Step One notions to help clients identify the negative consequences of both their chemical use and their survivor issues and examine patterns of denial and ineffective coping. Again, we try to maintain a balance between helping clients accept the reality of their situation and, at the same time, preventing them from being overwhelmed by it.

Core Issues Anchored to Safety

Every client has some core issue, some basic negative consequence he or she fears most. Some clients truly fear going crazy or becoming like their abuser. We try to identify this issue and make use of it.

Some clients enter recovery "for the sake of the children." Others do so to save a marriage, a job, or even their own life. Some professionals feel that only if clients get into recovery for themselves is the recovery likely to be genuine and long-lasting. We agree that lasting recovery is more likely if this is the case. In the short run, however, we are more than willing to accept clients' willingness to enter recovery for the "wrong" reasons if this gets them started.

We try to establish a "conditioned connection" in clients' minds that links old ways with lack of safety and negative consequence and associates recovery with safety and positive outcome. For example, we finally connected with one angry and resistant client when we suggested that each and every time she drank and became suicidal, her abuser (her father) won.

Sometimes we discuss stepwork and issues of unmanagability and lack of safety with our clients in a direct way when providing diagnostic and treatment information. At other times we, listening carefully to what our clients say, weave these themes into our discussions with them as they raise them. We might also assign written "stepwork" exercises (as provided in the following chapters) or work in a client workbook we have written (10). At all times we are careful to explore these themes in a direct, matter-of-fact way, avoiding both heavy-duty confrontations and a glossing over of denial. We also try to maintain a balance between the reality of a client's disease and his or her need to maintain hope and avoid being overwhelmed.

When Safety Has Been Established

Most of our clients, as mentioned earlier, come to us clearly in the crisis stage. Some, however, come to us having had some clean and sober time, in no immediate crisis, and perhaps having already had some treatment for either their addiction or their PTSD or experience with 12-step or other support groups. Some clients may "look good" and appear to be at a later stage of recovery but may be minimizing their symptoms and concerns to us and themselves. Either way and at a minimum, we always establish the diagnosis and present the treatment plan, negotiate a safety and treatment contract, complete a fail-safe plan, and assess how much Step One-type work is needed. No matter what the stage our clients enter therapy in, we are always careful to make sure we assist them in developing skills to stay safe. The reason for this is simple: the high probability of relapse in our clients. Not only are both PTSD and other survivor syndromes and chemical dependence chronic disorders in which relapse is common, but neither we nor our clients can predict with certainty when they will encounter a "trigger." Triggers can occur as part of daily life experience or because a client is processing disturbing material during treatment. Establishing a safety framework and fail-safe plan at the start of therapy, no matter what the client's stage, helps us to accomplish several things. We are less likely to miss important symptoms and issues, such as more subtle forms of denial as well as suicidal thinking or thoughts of self-harm.

We have learned the hard way the importance of always starting treatment and case sessions with a safety check. For example, a client might reveal in the fourth session the fact that he or she has been having suicidal urges the whole time we have been working together, or clients who have admitted to being alcoholics later might reveal that they believe a little pot never hurts. We are also in a better position to keep potential crises from escalating, as when, for example, the client suddenly receives a phone call from the now elderly father who was the childhood abuser and who is now very ill and has asked if he can move in with the client, thus triggering a flood of feelings and memories and a desire to drink. Or perhaps, no matter how carefully we and the client have laid the groundwork, the client becomes overwhelmed and floods during the telling of his or her life story. We manage such an event by asking clients how they could stay safe and reminding them of their fail-safe plan. We receive remarkably few emergency phone calls from clients, and the calls we do get generally take just a few minutes to handle because we have always worked to put in place this safety net.

Case Managing to Prevent Further Crises

Throughout work in the crisis stage we sometimes feel we are case managers, nurses, and social workers as well as therapists and counselors. We are comfortable with this (while recognizing that we must operate within our scope of practice and refer to other providers when necessary) and understand that treatment that does not address these fundamental safety issues may be riddled with crises and is likely to be ineffective. The next chapter describes those interventions for the later stages of treatment that are included in our recovery model and that are closer to what many readers might consider psychotherapy.

REFERENCES

1. Brown, S. (1985). *Treating the alcoholic: A developmental model of recovery.* New York: Wiley.
2. Kofoed, J., Friedman, M. J., & Peck, R. (1993). Alcoholism and drug abuse in patients with PTSD. *Psychiatric Quarterly, 64*(2), 151–171.
3. American Psychiatric Association. (1994). *Diagnostic and statistical manual of mental disorders* (4th ed.). Washington, DC: Author.
4. Evans, K., & Sullivan, J. M. (1990). *Dual diagnosis: Counseling the mentally ill substance abuser.* New York: Guilford Press.
5. Picard, F. (1989). *Family intervention: Ending the cycle of addiction and codependency.* Hillsboro, OR: Beyond Words.
6. Marlatt, G. A., & Gordon, J. K. (1985). *Relapse prevention: Maintenance strategies in the treatment of addictive behaviors.* New York: Guilford Press.

7. Evans, K., & Sullivan, J. M. (1991). *Understanding post-traumatic stress disorder and addiction* [pamphlet]. Center City, MN: Hazelden.
8. Friedman, M. J. (1990). Interrelationships between biological mechanisms and pharmacotherapy of posttraumatic stress disorder. In M. E. Wolf & A. D. Mosnaim (Eds.), *Posttraumatic stress disorder: Etiology, phenomenology, and treatment* (pp. 205–225). Washington, DC: American Psychiatric Press.
9. Soloff, P. H., George, A., Nathan, R. S., et al. (1986). Amitriptyline versus haloperidol in borderline disorders. *Archives of General Psychiatry, 43,* 691–697.
10. Evans, K., & Sullivan, J. M. (1994). *Understanding posttraumatic stress disorder and addiction* [workbook]. Center City, MN: Hazelden.

Interventions in Later Stages of Recovery

Lost Hope

Memories are kept hidden and secrets aren't told.
Her father has lies and alibis, her mother possesses her own,
She makes life a reality, when she dreams it a fantasy.
Her scars cut deep.
Her father abandoned her,
Her mother ignored her,
She grew up too fast,
Now her childhood is gone.
Her face filled with laughter, her eyes with pain,
Her heart with confusion.
Now she has learned to forget lost hopes.

—GINA, age 14

In this chapter we discuss the four remaining stages of our recovery model—the stages of building, education, integration, and maintenance—including the indicators and therapeutic tactics associated with each stage.

THE SKILLS-BUILDING STAGE

Our clients are ready for a primary focus on the skills-building stage when they have ensured their immediate safety and health, are generally following the treatment plan, and appear to be committed to continuing their recovery work. They may still be relapsing, but if they show some ability and willingness to be sober and safe and to be honest about relapses, they are ready for the work of the building stage.

119

The goal of the building stage is to assist clients to learn skills for protecting and nurturing themselves or to make greater use of skills they may already possess but have, for whatever reason, failed to practice in their lives. As noted in Chapter 3, having and using such skills distinguish survivors who are less impaired from those who exhibit the more severe symptoms and consequences of abuse. In therapy what may appear to be resistance on the client's part may actually be a skills deficit or a fear-based suppression of a skill, yet such skills promote recovery and provide the basis for more advanced therapy work.

Many people have never learned these skills. We professionals must be careful not to take it for granted, for example, that a client knows how to set a goal, develop a plan to attain it, and modify the plan as needed or that a client even knows that it is possible to talk through a disagreement with significant others in a way that is safe and that leads to a negotiated solution. A remarkable number of survivors never had contact with healthy people who could model such life skills. Perhaps they were so busy surviving that there was no opportunity to practice such skills, or perhaps parents punished them for doing such things as being assertive. Linehan pinpoints an invalidating environment in the family of origin as one important basis for survivors' difficulties in managing strong emotions (1). Many people have been so caught up in their addiction and survivor issues that their skills (if they have worked them) have atrophied. The use of mood-altering chemicals has kept others from learning self-care skills; instead of learning how to relax in more constructive ways, they simply took a pill or fixed themselves a drink. Now abstinent, they need to learn how to relax without the use of chemicals.

The transition to the skills-building stage is gradual, not abrupt, and does not have any sort of crystal-clear demarcation. Many of the interventions in the crisis stage are based on the assumption that the client has a basic level of skill. For example, expecting clients to attend therapy and 12-step meetings assumes some minimal ability on their part to organize time and resources and to tolerate groups of people. Though often reluctant, most clients can accomplish these activities at some minimal level when given firm encouragement. Those who cannot maintain even a basic condition of safety and health raise the question of the need for a more intensive and structured treatment setting. However, treatment in the skills-building stage begins to shift the locus of action away from external support and containing and toward clients themselves, thus making safety more portable. A client's deficiencies and discomfort in implementing crisis stage strategies help both client and therapist to identify which skills might prove vital to the client's recovery.

Teaching New Skills

We introduce the concept of a particular skill to a client by discussing its importance and giving some preliminary examples. We then discuss the skill in terms of the protector/nurturer/wounded parts framework discussed in Chapter 3. For example, we might define being assertive and setting boundaries as another way that the client's protector part can help the wounded part feel safer. This approach provides a common language, or set of consistent verbal anchors, for discussing new skills and reactions to situations and also lays the groundwork for the later stages of recovery. We have found that since so many of our clients have a concrete thinking style, owing to their disorders, we can never be too detailed and concrete in our questions and instructions.

We explore our survivor clients' skill level sand evaluate when they are unable to access their skills consistently. Figuring out the basis for the blocks can be very fruitful. Quite often there are underlying beliefs that form these blocks that are important to unearth and examine, beliefs such as "I can't do anything right" or "I don't deserve to feel good." Persons who already have in place a good set of skills but who are blocked in this way can often move into the education stage and work to anchor the already available skill set into the "trance" state blocking access to the skill as described in the education stage section.

Many of our clients report a vagueness or forgetfulness about what happens in their therapy sessions. This suggests that some dissociation is occurring and that for therapy to be beneficial we need to provide some means for clients to transfer what they are learning in their sessions to their life beyond the therapy office. We might inquire, for example, if clients know someone who is especially good at being assertive; if they do, we might ask them to observe that person for a week. Or we might ask them to monitor and rate their anxiety levels at selected times and bring us a record of this in the form of a journal or some other written format. We suggest that our clients limit their journal entries to current issues in their lives and avoid prematurely processing material from the past. We might ask them to practice doing things differently in their imagination, for example, seeing and feeling themselves successfully implementing more helpful behaviors. We have also recorded part or all of a therapy session on audiotape and given it to clients to take home and review, and we have sent clients home with a written account of key words or phrases that capture the essence of a particular session and have instructed them to place this where they will be able to read it. Some addicted survivors who have found a safe place in 12-step meetings may find that their sobriety coin (which is given to celebrate various periods of sobriety) may serve as a helpful transitional object. When it is touched outside a 12-step meeting, the coin may be able to anchor a survivor to the safety and serenity of the recovery group.

Engineering a success is important. Assuming, and pointing out to our clients, that most of us learn to swim more easily in the shallow end of the pool, we assist clients to identify situations in which it is likely to be easy, medium, and hard to implement a new skill. For example, practicing relaxation techniques for the first time while having a panic attack is not likely to go very well. Instead, first practicing such techniques at times of low anxiety and in a safe place is more likely to go well and to give clients a sense of hope and efficacy. We might also ask clients to practice their skills within the safety of a therapy group or a 12-step group, where the atmosphere is less likely to be judgmental, and we remind them that the goal is progress, not perfection.

We often ask clients to purchase books or audiotapes about a certain skill and to study them and might also ask clients to attend classes on the skills if these are available in clinics, community colleges, and other local forums. The appendix contains a "Staying Safe" worksheet for clients to complete that will help assess clients' skill areas; orient them to new, more helpful, responses; and help transfer these skills to the world beyond the therapy office.

New Skills for More Than Surviving

Assertion Skills

Absolutely key skills that we always assess and help clients develop and fine-tune are their self-protection skills, many of which fall under the rubric of assertion (2). Assertion refers to a number of behaviors, including stating one's opinion, interests, and needs directly and clearly; saying no; and otherwise maintaining reasonable boundaries, physical or emotional. The term *boundaries* refers to the limits where one person's physical and psychological "space" comes into contact with the physical and psychological space of others.

The general verbal formula for being assertive is "I feel X when you do Y, and what I'd like to see happen is Z." A specific verbal pronouncement based on this general formula, combined with a direct gaze, a centered stance, and a firm demeanor, is the assertive way. Another aspect of assertion is the ability to calmly and rationally set limits on other people's demands on them after repeated and/or highly invasive violations of boundaries or negotiated agreements and to follow through with that bottom line. The formula for this is "If you continue to do X, then I will do Y" (e.g., as in "If you keep hitting me and refuse to go for counseling, I will move out"). We are always very careful to make sure that clients are ready to follow through on their bottom lines to avoid impotent gestures, which merely train others to further ignore and invalidate clients, thus further feeding their sense of ineffectiveness.

We have found it useful to help our clients become more assertive not only with other persons but also with their internal self. This internal "other" is the part of the individual that harshly criticizes simple mistakes the person has made, makes unreasonable demands for performance or compliance, and otherwise subjects the person to an overwhelming barrage of shoulds and oughts. This part can also include the thoughts and images that push for such unsafe behavior as chemical use, self-mutilation, or involvement in relationships where the client might again be abused. Having already been introduced to the notion of parts of the self in the early stage of treatment, clients can generally accept our suggestion to stand up to that part of themselves that constantly criticizes them if they are not perfect; they understand us when we say to them, "Say no to the part of you that holds your disease of addiction and remind it of all the trouble your drinking and using has gotten you into." As discussed earlier, talking about parts of the self ("the part of you that . . .") allows us to give feedback to clients in a way that typically feels less critical to them and is thus less likely to trigger a shame response.

Managing Feelings

We also help survivors learn to better protect themselves by learning skills for managing the negative emotions, thoughts, and memories that are part of their experience of flooding or are potential triggers for relapse. We continue to encourage "constructive avoidance" through planned time-outs and the seeking of safe people and places identified in the crisis stage. However, we now add internal ways to manage and contain overwhelming emotions.

We help our survivors continue to experiment with general tools for managing negative feelings and thoughts. Some clients find that music helps break aversive feeling/thinking states. Soaking in a hot tub, reading a favorite piece of inspirational literature, watching a video, or even doing housework can be helpful. We especially encourage clients to take up some form of exercise after consultation with their physician. We try to reframe the concept of exercise, particularly for those individuals with a long history of failed diets or those for whom exercise otherwise has a negative connotation, as something other than an activity that involves sweating and gasping for air. Instead, we say that it is "all about moving." Even encouraging clients to just go for a walk is a first step toward having them get back in touch with their physical selves and begin to feel good about their bodies.

These sorts of more general skills appear to help with both the flooding and the high baseline level of anxiety and/or anger our clients experience. We have found that physical interventions seem to be particularly important for clients who have a history of severe physical abuse and have a hard time early in treatment sitting still for more traditional relaxation training. Many times clients begin to use these interventions in a compulsive way by, for example, becoming addicted to pumping iron. We are comfortable with this level of adaptation at this stage; compulsive jogging beats compulsive drinking, at least for the time being.

We also take advantage of survivors' well-established abilities to use trance states by encouraging them to "fight trances with trances." That is, we teach our clients a simple breathing/focusing technique in which we ask them to relax in a chair either with their eyes closed or focused on something in the room. Some survivors are very uncomfortable keeping their eyes closed, especially when the therapy relationship is just forming. We then ask them to "take these next few minutes to let go of the past and worries about the future and come into this time and place." Next we suggest that they focus their attention on just their breathing and notice "whatever wants to be noticed" about "that breathing." We emphasize that they observe their breathing without judgment or efforts to change it, letting it be "whatever it needs to be." Timing these suggestions to either the inhalations or exhalations of the person helps to further the success of the procedure. Almost inevitably individuals relax naturally, and they report that the technique is easy to practice and use and takes very little time to implement. We then use a phrase like "Take a breather" or whatever makes sense to the client as a cue to use this relaxation technique. Such training also sets the stage for later work such as anchoring skills in imagination or for doing abreactions.

Another technique we teach our clients is something we call sensory counting (3). In this exercise we ask clients to first name one thing they can see in the room, then one thing they can hear, and finally one thing they can sense in their bodies; then we ask them to name two things they see, two things they hear, and two things they sense. We explain that they have to decide if they want to repeat things or try to find new things. We ask them to repeat this process again and again, increasing the number of items each time. By the time they reach four or five things for the three sensory channels, clients typically find they are back in the here and now, tuned outward and struggling to find the required number of things they can hear or sense (the visual part of the exercise is the easiest to do) and to decide whether or not to repeat objects. This technique is excellent for managing flooding and other forms of dissociation.

Containment

We also ask our clients to learn to vividly imagine both a safety "container" and a safe "place" in their minds. The safety container is a receptacle in which they can "put and lock away" unpleasant thoughts and feelings, and the safe place is somewhere they can go to "get away and rest." As part of the exercise used to develop these tools, we instruct our clients to vividly imagine their safety container and their safe place, encouraging them to notice what they see, hear, smell, and sense as they get to know their container and place. We ask clients to try to practice in the office first the techniques of using their container and going to their safe place and then to try the techniques at home when not experiencing any strong emotions.

Consistent with the goals of Step Two of the 12-step program, we say to the client, "Imagine a picture, symbol, or image that represents for you the hope and strength of you and your recovery." We then ask the client to make a place for this image in his or her safe place. Many clients can reconnect with a sense of God, as understood in most religions; some use an image of a "fairy godperson," an image based on someone they have identified as the loving person of their childhood. For example, one man who had experienced his grandmother as the only loving person in his life imagined her in this safe place and found this image helpful when his optimism wore off after several weeks and the reality of the continuing financial and legal consequences of his chemical use and assault conviction sunk in. Asking him to look at his grandmother's "picture" and to imagine what she would say to encourage him proved to be helpful. Some clients imagine symbols of AA. We try to discourage using an image of our office and of us as their recovery symbol, knowing that sooner or later clients will lose their idealization of us and possibly precipitate an abandonment crisis. People with little experience, past and present, of support from others are especially likely to temporarily adopt us as their special image.

A cornerstone of a successful approach to working the steps of a 12-step program is learning to avoid having expectations that are unrealistic. Unrealistic expectations of managing things perfectly or of failing miserably can set a client up to have a particular reaction to an event even before it takes place. Trying to live "one day at a time" helps prevent living in tomorrow and missing today entirely. Cultivating this attitude is a useful antidote for survivors who are stuck in a negative past and feel depressed or for those who feel burdened by the anxiety of contemplating a future full of "what ifs" and catastrophes.

Using Dissociation in a Positive Way

We encourage beneficial dissociation/trancing. We help our clients imagine themselves (in all sensory channels) in the future, that is, as further along in their recovery and able to experience "more and more, each and every day, the safety and serenity" of their healing. We encourage them to imagine that they are viewing their experience on a movie screen and that they have a remote control in their hands that can speed up, slow down, freeze-frame, or stop the picture on the screen as well as control the audio. We then have them practice reviewing and controlling "movies" of pleasant events in their lives. We later ask them to project their visual flashbacks on the screen and learn to fast-forward them, to reverse them, and finally to shut them off. We ask clients to see, hear, and feel being in the theater and to experience the relief of being able to shut off the movie. We also have them practice taking the role of reporter, that is, of deliberately stating just the facts and thus staying in their head and being numb. These techniques are all useful in helping a client cope with intrusive memories and flashbacks.

Self-Monitoring

Enhancing or redirecting the ability to self-monitor is another skill we teach our clients. Our clients' ability to be aware of their situational triggers and their BASK responses is almost always seriously compromised or directed toward too much external or internal monitoring.

We have found that it is very important to go slowly in our attempts to increase our clients' ability to observe themselves. Prematurely pushing for too much awareness leads to floods of anxiety or other intense emotions that can disrupt therapy and, in some cases, prompts a relapse back into the crisis stage. Instead, we gradually work to increase client's awareness, focusing first on encouraging clients to track external triggers and their general reactions to them. Some clients are focused too much on themselves and are overly preoccupied with their own internal experience; we might ask these clients to monitor others' reactions in an attempt to get them out of themselves.

We encourage increased self-monitoring both directly and indirectly. We start the therapy session with a general check-in by asking how the client is doing today. We assist our clients in staying present in the session and working on dissociative behaviors by asking where, when, who, and what questions about important problem areas in the client's life, encouraging the client to be more and more specific in his or her answers. We suggest to clients that they might want to notice, for example, when they do feel anxious or when they have trouble setting boundaries. We might ask a client to keep a log of specific issues and write down what happened either in the evening of each day or at some other regular interval. We are careful to instruct clients to limit their journal writing to current issues and to avoid any processing of past traumatic material. We take it as a sign of progress when clients begin to say, "I noticed that . . . ." We then ask the client to begin to notice specific things, for example, how things are different or how it feels when he or she begins to think about asking for help or whatever noticing needs to take place to help that particular client change his or her response style and pattern.

Nurturing the Self and Preventing Relapse

One framework that we use to teach clients nurturing skills is the acronym HALTS. Used in AA to identify high-risk relapse triggers, the H stands for hungry, the A for angry, the L for lonely, the T for tired, or S for sick. In our experience these are also common triggers for relapse into trauma-based symptoms. We explore with clients their status in these areas and spend a great deal of time developing specific ways they can take preventive and proactive action in this area through self-care activities.

Relapse as a Videotape

The best experts on relapse are the persons who have relapsed. Their relapse can be rich with information on how to prevent relapses in the future. We ask clients to play back their last relapse as if it were on a videotape. We rewind it, replay it, make it pause, and fast-forward it several times. Poring over the relapse in this way is very informative for both therapists and clients.

It never ceases to amaze us how the disease of addiction tends to cause survivors to edit out key information about themselves when they are susceptible to relapse. When most alcoholics and addicts are contemplating resuming their use of substances, their disease leads them to glamorize and romanticize the chemical and its effects and to have thoughts like "I just want to escape the pain for one night" or "I just want to get loaded one more time." The disease makes survivors lie to themselves and believe that they will feel better or be happier if they return to their old long-lost friends—drugs and alcohol. Unfortunately, most people relapse because the "tape" in their heads tends to stop at the point of consumption of the mood-altering chemical and fails to continue beyond it, to the consequences of relapsing. The guilt and remorse that follow a relapse, along with the feeling that they have failed once again, are devastating for most survivors. These feelings can be powerful enough to turn a one-time relapse (or lapse) into a permanent return to active drinking and using and an abandonment of all attempts to work on any recovery issues. Learning to think through the sequence of events that occur after using the chemical can help prevent a relapse and combat the immediacy of the urge to relapse.

Gentle Parenting

Many of our clients work hard at being supportive parents. We point this out to them and ask them how they respond to their children when they have an accident or make a mistake; when we hear the tolerance and understanding in their answer, we wonder aloud how they can be so supportive of their children but not of themselves and how they might do for themselves what they do for their children. We work with clients both to acknowledge the occasions when they could have done better and to forgive themselves for not being perfect. The coining and sobriety birthday ceremonies found in AA and related 12-step programs model and reinforce the importance of celebrating accomplishments and not just taking them for granted. Although truly exorcising the shame demons usually requires the interventions in later stages of our recovery model, we know we are making progress when they say to us something like "I know you'd say I need to be kinder to myself about this." We promote the acknowledgment of true and legitimate achievements and of small but steady increments in true competence.

We constantly model and encourage improved problem-solving and goal-attainment abilities in our clients. Some of our clients are literally unaware that alternative solutions might exist for a given problem. For example, some clients might express a great deal of fear and concern about how they are doing at work; since they have had experiences with parents who were absent or actively abusive, the notion that one could ask an authority figure for feedback and that this would not necessarily be a horrible experience is foreign to them.

Other clients have a difficult time breaking down goals into discrete, attainable objectives. Clients often trigger in certain situations, and the anxiety they experience tends to lead them to be vague on the exact nature of a problem, to prematurely close off options, to see things in either/or terms, or to impulsively choose the most immediately available solution—or they feel so overwhelmed that they simply stay stuck.

Reaching Out for Support

Utilizing social support is a core issue for our clients. Their experiences in their formative years have almost always distorted their beliefs about others and the ways they relate to others. Whether they are compulsively independent or codependent or alternate between the two, our clients inevitably have difficulty both accepting support from others in a healthy way and changing this pattern. They are often isolated or alone, perhaps because they have consistently distrusted others or have alienated them by their behavior or because they have taken the "geographic cure" of moving away from former friends in the mistaken belief that in a new location they would not encounter interpersonal problems. Perhaps they are in relationships that are damaging or that are superficial and lacking in true intimacy (often an issue for survivors). Or perhaps their previous social contacts all revolved around partying and using chemicals and they have had to give up these friends in order to maintain abstinence.

Sometimes, however, clients only need a little encouragement to make better use of the social support they already have (e.g., they can be easily persuaded to call a friend) or to give a 12-step program a try. With the client's permission, we often hold a conference with his or her spouse, parents, friends, or sponsor to explain what is going on with the client and to elicit commitments of support from them. This is also an excellent time to encourage family members to do whatever recovery work they themselves might require.

More often, however, the addicted survivor has serious barriers to building and using safe social support. Some clients have difficulty deciding on who might be truly safe and supportive. Others have unrealistic expectations of what social support is all about, believing either that a supportive relationship must always be completely free of risk and disappointment or that no one can ever be truly supportive. Some clients have had little experience in socializing and having fun without chemicals. Others are hypersensitive in social situations, feeling that others will judge them or find them a burden.

AA and related 12-step programs are an excellent source of social support and provide their members with opportunities to practice various social skills. The atmosphere is generally warm, accepting, democratic, and oriented toward "living in the solution and not the problem." Members model sharing openly and honestly, and the sharing times—during which members, who are free to share or not, can opt to merely sit and listen if they so desire—provide occasions for practicing this skill. Social support in the form of a special mentor relationship is an integral part of the program, and 12-step groups organize recreational events, such as cookouts and dances that are "clean and sober," and in many locations also operate ALANO clubs, which provide a place for members to drop in and socialize.

Unfortunately, the special sensitivities and issues of survivors often stop them from using 12-step programs. Some survivors have had a bad experience in a group—some report that they flood when they hear others' stories, which may make them feel anxious and paranoid—thus reinforcing their tendency toward avoidance. Others, feeling abandoned by, unworthy of, or angry at God because of their childhood experiences, have a difficult time with the spiritual aspects of the program. Some survivors reject the program because they have heard an AA member inveigh against medication or psychotherapy, insisting that if people just worked the program, everything would be fine. The newly recovering survivor is especially vulnerable to revictimization in just about any setting, even a 12-step meeting.

We typically recommend that our clients not only begin individual therapy but also participate as soon as possible in the alcohol and drug groups in our clinic and then move on to a same-sex relapse prevention survivor recovery group. This gives them an opportunity early in recovery to become more comfortable with groups in general and to meet group members who are further along in their own recoveries and are attending 12-step meetings—and who often spontaneously offer to take newer members to these meetings. We also try to have a sense of the atmosphere and style of various groups available in the local area so that we can direct clients to groups with which they would feel most compatible. We encourage clients to try at least three different types and locations of 12-Step meetings before making up their minds about whether these self-help groups can be helpful to them.

Shuttling

After they practice their skills in less stressful situations, we then assist our survivor clients in learning "shuttling," an advanced skill that can help them keep themselves safe and manage anxiety in a variety of situations.

Shuttling involves learning to move in and out of the trance/state/part that gets triggered and involves distressing emotions or blocks one's ability to utilize more helpful protection and nurturing skills. Since clients can typically re-create troubling states in the office when prompted to do so, they can also be taught to shuttle. And although the emphasis in the skills-building stage is always on currently experienced difficulties, shuttling facilitates the abreaction work in the integration stage.

We start our instruction in this area by establishing with clients the premise that whatever happens during the shuttling exercise—that is, if flooding occurs or if they have difficulty doing the exercise—is useful in helping them avoid a potential fear or shame attack. We then ask our clients to re-create the problem feeling, state, or reaction in a very small way; we might, for example, ask them to feel just a drop of the fear or one snapshot of the visual flashbacks. We let them know that they can always say no or ask for help during this process. We view this client limit setting as a sign of their progress in recovery. Most survivors take a few minutes to create a stressful situation at first in their minds, but become increasingly adept at generating the troubling feeling, state, or reaction over time.

Usually clients can come out of their re-created state when we ask them to, and they can do so without our help. We prefer to see if they can generate their own solution at this stage. This approach has two advantages: Clients sometimes come up with a helpful response that is unique, and generating a solution themselves makes clients feel that they "own" the solution, a feeling that increases their sense of empowerment. If clients have difficulty doing this, however, we suggest that they open their eyes, use deep breathing, go to their safe place, or even stand up and walk around.

We then ask our survivor clients to shuttle back and forth a few times between the observer position and their re-created state. We ask them to observe what is occurring in all the BASK components and to notice the color, texture, size, and shape of the state. We then ask them to change each of these aspects and again notice who is observing this state and creating these changes and how they are doing this. Clients are often quite amazed to discover the control they have over their own experience. We then ask clients to go back into the state and repeat the process of exploring the BASK components and other aspects of the state; we again ask them to change these aspects as much as they can, and we give suggestions as needed.

As survivors learn to shuttle in and out of trauma-induced trance states, they build self-confidence and can feel certain in their ability to keep themselves safe. Shuttling also provides an opportunity to practice new skills even when triggered and overcome state-dependent blocks to accessing these skills. When originally in these states, survivors will have difficulty accessing alternative and more skillful responses. For survivors to activate their new skills when they are in the triggered state means that the new responses must be introduced into that state so that they are more accessible. Thus, we might ask clients to "feel just a little bit more of that anxiety," observe it, put it in the container, and then go to their safe place. We then ask them to re-create no more than a medium amount of the anxiety and repeat the process; we might, for example, ask them to see more of the flashback scenario, but to fast-forward it so that it ends it ends quickly, and then shuttle to their safe place. If the client is flooding, we might deliberately break the state into BASK components to help make it more manageable; for example, as a way to teach the positive uses of dissociation, we might ask the client to use just the thinking process that goes with that state.

Shuttling helps the survivor to develop an observing ego in the triggered state, an ego that is likely to be more aware of what is happening as it happens and of what is responsible for creating these states and how. Clients especially prone to dissociating, including those suffering from DID, often appear to already have a strongly developed and differentiated observing part of the self that has a life of its own (4). As the therapeutic alliance develops, this part of the client is more likely to present in the session, either on its own or at the invitation of the therapist, and it can provide a treasure trove of information about the client's various parts and act as an ally in exploring these issues. Nonetheless, this "master observer," while perhaps having an overview of what is occurring and knowledge about how it works, is typically not accessible to the client (and therefore the therapist) when another part of the self is in operation. Part of the goal of shuttling is to tap or develop the observer part associated with each of the client's parts to supplement the observer created earlier in the building stage. Learning to access new skills when in various states or when various parts of the self are dominant is another aspect of the therapeutic goal. Shuttling also helps to truly move skills available when triggered.

Self-Defense Classes

Our local police departments offer free two-night workshops for women to teach them basic self-defense techniques and to help them become more comfortable fighting back. More extensive self-defense classes of various kinds are also available for both men and women. Clients who attend these workshops often report a very positive experience, including male survivors who are often haunted by fears regarding their masculinity and who find their ability to fight back reaffirming.

We sometimes encounter in our clients a resistance to the learning of self-defense techniques. Influenced by the culture to regard physical defense as uncivilized, apprehensive that it will be too physically demanding, or fearful that forcefulness means they are in danger or are like their perpetrator, some survivor clients balk at first at the suggestion that they take a course in self-defense. We have found that it is helpful to explain the rationale behind our suggestion, to ask clients to take it one step at a time (e.g., "Why don't you just call to get some basic information?"), and to point out that their strong protestations against the idea suggest that they may indeed have a need for such self-defense skills. Parents of adolescent male survivors with acting-out problems or those who were themselves abused as children often envision turning their sons into trained assailants and are quite reluctant to follow through on this sort of suggestion. It sometimes helps parents deal with their fears when we explain that the aikido school of martial arts emphasizes defense and that most self-defense training stresses self-discipline and obedience to proper authority and emphasizes that the best fight is the one that is not fought. We have found that some survivors become so dissociated or so flooded when taking such classes that the instruction does little good. We encourage survivors to take these classes only when we feel they possess enough of the other aforementioned skills and can remain sufficiently focused in the present to benefit from the instruction.

It is very important as part of the process of helping clients establish a recovering identity to take the time to build, strengthen, and link their protector and nurturing parts. It decreases the likelihood of serious relapses and continued unsafe behavior and makes later work much easier and more complete. This process begins in the building stage and continues into the next two stages.

THE EDUCATION STAGE

The goal of the education stage is to transform survivors' deeply felt sense of themselves from victim and drunk/junkie to recovering survivor and alcoholic/addict. Establishing a recovering identity involves more firmly rooting the skills one has learned in the building stage so that these new ways to respond become more integral to one's sense of self. It also entails knowing and accepting all the parts of oneself and one's history without shame and other crippling emotions and feeling firmly a part of the recovering community.

Although we we teach such things as the signs and symptoms of addiction and PTSD and the elements of a recovery program all along during the treatment process, we wait until the education stage in our clients' recovery to do education-type work because our experience has been that clients are certain to intensely trigger as they deal with these issues. Most standard psychotherapy approaches assume that survivors are able to contain and tolerate strong emotions and impulses and that they can then work within the frame of the therapeutic alliance to achieve insight, behavior change, and integration. Basically, these approaches assume that clients are already at the education stage when they enter treatment, an assumption that is sometimes correct for high-functioning survivors who are merely abusing chemicals and whose history of trauma is relatively minor. However, initiating education-style work as the first stage of treatment is very often inappropriate for chemically dependent survivors with a history of serious trauma. For example, asking chemically dependent survivors to write a letter to their abuser is premature unless they have achieved the ability to feel safe and skills to stay safe. Until they are clean and sober and have the necessary skills, survivors will simply skim through the education stage and, because they remain disconnected, will derive no deep or lasting benefit from it. Or they may flood so strongly that they resist further growth in this area or even revert to the crisis stage.

Most of our clients at this point in their recovery find that they are generally feeling and doing better. They are clean and sober, are in no immediate danger of harming themselves or others, are taking better care of themselves, and have enhanced protection and nurturing skills. By this stage they are also somewhat more connected with others and with themselves, and they are functioning better at home and at work. However, our clients generally still report persistent difficulties in certain areas or with certain issues. They typically continue to flood and experience strong feelings of confusion, fear, or anger in response to particular triggers. Generally, they also still show the behaviors associated with these emotions, such as escape and avoidance. For example, a female client might report that she continues to avoid sexual contact or bursts into tears at the slightest criticism. Our clients also tend to persist in responding with old behaviors and have trouble using their new skills. A survivor might say such things as "I still can't slow down" or "My wife still thinks I'm a demanding son of a bitch." Furthermore, as they enter this stage, many of our clients remain unable to remember aspects of their past or continue to experience explosive levels of negative emotions or complete numbing when recalling the past. This in turn can prompt a reversion to the kind of thinking that attempts to justify a return to chemicals or other unsafe behavior. The wounded part of the self, for example, can return to believing that the painful feelings and memories cannot possibly be tolerated and that instant relief is needed; the nurturing part can once again mistakenly believe that chemicals will help soothe the pain and that they carry no risk; and the protector part begins to rationalize the use of chemicals and can become angry and withdrawn which can lead the client into a relapse of drug and/or alcohol abuse.

Survivors of childhood physical and sexual abuse struggle not only with issues related to their experience of trauma and abandonment but also with issues related to shame, issues that need much attention at this stage. No matter what most survivors who are ready for this stage say, they still have tremendous shame issues. Some survivors have had the experience of hearing their perpetrator or an enabler of the abuse literally tell them they were bad and deserved what happened to them. More often, however, survivors have concluded this in the egocentric and grandiose fashion of children who struggle to understand the reasons for their pain, and it is a conclusion that becomes more firmly established in the survivor's mind in the absence of any support from significant others who could absolve the survivor of responsibility for the abuse and provide input about what normal behavior is. Even if and/or when children cease to blame themselves for the abuse, even when, as they get older, they come to understand that what is occurring (or has occurred) is abuse, survivors often feel ashamed about how they coped with their situation.

A core sign of chemical dependence is the conflict between the addict's moral and ethical values and beliefs and the reality of his or her actual behavior when drinking and using. Addicts inevitably violate their own values and create a trail of ruin as they practice their disease. Once they are drug free, this guilt can be overwhelming. Chronic lying, angry tirades, broken promises, one-night stands, neglected children, resentful spouses, forged checks, and lost jobs constitute the legacy of chemical dependence, and the lament "I really screwed up" is one of the themes that individuals recovering from chemical dependence have to grapple with and resolve.

Substance-dependent survivors, who are already saturated with shame and primed from an early age to readily equate doing "bad" things with being "bad," now have additional confirmation of their low worth. In the past, many survivors took vows never to be like their abusive/abandoning parents; to now find themselves acting in ways that sometimes remind them of their parents' behaviors—that is, to now recognize that their pledge to do things differently has been broken—is an additional burden of shame.

Staying with this shame at best makes for a less than satisfying recovery and at worst sets survivors up for a relapse. A pervasive and lingering sense of being "bad" robs their life of joy and a sense of self-esteem. As one survivor client with one year of sobriety told us, "I always go around feeling that I should apologize to people just for being alive."

Unresolved shame can contribute to the development or acceleration of other compulsive behaviors, such as an eating disorder or workaholism, in an attempt to feel good on the inside by looking good on the outside. Standing shamefaced before others, figuratively if not literally, with eyes downcast and checks reddened with embarrassment, contributes to a continued sense of being alienated from them and forestalls the possibility of true eye-to-eye validation and mirroring. Besides exerting an ongoing pressure to remain reclusive and seclusive, shame provides an incentive to remain secretive and hence less than honest with self and others. Secrecy is one of the elements that breed and perpetuate the denial associated with both abuse and substance dependence, and a variety of conditions can easily fan the embers of any remaining denial into the flames of renewed drinking and using, suicidal feelings, acceptance of unhealthy and unsafe relationships, and so forth. Therapists must learn to handle this shame with care from the very first session, or their clients will either remain superficially involved in the treatment or bolt from it. Substance-dependent survivors are not just ashamed about what happened and what they did; their very identity is shame-based. Unless they deal with the shame, these clients will remain disconnected from self and others and at risk for stalling or regressing in their recoveries.

People in the education stage work on developing a greater ease and sense of responsibility (as well as "response-ability") for their history, their diseases, all the parts of themselves, and their recovery. We assist clients to protect and nurture themselves even more easily, competently, and flexibly, with enhanced communication between all their parts. We assist our clients to tell their story fearlessly, openly, and honestly while literally looking directly at others. We want survivors not only to know the true causes and remedies for their diseases but to also accept responsibility for being in recovery and no longer sick. We help clients learn to accept responsibility for their own behavior without shame and to learn that making amends is a sign of strength and a means of healing. And we encourage them to honor their suffering and the incredible strength they possessed in order to survive an insane situation.

Written and Other Materials

During the education stage we encourage our clients to take advantage of the books and tapes available on such topics as codependence and sexual abuse healing. We also might suggest joining an AMAC (Adults Molested as Children) group in addition to their 12-step group to supplement their recovery support system. Our experience has been that only at this stage of their recovery are clients likely to benefit from doing these sorts of activities.

Mapping

Survivors seldom have only one, simple reaction to a trauma-related trigger. Instead they are very likely to have developed a series of trance states, each with their own function, feelings, logic, set of behaviors and even chronological age. These states or parts are dissociated and hence are likely to play out in an unconscious and unhelpful manner because each state is likely to be highly reactive, extreme, and limited in its flexibility and range of options. Quite often these states represent polar extremes such as perfectionism or shame, codependent clinging or abandonment depression, and rage or terror. These parts range in complexity from relatively simple ego states to the highly developed "personalities" of DID. Sometimes states are linked, and if one of the states is triggered a series of states play out with only partial awareness. At other times, there is little or no connection between parts as with DID.

For example, we worked with a female client whose father was extremely emotionally and physically abusive. Her presenting problems included anger blowups, avoidance of touch from her husband, and anxiety. This person's primary state was relentless perfectionism. However, when things became out of her control and she became "imperfect," she would experience shame, followed by anger, anxiety, depression, and frantic efforts to "make up" with others. Then the cycle would begin again. In another example, we worked with a client with DID who had experienced severe physical and sexual abuse and neglect as a child. She had three parts. "Jason" was the adolescent protector who was intelligent, strong, in control, without feelings, and was the primary state. "Elizabeth," an older woman, was the nurturing part. She was very underdeveloped, seldom present, and distrusted by both Jason and "Mary." Mary was a 5-year-old female part who had most of the feelings for this client, both positive ones, such as being playful, and negative ones, such as fear when touched by men or when dealing with angry women. When Mary was "out," neither Jason nor Elizabeth were available as resources.

Assessing all the survivors' states or parts and their interrelationships is essential for treatment to ultimately be effective for a variety of reasons. Unless therapy addresses a part (especially if it is an important one), this part is likely to continue to trigger. This might take the form of a single, troubling state. Or, if the part is included in a chain of reactions as in the first example above, the unresolved state can reactivate other states in the chain even if these connected states have been processed in therapy. A final consideration is that each state often has a piece of what is needed for healthy functioning, and helping these parts work together can be an important part of progress in treatment. This requires knowing some of the "interpersonal" dynamics between parts. For example, as per the second example above, we explored and worked through Jason's and Mary's distrust of Elizabeth, a distrust based on the earlier experience of this client's drug-addicted mother who could be alternately nurturing and abusive. After building up Elizabeth's nurturing skills, we taught Jason to call on Elizabeth to help comfort Mary when Mary was scared and after Jason had taken protective action.

Mapping is the term used to describe the process of taking an inventory of each state and an in-depth analysis of a client's trances and parts. This analysis includes both the intrastate dynamics of the part as well as the interstate dynamics between different parts. The term mapping is appropriate because of the notes that we keep during this assessment process. We find that taking notes is helpful because of the quantity and importance of the information generated. This is particularly true if the client has elaborate, branching chains or states that are personalities who might get offended if we do not remember their names, ages, and other important information about them after a "meeting" or two. Literally drawing out the parts and their relationships by using circles and lines and jotting down the information gained about each state/identity helps keep sessions on track and important information in mind. Mapping also lays the foundation for integration stage work as described later in this chapter.

We usually start by discussing troubling states that bother the client or that we have noticed as interfering with the client's functioning. We then use our protector/nurturer/wounded part framework (as described in Chapter 3) to do a preliminary probe and organization of the client's material. We then ask the client to review in a detailed, step-by-step fashion the nature of the trigger cues for each of these states. We use the BASK model to inventory the "how" of the reaction. We may give the client the homework assignment of noticing, even more precisely than before, when a certain state or sequence of states triggers outside the session and to report their discoveries back to us. In addition we try to develop a historical context for the development of the state based on what we know about the client's history. We encourage clients to give a name or label for the trigger that fits for them, for example "one of my abandonment triggers" or "my incompetent authority button." We also encourage our clients to remain both honest about themselves and accepting of their reactions and to avoid shame attacks and judgmental, black and white thinking about their states.

We typically ask a number of specific questions to explore triggered states in this way, including:

1. What word or phrase best describes this state for you?
2. What is the who, what, where, and when of the trigger for this state?
3. What do you do, feel, sense in your body, and think (BASK) in this state?
4. What positive goal or purpose does this state try to accomplish for you?
5. What strengths does this state have for accomplishing this purpose?
6. What limitations?

7. What might be a more helpful response that takes advantage of these strengths and compensates for these limitations?
8. How old do you feel when in this state?
9. Why do you think you might have learned to react this way?
10. What state comes before and after this state?

We sometimes send home with clients a summary of their maps and ask them to observe their reactions more closely and fill in details. We also use the maps to explore ways in which the survivor's protector, nurturer and wounded parts interact to further pinpoint problems and solutions. For example, we might point out that the survivor's need to be perfect leads to a very critical stance toward the self and that this probably makes the wounded part feel very badly when a mistake is made; we might then discuss ways to nurture the self when a mistake is made while still keeping some sense of wanting to do things "as best as you can." Or we might point out to the person that when the protector part blows up at others with little cause, the end result for the wounded part is likely to be increased shame or loneliness; we then might discuss other ways to protect the self, such as using the assertion skills the person has been practicing but has been having difficulty using in trigger situations. Sometimes we point out that another state would be a helpful "ally" and discuss ways that, for example, the fearful state could let the person know something might be amiss, the protector state could begin to mobilize and, with a little help from the nurturing state, set boundaries in a more diplomatic way with a family member. A standard intervention that we use labels chemical use as a misguided attempt to help the wounded part feel better. Asking parents if they would counsel their 6-year-old daughter to get drunk in order to handle being teased at school typically elicits a horrified "No!" and leads quickly into a discussion about more helpful options for handling the rejection and shame that the "child" part of you feels when faced, for example, with a critical boss. We would then add the new options to the map to serve as reminders to ourselves and clients.

We make use of the survivor's shuttling skills to deepen our joint understanding of each state, to anchor new response options and, if ready, to begin preliminary integration work. After preliminary mapping of a state, we might also ask the client to actually recreate the state right in the session "if it feels safe to do so." We then explore the state using the same questions outlined above and then have the client practice the new options in session or imagine themselves responding differently when the cues occur from within the state itself. Recreating the state helps to insure that we have not missed important aspects of that state and increases the chance of the new options being elicited even when the client is triggered. Clients with strong dissociative defenses (most particularly those with

DID) will require the shuttling approach to do mapping because they have so little general awareness of their states. If the client begins to experience strong flooding when recreating the state, we ask them to use their various safety skills or simply give a suggestion that they dissociate the feelings. If the client can experience the state without strong flooding, we might even begin to ask them to recall memories associated with this state, always "erring" on the side of safety.

Case Illustration

An example of this process in action might be helpful. We worked with a mother we shall call Sheila who triggered very strongly to her angry daughter's tirades. Sheila's first response to this was to go into a hyper-reasonable, placating state. When that did not work, Sheila would blow up and rant and rave at her daughter, but then feel very ashamed at her reaction. Sheila had been emotionally and physically abused by her father and by her first husband. We had already worked with Sheila on assertion and boundary setting, but she had a difficult time using these skills when triggered and, as an insightful person who had done a lot of self-help reading, Sheila had an overall sense of her reaction sequences. We asked her to re-create the anger "in a small way" and notice what that state was about. She noticed a distinct sense of fear in her stomach as well as a tightening in her throat. As it turned out, the fear followed the placating and preceded the anger. This was a new insight for Sheila. Exploring the fear revealed themes of being both unlovable and beaten, if not perfect, which Sheila connected to her father. We worked to connect the fear "by sending a message up to her throat" to the angry protector state. We then worked with the anger in terms of "saying what needed to be said and doing it in an assertive way." Sheila went on to work on the shame that followed the anger by identifying thoughts of being unworthy of love and learning to dispute these "lies." She practiced self-acceptance with self-statements like "progress not perfection," and by saying out loud what she had needed to say to her father and husband but was unable to at the time.

Learning to Ask for Support

At some point, whether and how to reach out to friends and relatives to share their stories and seek support becomes an issue for survivors. We try to help clients clearly understand their motives for doing this and encourage them to explore their fears and hopes. Some survivors have unrealistic, childlike fears of negative reactions from others, and many have unrealistic fantasies that they will finally get the support and validation they always wanted. We must very often clarify for clients that the primary goal is to speak their truth honestly and without fear and shame and remind them that the secondary goal of getting what they want from others may not be met. Survivors must have their fail-safe plans in order and need to learn to identify and distinguish between those friends and relatives who are likely to be supportive and those who are not.

Some survivors, on the one hand, still feel deeply ashamed or afraid to talk to significant others about their issues. They then fail to receive the enormous support and validation that may be available to them. They often fear the worst and unrealistically retain old, shame-based defenses that continue to keep them disconnected. On the other hand, there are many survivors who find they have almost a compulsion to practice rigorous honesty and self-disclosure and to tell everyone everything about themselves and their issues. They get swept up in the torrent of relief that can come from finally feeling free to speak their truth. Unfortunately, they sometimes find themselves disclosing information in ways that make them vulnerable to revictimization, which can range all the way from having their constant disclosures finally reacted to with indifference and/or fatigue, to being seen as the weird or obsessed one in the family or at work, to being told by relatives that they are making up what happened. Most often, clients have a good sense of what the general reaction is likely to be for individuals they know well but will tend to magnify or minimize the intensity of both the validating and the invalidating responses they are likely to receive.

For a client to reveal the secret of the abuse to members of his or her family of origin is a high-risk–high-gain strategy. Sometimes family members readily admit to what happened, express sorrow, and ask what they can do to help. This is especially likely to happen if a sibling who was also abused discloses their abuse to family members. Sometimes family members rally partially but then get so caught up in their own guilt or anger that the survivor perceives another abandonment. This is especially likely to happen when the parent or parents not directly involved in the trauma itself respond with comments like "How could I have been such a terrible parent not to see!" or "Why didn't you tell me or run away!" While ostensibly supportive, the subtext of such comments is that the family member's own needs once again become more important to him or her than the survivor's needs. Sometimes family members continue to live in denial and blame the survivor. This is especially likely to happen if the perpetrator is still in the family and/or if family members are chemically dependent or otherwise in denial themselves. Statements like "Oh, you don't have a problem with drinking" or "That never happened; you're just trying to stir up trouble" are hardly likely to result in a reduction of fear and shame.

Confronting the perpetrator who is still alive is the ultimate "coming out" and extremely empowering. However, many clients, we believe, do this prematurely, either on their own or at the insistence of well-meaning therapists. We believe that such a confrontation is best done at the very end of the education stage of the recovery work, when clients are more likely to be able to do this safely no matter what the response of the perpetrator. We are also aware of the recent controversy around the so-called false memory syndrome, a topic discussed in more detail in Chapter 1. As ultimately healing as such a confrontation can be, clients and therapists need to be carefully prepared to handle a wide variety of counterattacks, ranging from denial to physical assaults and lawsuits. Survivors can still attain the highest quality of abstinence from chemicals even if they are unable, for whatever reason, to confront the perpetrator. Perhaps the perpetrator is no longer around owing to death, imprisonment, or some geographic barrier. Or perhaps he or she is so frightening and unsafe that it would do the client more harm than good to have any contact at all. The issue of whether or not confrontation needs to occur directly must be resolved according to the individual survivor's unique situation. We want to make it clear that we are not suggesting that highly sensitive and suggestible survivors have not worked a good enough recovery program or cannot do complete integration work unless confrontation occurs. Sometimes returning to the city, state, or location of the abuse is enough confrontation. Returning as an adult, with an adult's power and maturity, can help the wounded part of survivors see that they no longer have to feel afraid of being vulnerable and small.

We encourage clients to use labels like "alcoholic," "addict," and "survivor"; phrases like "my addiction" and "my sexual abuse"; and statements like "That's my disease talking," "That's the part of me that thinks like a victim," and "That's my abandonment stuff." We then explore their reactions to this, for example, by asking clients to notice and report on how they feel when they use these labels; or we might point out to our clients that we noticed that they speeded up and looked away when they called themselves these "names" and then explore what was happening in them as they did this. We constantly promote the perspective that these are diseases and that responsibility lies not in having a disease or in being a victim but in being an alcoholic and a survivor *in recovery*. Our stance toward relapse, for example, is not that relapsed clients are "bad" but that they need to examine what is missing in their recovery program and must then, with whatever assistance is necessary and available, add this missing element. We also characterize symptoms as the best possible means by which our survivor clients were able to stay safe and cope at the time of their trauma, and we encourage them to consider what other coping mechanisms might be helpful now that they have more options.

We state over and over again that there are no failures in the recovery process, only lessons!

Reframing Being a Survivor as an Asset

We constantly emphasize throughout the process of treatment that the symptoms of PTSD represent their creative and sane solutions to an insane situation. For example, we might point out to a hypersensitive client that while this trait may cause hurt feelings at times, it also has strengths; as hypersensitivity is also intuition and is a skill they might find useful in people-oriented jobs such as sales, teaching, and counseling. Or we might focus on a client's hyperawareness of injustice and point out that this trait, suitably channeled, can help create a personal and social environment that is more fair and just. Survivors frequently have excellent artistic abilities, a reflection of their extensive use of right-hemisphere survival strategies and of their ability, as recovery proceeds, to more and more easily access the child part within themselves in healthy ways. We encourage them to use these creative abilities not only in their recovery work but as a source of personal satisfaction and perhaps even as the starting point for a career.

An analogous technique is to ask clients to specify what positive and helpful functions are being served by negative states like fear or shame and what limitations a positive condition, such as being independent, might entail. These exercises help reduce black-and-white thinking about the survivor's states or parts. Our constant message to our survivor clients is that they are survivors, not victims; that only the strong survive what they have gone through; that their experiences, properly seen, are sources of growth that nonsurvivors will never be able to tap; and that they are complex human beings.

Telling a New Story

The education stage of recovery is also an excellent time to help clients rewrite their life story and correct the misconceptions in their understanding of themselves that crop up in the telling of their stories. For example, one male client with polysubstance dependence and severe PTSD symptoms who had a history of horrendous physical abuse (including being shot at and thrown out a window) for the slightest infraction of house rules constantly wondered why only he and not his siblings had received this treatment. When exploration revealed that his mother had conceived him during an affair and that he was not the biological son of his father, we were able to point out to him that his "father" (i.e., his stepfather) had displaced all his rage at his mother onto him. This rewriting of his history proved very helpful in answering this young man's "why me?" question and in disputing his "it must be my fault" thinking.

A classic element in the histories of many survivors of sexual abuse is the confusion and shame they feel around the fact that they may have became sexually aroused during the abuse experience and may have enjoyed the physical contact. Explaining that humans have a strong instinct for sexual arousal and that offenders exploit this and use it as an excuse for their own behavior is often helpful here, as is pointing out to survivors that they received little physical or emotional affection other than from the offender. Asking them to pay attention not to what they told themselves about the abuse but to what their bodies felt—that is, making the point that our minds can fool us but our bodies do not lie—is helpful if survivors are still struggling with the question of whether the abuse was that bad; we are often able to make this particular point by drawing clients' attention to their own body language, namely, such automatic body reactions as crossing their legs or folding their arms when discussing the abuse in a therapy session. Some people also seem to benefit from our repeatedly stressing that abuse is not only about sex or beatings but about violations of power and trust and that children inevitably blame themselves for events out of a naturally occurring but misguided and egocentric grandiosity. They also seem to benefit when we explain the brainwashing paradigm and review the fact that offenders have the ability to rationalize the most outrageous behavior.

Stating that addiction is a matter of genetics and chemistry and not willpower or strength of character is another useful refrain. We also try to challenge survivors' childlike notion that there was some way for them to magically stop the abuse and the abuser by pointing out that it is unreasonable to think that a child can take control of a larger and stronger perpetrator and get him or her to stop the abuse. It is important to remind all survivors that abuse is by definition a power relationship; that the perpetrator has power over the victim, thus making the enforced behavior a matter of abuse; and that without the power differential, there would be no abuse.

Chemically dependent survivors in particular are doubly prone to feelings of shame and black-and-white thinking. Our clients often drown in excessive mortification and lose all sight of any strengths they possess. The extensive probing of sexual acting out and/or early childhood issues that is commonly available in some written Step Four inventories, such as child masturbatory experiences, promiscuity, or details of their sexual abuse, can trigger severe flooding in survivors. Some clients dutifully work these steps but fail to feel any relief and renewal; most likely, these clients remained dissociated during the process or had an attack of shame rather than guilt, which is relieved by working a Step Four self-abuse inventory. It is important to help clients do balanced Step Four work, with an equal emphasis on strengths and limitations (see Chapter 7 for a further discussion of tailoring step work to the survivor and the appendix for specialized step work). Steps Five through Nine provide additional opportunities to help clients learn that forgiveness of themselves is possible and that making amends to others need not be an exercise in shame.

THE INTEGRATION STAGE

Resolution of the past and acquisition of the ability to live in the here and now are the goals of the integration stage. Having acquired new skills, having reconstructed his or her life story, and having begun to reconnect with self and others without shame, the survivor is now ready to integrate these new beginnings in a cohesive fashion. Achieving integration allows clients to move through and beyond the recovering alcoholic or addicted survivor identity constructed in the last stage and into "living life on life's terms" and truly taking things "one day at a time."

Three Tasks of Integration

Survivors focus on three tasks when doing integration work. The first task is to "burn off" the intense emotions and feelings associated with trance states. Only by working through and beyond the issues of the trances/parts, through such processes as abreaction of emotions and exposure treatments, will all parts of the personality of the client be reunited and the problems of the past laid to rest.

The second task for survivors is to continue to work at being "detranced," that is, to diminish the readiness and intensity with which they respond to focal triggers by means of automatic trance states or split-off parts. Examples of such progress are evident in the following client statements: "I only obsess for three days rather than three weeks after I get criticized at work"; "I can now control my anger when someone lets me down, but the intensity of my feelings still sometimes scares me"; "I know I was abused and why I'm so scared of men. I still freak out sometimes when dating, but much less often now." Survivors may also still report or evidence dissociative symptoms, such as feeling numb at times or having difficulty recalling their childhood; or after stating in a therapy session that they are merely seeking help for their depression, they may suddenly turn "robotic," stare into space, and report that they have dealt with the fact that their stepfather raped them repeatedly. Survivors in the integration stage are usually still struggling to some extent not only with issues of fear, abandonment, and shame but also with the associated defenses of fight, flight, and freeze. They may also still feel the siren call of chemicals.

Grief work is the third task of this stage of recovery. The literature on grieving commonly identifies several stages: denial/numbing/shock; preoccupation/yearning/searching; rage/despair/disorganization; and acceptance/reorganization/resolution (5). Grieving in reality is seldom so tidy but such schemas provide a framework for understanding the grieving process.

The intense affects associated with the abreactions and the working through process involved in de-trancing are different from those of grieving. The kind of grieving that survivor clients must accomplish focuses not only on the pain of what did happen but on the pain of what happened as a result of what did not happen. Grieving does not grapple with the issue, for example, of what father did but with the fact that the client never had—and will never have—the kind of parent–child relationship a father is supposed to provide. In grieving, clients wrestle not so much with their history of addiction as with the fact that they lost career opportunities, a marriage, or even health as a result of the addiction and with the fact that this loss is irrevocable. Abreaction is likely to be rageful and full of explosive tears; grieving, in contrast, is more likely to be characterized by resentment and/or gentle weeping. As one client told us, "I was watching a documentary on the seventies, and I started quietly crying for all those nightmare years of drugging and endless relationships that never worked. I just recently have begun to realize that I had downplayed how much I've lost." Until people grieve, there is still unfinished work that absorbs their energy and keeps them subtly stuck in the past. Clients who have done their grieving tell us that they literally feel lighter and are less preoccupied with the past.

Survivors, whether chemically dependent or not, present some unique issues when it comes to grieving. We try to be alert to whether our clients have, in fact, truly grieved the past and not just skimmed through this process—or skipped it altogether. Many clients claim they have grieved, but often we discover that their experience was dissociated or premature. Our clients also often confuse forgiving the perpetrator with acceptance of the past. In our experience this forgiveness is often premature and misguided and represents continued denial about the impact of what happened on the survivor's life. We try to distinguish between forgiving the perpetrator and letting go of the past. We are strongly opposed to trying to force the survivor prematurely to "forgive" their abuser. One can let go emotionally of the pain, however it is the abuser *not* the survivor who needs to be making amends and taking responsibility for the abuse. The advice to quickly forgive the abuser, often given by family, friends, and counselors, can be well-meaning and can represent an earnest attempt to help survivors move on with their lives, or it can represent denial in another form. Either way, we believe this advice is not useful. On the other hand, we are also very much against survivors remaining endlessly stuck in rage and resentment; this means that the perpetrator still has power over the survivor and that the survivor still has energy tied up with the past that could be used for growth. Keeping resentments is like "swallowing poison and expecting the other person to die." The goal is not to forgive and forget, but to grieve and let go. Once that is done, working the 12 steps on all issues, including those related to trauma resolution, becomes possible.

These three tasks—burning off intense emotions, continuing to work on being de-tranced, and grieving—complement one another. Different parts of the self, even after they have abreacted, very often still want the missing experiences they never had and therefore still remain. For example, the wounded child part often still wants to have the parenting it never got. This part needs to have that wish both validated and disputed; that is, the message to that part of the self needs to be that the wish is acceptable and that it is unfair and sad that good parenting never happened. That part must also be given permission to grieve, and then it must let go and allow the older, stronger, more nurturing part of the self to gratify those needs as much as is possible today, taking one day at a time. At the same time, the self parts that clients created to deal with the trauma will not relinquish their duties and feel free to go unless they are fully convinced and accepting of the fact that the self now has more helpful trances/parts/identities to help it stay safe.

Therapeutic Strategies and Interventions

We use general sets of strategies to accomplish the working through of issues in the integration stage. The first goal is to assist the survivor to connect the present to the past in a direct, experiential way. Up until now, the survivor has focused on the past only in an intellectual manner during the education stage. The second goal is to help the survivor abreact the past. Abreaction, which refers to a reliving of emotions in order to relieve them, includes both the intense affect and the grief associated with the trauma and the chemical use. The third goal is to defuse remaining triggers by helping survivors have the missing experience they needed at the time of the trauma. While people at the integration stage of recovery have had numerous corrective experiences, they benefit from having one anchored in both the past and the present and experienced through all BASK components. Many traditional therapies are appropriate for this stage of work. Our intent in this section is to describe the procedures we generally use, especially those that operate within the trance paradigm we have incorporated into all stages of our work so far.

We use several general tactics in this stage. We work with survivors on their shuttling skills so that they can move easily not just among current states but back to the past in their memories. For example, we might ask clients to go back to the first time or one of the first times they felt a certain way, if this feels safe. They are then able to connect current responses to past adaptations and to truly know what happened and who they are as a result. In the re-created past state clients can utilize new skills and identities and further "rewire" their neurophysiological states. We might also encourage clients to give themselves the missing experience in their memories to truly re-create the past in a way that is likely to defuse triggers or to re-decide old childhood decisions about who was to blame. We also try to help survivors revisit the past by doing such things as writing a letter to a dead perpetrator or visiting their childhood home. With some clients we might actually begin to encourage extinction of cues associated with chemical use; for example, clients might now be ready to meet friends in a bar or other "slippery" place if we and they feel they can do so without relapsing.

We use the principles and behavioral techniques of desensitization here to guide us in our work with our clients' abreactions and behavioral assignments (6, 7, 8). Desensitization procedures call for organizing feared or risky situations into a hierarchy of steps or scenes from least feared to most feared, according to subjective ratings given by the client. For example, using a rating scale of, say, zero for "no fear" and 10 for "maximum fear" and starting with the least feared scene, clients experience each scene either by talking about it, imagining it, or actually repeating it (i.e., by going to the scene itself). Clients then move on to the next level of the hierarchy when they report that they only feel a low level (e.g., zero to 2, in this example). Extensive research has shown that the key elements leading to erosion of the fear response are simply "safe" exposure and not responding in the old conditioned way, which gradually produce an extinction of the conditioned fear or response. However, although using anxiety management skills such as deep breathing is not absolutely necessary, most people seem to be more willing to go through the process if they have some procedure they can employ. As a general guideline, people benefit most from experiencing intermediate levels of anxiety or "urge." We constantly monitor the intensity of the emotions to assist clients to stay in this more therapeutic intermediate level.

Eye movement desensitization and reprocessing (EMDR) is a recent development in the field of exposure techniques (9). This procedure involves having clients imagine and tell their story of the trauma while simultaneously tracking with their eyes a target such as a pencil being moved back and forth laterally by the therapist. The theory behind this procedure is that it disrupts the conditioned pathways, possibly by engaging both hemispheres in the working through of the traumatic memories. The results of prelimiary studies are encouraging. Shapiro, who discovered the technique, cautions against the untrained use of this technique and now offers workshops in EMDR to credentialed individuals (10). We have talked with many clinicians who are quite enthusiastic about this technique; others have found it to be less effective with persons who have heavy dissociative defenses.

As part of the memory work, we make sure to work within the BASK model, both to titrate the experience and to make sure the desensitization is complete. We might start memory work by asking clients to think about a past traumatic event in their life and only report on the behavior (of the BASK components) part of what happened, or we might ask the client to use the movie screen technique to report on what they experienced by viewing their life drama in a more safe, depersonalized fashion. We make sure that we recapture all BASK aspects, correct any cognitive distortions (e.g., about responsibility) that they uncover, and, in some cases, even provide the missing experience. We might, for example, say to a client, "Imagine that the older you was there and provided protection and nurturing." By this point people can usually generate the missing experience, but they sometimes still need prompting from us. Before we provide a reframing and nurturing statement, we might, for example, say to a client, "Ask that part of you that is still that 5-year-old to listen to me." In some cases we invite other members of the survivor's recovery group to provide the missing experience, such as interrupting the trauma or coming to the survivor's assistance. In others we arrange for the survivor to meet the perpetrator in our office for a clarification or confrontation session—with one or both of us present—although this scenario is fairly rare since the perpetrator may be unavailable or unwilling to participate.

With the appropriate foundation in place, most people can usually tolerate this work. Typically, survivors report a tremendous sense of relief and calm after abreacting and obtaining the missing experience. Sometimes, however, they flood too strongly. In this case we simply fall back to safety skills and then try again later, once safety is re-established. In other cases clients quickly lose the trance state before all the work is done. Because our experience is that working within the state is the most effective approach, we simply ask our clients to re-create the state and proceed. Sometimes clients are unable to produce a state. We then ask them to more intensely re-create the block interfering with their re-creation of the state and simply treat the block as one more part that needs work. The block may indicate the existence of a new trauma state in the sequence that still needs work.

Sometimes clients continue to report very focal episodes of triggering and flooding involving unexpected tears or an attack of other feelings, such as fear or rage. At such times clients feel that their feelings, which tend to be an overly exaggerated response to a given situation, have taken over. This type of flooding is a sign of unresolved issues.

Thirteen-year-old Lisa had been in therapy for over a year, in both a women's group and in individual treatment with us, to work on her experience of sexual abuse by her grandfather. In August she reported that she was beginning to fear and dread the coming Christmas season and that she was having nightmares about her grandfather and his molesting her. She felt that it was time to write her grandfather a letter, and her individual therapist as well as members of her therapy group agreed that this would be helpful. It took Lisa a week to complete the following letter, which she gave us permission to publish:

November 9, 1992

Dear Ray,

I didn't write to you as my grandfather, because what you did to me isn't what "normal "grandfathers do to their granddaughters.

I am writing you because I want you to know how much you have hurt me and how you continue to hurt me by not admitting to what you have done.

I have been in counseling for over a year trying to deal with the hurt caused by your actions. It is hard to relive the pain, but I am doing it so I can put this all behind me.

It continues to be hard because you and your behavior have affected my relationship with my mother and grandmother. I used to laugh and feel comfortable with them; now they feel distant toward me.

Before I told about what happened to me, I was starting to get close to my mom. You taught my mom to keep the abuse a secret; she learned that very well. When I told your secret about the abuse, my mom got angry at ME for telling about the abuse, not you for doing the abuse!

My mom and I still cannot talk about the abuse. I don't know if we ever will be about to. Your molesting me has also hurt my ability to have a normal relationship with a boyfriend. When I start to get close to a guy and he touches my hand, I feel sick and scared and pull away. I get worried that no man will ever want me because I am not "pure." I feel as if I have been dirtied by you.

What you did to me not only sickens me but makes me hate you! I usually can't hate someone this much, but I do. I don't always hate you but I also can't love you. Not after what you have done to me.

I think of how you used to ask my mom if I could go out of town with you. I hate to think what you would have done to me if she had let that happen!

Writing this letter has been very helpful to me. I am glad I found a way to tell you these things without having to see you!

Signed,
Lisa

In Lisa's letter there is mention of several trigger points: (1) when a boy touches her hand, (2) when her grandmother seems distant, and (3) when her mother cannot discuss the abuse with her. Lisa's final abuse took place on Christmas Eve, and the abuse was discovered on Christmas Day, causing police investigators to have to speak to Lisa alongside her Christmas gifts. This explains her fear and dread of the Christmas season. Lisa was able to work through her triggers by going back in time to the last time her grandfather molested her. For the first-mentioned trigger we worked with her memory of the last time a male touched her and suggested that when a boy touches her hand in the future, she will feel the youthful excitement of first love and that the harder she tries to feel dirty, the more pure she will feel. For work on the second and third triggers we had Lisa imagine a situation in which she was able to get the love and support of both her grandmother and her mother. The Christmas trigger was handled in a similar way, namely, by introducing a positive Christmas experience to counteract the trigger response.

Focal trigger work builds on the client's increasing ability to shuttle and "work inside" and depends on the client's ability to associate new, more helpful, responses to old triggers. We use the client's new skills, his or her feelings of being in the presence of a higher power, images of 12-step meetings, the supportive voice of the "fairy godperson," and whatever other resources, old or new, are available to the client. Yapko's book on hypnosis provides other examples of reworking the past and establishing new associations to triggers (11).

Veterans visiting various Vietnam war memorials exhibit a prototypical healing ceremony for trauma. Many Vietnam veterans find that by visiting a memorial and leaving a gift for a friend lost or killed in combat that they are able to access and work through painful feelings and memories. We have visited the Vietnam memorial in Washington, D.C. and found a number of metals, photos, flowers, and other tokens of love left to honor the memory of those lost or killed. This ritual also honors that part of the surviving veteran that was killed by the experience—the innocent youthful 18-year-old boy who was sent halfway around the world to watch and participate in the killing and maiming of other human beings. That lost part of them needs a chance to be acknowledged before it can let go and grieve completely. Other veterans return to Vietnam to see through adult eyes what they survived as youth. We encourage our clients to pick out a strategy that works for them to symbolize the recovery of the whole self. As mentioned earlier, revisiting the place of the trauma and, when it is possible and safe to do so, confronting the perpetrator and/or telling other family members are especially healing. AA birthdays, celebrated on the date marking the first day of sobriety, also represent healing ceremonies and can serve this purpose. Since each person is unique, the way of healing will need to be individualized to fit a person's own needs.

Once clients have worked through all their states, in whatever number of therapy sessions is necessary, they report a lasting sense of calm with no further troubling emotions. We then use one final set of integration tactics, which is based on the work of Wolinsky (12). We ask people to re-create each state in the sequence; to take away any and all story lines, old and new, in each state; and to notice what happens. Our clients generally report a lessening of feelings. We then ask them to take away the label for the state (e.g., fear) and just feel the feeling. Again, they report a lessening of the feeling. We then ask them to merge with the feeling and simply experience it as energy in the body. Survivors generally report that they can do this and that they experience the energy as positive or (paradoxically) as calm. If someone experiences a negative feeling, this typically signals another linked state. When clients are finally in that completely calm state, we ask them to "turn around and see or feel or hear" each state in the sequence. We then ask them what part of them is now being experienced and invite them to imagine those states as being made of the same substance as the safe, calm space around them. We ask them to notice what happens as they imagine this. Typically, people report that all those former states simply evaporate and that they are left just with a me. We finally ask them to set up the states again and ask them who is doing this; after they say, "I am," we ask them to simply dissolve all those states and reabsorb them. When clients can take, create, and dissolve all the states/parts/identities at will, they have achieved integration. Other ways to achieve fusion involve asking the different parts of the self to "breathe together as one," imagining the merging together of visual images, and following other suggestions pertaining to flowing, blending, and moving together as one united self (13).

THE MAINTENANCE STAGE

Chemical dependency is a chronic disease. PTSD and related survivor syndromes may also may be chronic, or they may recur. Addicted survivors are always recovering, never recovered. Relapses, while less probable at the maintenance stage of recovery, are still possible. While we are not advocating that clients stay fixated on the past, our experience is that complacency can be dangerous.

Twelve-step approaches recognize this and provide mechanisms for assisting persons to stay in recovery. The tradition of telling one's story at 12-step birthdays and being a sponsor are examples of such mechanisms. Steps Ten through Twelve—which provide for the continued taking of a personal inventory, progressive development of spirituality, and commitment to practice the principles of the 12-step program and carry its message to others—also address the need to continue to work a recovery program. We are always careful to support our clients as they develop a maintenance program prior to their terminating treatment. We review where they were, where they are now, and what was most helpful in getting them to this point. We then work in partnership with clients to establish some sort of ongoing review and recommitment program, preferably in written form.

Recovery is a spiral. People may experience triggers regardless of the quality of their recovery program. The ability to consistently and effectively manage these triggers and a deep understanding of all the parts of the self are earmarks of maintenance stage recovery work.

It is important for all survivors, not just recovering addicts, to "carry the message," that is, perform service work. Such work can take a number of forms, including being a sponsor, working on a hotline for survivors of trauma, lobbying legislatures for laws and funding to combat abuse, and working within an organization such as *Survivor Connections* that provides networking for those who are survivors of sexual abuse (14).

REFERENCES

1. Linehan, M. M. (1987). Dialectical behavior therapy for borderline personality disorder. *Bulletin of the Menninger Clinic, 51,* 261–276.
2. L'Abate, L., & Milan, M. A. (Eds.). (1985). *Handbook of social skills training and research.* New York: Wiley.
3. Dolan, Y. (1990). Oregon Psychological Association annual meeting workshop, Newport, Oregon.
4. Horevitz, R. P. (1983). Hypnosis for multiple personality disorder: A framework for beginning. *American Journal of Clinical Hypnosis, 26,* 138–145.
5. Rando, T. A. (1984). *Grief, dying, death: Clinical interventions for caregivers.* Champaign, IL: Research Press.
6. Wolpe, J. (1958). *Psychotherapy by reciprocal inhibition.* Stanford, CA: Stanford University Press.
7. Wikler, A. (1973). Dynamics of drug dependence. *Archives of General Psychiatry, 28,* 611–616.
8. Powell, J., Gray, J., & Bradley, B. P. (1993). Subjective craving for opiates: Evaluation of a cue exposure protocol for use with detoxified opiate addicts. *British Journal of Clinical Psychology, 32*(1), 39–53.
9. Shapiro, F. (in press). *Eye movement desensitization and reprocessing: Principles, protocols and procedures.* New York: Guilford Press.
10. Shapiro, F. (1991). Eye movement desensitization and reprocessing: A cautionary note. *Behavior Therapists, 14,* 188.

11. Yapko, M. D. (1990). *Trancework: An introduction to the practice of clinical hypnosis* (2nd ed.). New York: Brunner/Mazel.
12. Wolinsky, S. (1990). *Quantum consciousness: The guide to experiencing quantum psychology*. Norfolk, CT: Bramble Books.
13. Hammond, D. C. (Ed.). (1990). *Handbook of hypnotic suggestions and metaphors*. New York: Norton.
14. Survivor Connections, Inc., 52 Lyndon Rd., Cranston, RI 02905-1121.

Depression, Anger, and Dissociation

Confused

You cannot cry,
Punishments don't hurt.
You cannot laugh,
It angers my drunken rage.
You cannot yell,
It aggravates my hot temper.
You cannot transgress,
For I will be forced to beat you.
You cannot seek the help from others,
I forbid you, because nothing is wrong.

—SHANE, age 16

The previous two chapters discussed our general integrated model for treating addicted survivors. No matter what a client's specific presentation is, we always use our general model to guide our treatment of addicted survivors. However, some clients have presentations that raise additional issues of diagnosis and treatment and suggest a need for different emphases and modifications in our general treatment approach. This chapter discusses specific issues that arise when treating addicted survivors whose presentation has strong and pervasive elements of anxiety/depression, anger, or dissociation.

THE ANXIOUS/DEPRESSED SURVIVOR

Addicted survivors often present with serious depression and anxiety as part of their symptom picture (1). We discuss depression and anxiety together not only because they fit within an "acting in" cluster but because addicted survivors often present with anxious depressions and depression associated with their anxieties.

The DSM-IV defines several different affective and anxiety disorders (2). The criteria for major depression include a period of 2 weeks or more of at least five of the following symptoms (either symptom 1 or symptom 2 must be included): (1) depressed or irritable mood, (2) diminished interest or pleasure, (3) significant weight loss or gain or decrease or increase of appetite, (4) trouble sleeping or oversleeping, (5) agitation or slowing, (6) constant fatigue or loss of energy, (7) strong feelings of worthlessness or guilt, (8) impaired concentration or indecisiveness, and (9) recurrent suicidal ideation or thoughts of death. The criteria for a diagnosis of mania include a distinct and persistent period of elevated, expansive, or irritable mood and at least three of the following: (1) inflated self-esteem or grandiosity, (2) substantially decreased need for sleep, (3) pressure to keep talking, (4) racing thoughts or flight of ideas, (5) distractibility, (6) agitation or highly increased activity level, and (7) excessive involvement in activities with potentially negative consequences such as spending sprees. Bipolar disorder includes swings or alternations between major depression and mania with bipolar I characterized by predominantly manic episodes and bipolar II by depressive episodes. Dysthymia refers to a "minidepression," which is characterized by depressed mood and two or more of the symptoms of a major depression, that lasts for at least 2 years. Cyclothymia is a "mini-bipolar-disorder" lasting for at least 2 years. And, to make matters more complicated, persons experiencing a major depression or a bipolar disorder can also have psychotic symptoms.

In addition to acute stress disorder and posttraumatic stress disorder, the DSM-IV recognizes several other anxiety disorders characterized by such somatic symptoms of fear as muscle tension, shortness of breath, sweating, and feeling keyed up and on edge; by persistent, unrealistic worry and fear; and by intense efforts to avoid or escape from the feared situation. These include various specific phobias, such as fear of snakes or of social situations. Panic disorder involves discrete periods of unexpected attacks of intense anxiety that is not associated with a specific phobic situation but may be associated with the person's being the focus of others' attention. Panic disorder may or may not be accompanied by agoraphobia, the fear of being in a situation in which escape might be difficult or embarrassing or in which help might not be available if the person experiences a panic attack; sometimes agoraphobia occurs without panic attacks. Obsessive–compulsive disorder involves either ritualistic behavior the person does not want to do or persistent ideas, thoughts, or impulses he or she does not want to think about, yet the person feels forced to behave or think in these ways to avoid the anxiety that would otherwise result. Generalized anxiety disorder involves severe symptoms of anxiety but does not have the specific focus of the other anxiety disorders.

Individuals suffering from chemical dependence commonly present with symptoms of anxiety and depression. Withdrawal from chemicals is also associated with anxious and depressed feelings. In the majority of cases these symptoms are transient and do not exist independent of the substance use; however, in some cases they do represent an independent coexisting disorder (1). This seems particularly true of addicted survivors. The DSM-IV considers PTSD an anxiety disorder, so to say that individuals are suffering from this disorder is not to say much. However, the DSM-IV also states that PTSD is commonly associated with a high risk of psychoactive substance abuse and that features associated with PTSD also include major depressive disorder, other anxiety disorders, and somatization disorder (2). Studies of veterans suffering from PTSD indicate high comorbidity rates not only of substance abuse disorders but also of major depressive disorder (MDD) and panic disorder (3). Research on survivors of rape find that even several years after the sexual assault, survivors evidence high rates of PTSD, major depression, substance use disorders, generalized anxiety disorder, or obsessive–compulsive disorder, often simultaneously (4). One report in the literature suggests a connection between multiple personality disorder and obsessive–compulsive disorder (5). We have treated several addicted survivors who also suffered from a coexisting bipolar disorder as well as survivors who appeared to suffer from a bipolar disorder but who showed severe levels of anxiety but not mania on psychological tests and suffered from an anxiety disorder. To make matters even more complicated, some research suggests that some MDD associated with PTSD might be qualitatively and biologically different than MDD alone (3, 6). Finally, anxiety is often a part of MDD (7). Perhaps some of the associated symptoms are just part of the underlying PTSD and are more a reflection of the difficulties sorting out differences between PTSD, depression, and anxiety diagnoses, except by means of very expensive and hard to access lab studies such as sleep lab monitoring (3, 8).

There may be several different reasons for this multiplicity of diagnoses. Perhaps the field's decision rules do not sort multiple symptoms correctly. Perhaps the stress of the survivor experience is a nonspecific cause of multiple disorders in individuals who are otherwise vulnerable because of genetics or developmental factors (9). Or perhaps some of these "complications" are simply independent processes that some individuals may have developed even if they had not experienced trauma. No matter what the etiology, however, certain conclusions are clear:

Addicted survivors may have three or more diagnoses, and many survivors experience not only substance use disorder and a PTSD-type disorder but also affective or anxiety disorder.

Our own experience confirms these diagnostic difficulties. Several different diagnostic situations exemplify this. The so-called melancholic symptoms of a major depression (2) are highly associated with a positive response to somatic treatments (most often medication) for major depressive disorder (1). These symptoms include either loss of interest or pleasure or lack of reactivity to usually pleasurable stimuli, and three of the following: (1) depression that is regularly worse in the morning, (2) early morning awakening, (3) psychomotor retardation or agitation, (4) significant anorexia or weight loss, (5) excessive or inappropriate guilt, and (6) distinct quality of depressed mood. These diagnostic criteria are difficult to apply with complete confidence to addicted survivors. Apart from the somatic disruptions caused by significant chemical intake (1), many survivors report a lifelong history of such symptoms as anhedonia (lack of pleasure), which could be part of psychic numbing and sleep and appetite disturbances, which are often found with PTSD. Given that addicted survivors, even when abstinent, often evidence mood swings, pressured behavior, distractibility and impulsive acting out, ruling out a diagnosis of bipolar disorder can become difficult. Addicted survivors, especially when in denial or amnestic for their trauma, often evidence symptoms that could be consistent with a generalized anxiety disorder. They also sometimes report symptoms consistent with panic disorder and agoraphobia, which, on questioning, are often found to occur in conjunction with their chemical use; for example, hiding in the house out of fear that others may cause one harm or several days of intense anxiety about having a heart attack are behaviors sometimes reported by individuals who are doing stimulants.

An additional complication is that the experience of depression or anxiety is very often the basis for motivating clients into treatment. A professional is likely to see clients when they are at their most anxious and depressed. "Hitting bottom"—whether from an internal collapse or from external pressures—provides a window through the denial associated with chemical dependence and often with the various survivor syndromes. Ironically, some anxiety and depression is actually desirable to motivate a client to engage and persist in treatment. We would be making a mistake if we could wave a magic wand and relieve all the client's distress in the first session unless this was a permanent cure, something that is unlikely.

Various kinds of depression and anxiety are common among single-diagnosis alcoholics/addicts when using and in early recovery (3, 10). Withdrawal produces a range of distressing somatic symptoms even when detoxification protocols are carefully followed. Having used chemicals to deal with distressing feelings and perhaps to provide social contacts and even an identity, newly recovering addicts/alcoholics now face the world without their trusty friend and main coping device. Feelings of anxiety to the point of panic can result. Grief reactions are also common: first is the grief over loosing one's best friend, namely, the chemical itself; then there is the emergence of grief over various losses, both recent and remote ones. Some of these losses are likely to be part of the crisis that prompted the person to seek treatment. Other losses, however, may be much earlier in time, even from childhood. Clinical lore suggests that chemical use interferes with the usual grief process, preventing the chemically dependent person from working through them. Of course, some chemically dependent individuals, even those who are not survivors, may also have other coexisting psychiatric disorders.

Alcoholic/addicted survivors in early recovery are very likely to have these same issues to an even greater extent. Chemically dependent survivors are typically awash in depression and anxiety; likely to be suffering from classic PTSD; at high risk for other DSM Axis I disorders; and with additional, early, or severe losses or deficiencies in coping skills. As with other depressed individuals, a key theme for the addicted survivor with depression is helplessness/hopelessness; for the addicted survivor with anxiety, as with other anxious persons, a key theme is fear. Very often these two themes are present at the same time and are quite evident. Anxious, compulsive efforts to control their chemical use and other aspects of their experience through denial, avoidance, and other coping mechanisms often characterize the addicted survivor (11). While almost anyone would feel depressed under these circumstances, survivors experience their situation as a recapitulation of the helplessness associated with their trauma. Consequently, we very often find that our clients alternate between periods of anxiety and depression. Biochemical depletion of important brain chemicals such as serotonin due to chemical use and to chronic levels of anxiety is often the physiological parallel of this psychological process of depression. We have coined the term "stression" to describe the state associated with this psychobiological process. Individuals with a stression typically present with a recent history of serious and ongoing stressors, although they rate their mood within normal limits, possibly because over time they have lost a sense of what a normal mood is. They report numerous signs of depression, most important of which are a loss of pleasure, low energy, and concentration difficulties. Stressions are very common among our survivor clients, whether they are addicted or not.

Given all this, the task for clinicians is to be alert to symptoms of serious depression and anxiety and to assess and include them in the overall treatment plan for addicted survivors. We do this in several ways.

Using the questions illustrated in the dual diagnosis tool and the decision rules provided in an earlier chapter, we are careful to assess symptoms of depression and anxiety at intake to make a differential diagnosis. If the depression or anxiety is moderate in intensity or a general one without the specific symptoms, such as compulsive rituals, associated with discrete syndromes, we prefer to wait for clients to have 4 weeks of abstinence before converting a ruled-out diagnosis into a probable one. If the depression or anxiety is severe in intensity or shows highly distinctive symptoms, we consider the additional diagnosis as highly probable and act accordingly. This intensity decision rule is consistent with studies that have attempted to identify indicators of the need for dual diagnosis treatment (8). Questions like "If you do have a chance to do something enjoyable or fun, is it pleasurable?" help to distinguish between a serious so-called reactive depression and one that has melancholic symptoms and is likely to respond to medication. If clients in a session report that their thoughts are scattered rather than racing and if they can calm down for periods of time with encouragement, we are more likely to suspect an anxiety rather than a bipolar disorder. If we note the clients behavior as being pressured, pushed, or energized throughout sessions, we suspect some sort of bipolar disorder. Observations of psychomotor retardation, as opposed to agitation, point toward a serious depression. Reports suggesting compulsive ("I have to") rather than impulsive ("I want to") patterns, even in acting-out periods, help make the same distinction between the energy driven by mania from that driven by anxiety. Taking into account the tendency for withdrawal from stimulants to result in depression and for withdrawal from depressants such as alcohol to result in anxiety and agitation (the principle of rebound) can also help to sort out the symptom picture. We use the Minnesota Multiphasic Personality Inventory (MMPI) to assist with this process (12) and encourage readers who have access to psychological testing to make use of this tool.

Depressed and anxious survivors often turn to the use of addictive chemicals. Many people use chemicals to help numb the pain of daily living. They attempt to trade in their painful reality for one that is more warm and "fuzzy." The survivor who is already overwhelmed with intense feelings of abandonment and emotional pain finds the immediate and "easy" relief and respite that chemicals can bring very enticing and is especially eager to attempt this trade.

We ask our clients to take an MMPI to make certain that we have not missed important symptoms and to get a baseline functional assessment. We have found this instrument to be particularly helpful in picking up stressions. The majority of the addicted survivors we treat take antidepressants, starting very early in recovery, unless otherwise indicated. Because antidepressant medication can make psychosis and mania worse, we do try to make sure that these are not part of the diagnostic picture. Whether or not they truly have a third diagnosis, most of the persons we treat have sufficient levels of anxiety and depression, sleep and appetite disturbance, difficulty concentrating, and other related difficulties as assessed by clinical interview and psychological testing that antidepressants appear warranted. Sometimes clients express confusion that we are requiring them to abstain from chemicals at the same time that we are sending them for medication; whether they lack information or are in denial, we attempt to educate clients about good drugs and bad drugs when we recommend antidepressants. When working with medical consultants, we express strong reservations about prescribing any addictive medications.

Evaluating benzodiazepine use among survivors, especially those with anxiety disorders, is very important. Often, well-meaning physicians have prescribed such tranquilizers as Valium or Xanax for people who complain of anxiety, which can either feed or set off an addiction for survivors. Extensive use of the minor tranquilizers sharply increases the need for medically supervised detoxification. In our experience, individuals with prescription drug dependence also present some special challenges. One is their tendency to think that these drugs are medications and that if they are prescribed by a professional, they present no problem.

When constructing fail-safe plans early in treatment, we pay particular attention to the potent relapse trigger of helplessness/hopelessness for depression and of fear for anxiety. Explicit conversations about these triggers and early fail-safe contingency planning reduces the likelihood of relapses. Consistent with our general model, we frame these discussions as safety issues and try to pinpoint specific, concrete possible alternative responses to these feeling states. This appears to be especially important for those clients with strong anxiety symptoms. Chemicals provide such immediate relief from anxiety that their use becomes strongly reinforced. Consequently, suggestions of alternatives that are almost as quick and that certainly have a strong somatic component, such as exercise or hot baths, are more likely to be heeded than is advice to simply "hang in there." Theoretical speculation that withdrawal from chemicals might be a conditioned emotional response triggering PTSD symptoms emphasizes the importance of early attention to relapse issues (13).

We point out to clients and ask them to observe how they repeatedly hypnotize themselves day in and day out with words and images having depressive and anxious themes. These negative trance states include thoughts such as, "My life has been awful and will always be awful, and there is nothing I can do about it," and "Awful things are sure to happen, and I must always stand guard to avoid this." To theorists using a trance framework, depressive thinking is an example of a trance oriented toward the past whereas anxiety is an example of a trance oriented toward the future. Twelve-step programs recognize this by encouraging members to avoid self-pity and "future-tripping" and remain in the here and now, one day at a time. Addressing codependency issues, especially through assertion training in the skills-building stage and as part of the education phase, appears to be very helpful for those with anxiety disorders. Mapping work in later stages of therapy almost always reveals that anxiety states precede depressive ones, supporting the notion that these two states are closely allied and that both typically require attention from the start. By the same token, our experience with clients who suffer from melancholic depressions and chronic, ingrained levels of PTSD-based anxiety is that they are often unable to simply resolve and dissolve these states and that medication is necessary. They can, however, resolve the stress-inducing states that feed the anxiety and depression, such as frustration and anger, and this capacity does tend to decrease the secondary overlay of the more physiological components of the anxiety and the depression.

Attention to addictive thinking is also important. Addicts and alcoholics typically evidence psychological dependence on chemicals. This involves thinking that revolves around the belief that the only way to have fun or feel good is to take chemicals. There is also an urgency to the thinking, as in "I must feel better *now* and I *cannot possibly* wait for relief." Such thinking is often found in the addicted/alcoholic survivor who is depressed and anxious. It is crucial to point out this thinking to such clients, discuss it with them, and help them practice alternatives.

Working the 12 Steps

Step One can be an early stumbling block for many addicted survivors who are seriously depressed and/or anxious. Step One states: "We admitted that we were powerless over our addiction, that our lives had become unmanageable." This apparent admission of defeat can cause most survivors to turn and run in the other direction to escape their fear of helplessness. Many survivors have used control as a way to hold on and to survive difficult, dangerous, and even life-threatening situations. They may confuse powerlessness with helplessness, and a tendency toward concrete and black-and-white thinking can compound difficulties with this step. As mentioned earlier, it is often helpful to these clients to explain that Step One is a paradox, namely, that by admitting that we cannot control those things that are beyond our control we can become empowered to live our lives with reduced stress and an enhanced sense of well-being.

We have found that the intense confrontation sometimes found in some drug treatment programs to combat denial and force the addict to surrender to Step One is counterproductive for depressed and anxious survivors. In our experience, pounding the survivor into a state of surrender only strengthens resistance to the idea of working the steps and typically increases denial.

Framing our approach in terms of psychological safety circumvents this resistance and makes work on Step One-type issues easier and more productive. Looking at drinking and using drugs as unsafe behaviors allows us to join with the survivor's need for safety rather than fight with his or her denial. Using the perspective of this frame of staying safe, we ask clients to consider how their chemical use has dominated their thinking or caused them to behave in ways that are outside their normal character. Step One work with this group of survivors can help them turn from self-defeating thinking and behavior and lay a foundation for comprehensive recovery.

Step Two states: "We came to believe that a power greater than ourselves could restore us to sanity." The goal of Step Two is to offer a glimmer of hope and faith, commodities lacking in the lives of most alcoholics/addicts at the time they enter recovery. Needless to say, most survivors, especially those suffering from depressive symptoms, are far from hopeful. Twelve-step recovery slogans such as "One day at a time" and "First things first" suggest the notion of breaking the concept of faith into small digestible bites. Gently challenging depressive thinking is essential to recovery. Traditional recovery counseling may include sayings like "Get off the pity pot" and "Stop stinkin' thinkin'." While these slogans may seem at first glance to be applicable to depressed and anxious addicted survivors, such direct attempts can be perceived as strong criticism, a perception that causes regression and even more feelings of fear and sadness. The hypersensitivity of survivors makes them perceive such challenges as statements that they are making a mistake or are "bad," and they will respond with an increase in defensiveness. A survivor's stubborn part may come to the fore, preventing further progress with step work or any other clinical intervention. Reviewing with these clients that things are at least a little bit better since they began abstaining from chemicals and promoting the issue of safety helps to further the goals of Step Two, and inducing a positive future-oriented view by asking them to imagine how things are going to be at least somewhat better as each and every day goes by can fight the negative past-oriented nature of depressive thinking.

Step Three states: "We made a decision to turn our will and our lives over to the care of God as we understood him." Step Three encourages the person to let go of the need for absolute control all of the time and is particularly pertinent to matters associated with anxiety. Most survivors find this a very frightening notion; trusting that letting go of control and turning things over to a higher power (however defined) goes against their grain. The strategy is to help the survivor learn to let go of things one small piece at a time, being careful to always associate the concept of letting go with the notion of staying safe. The focus of these discussions is the paradox (especially for survivors) of safely letting go.

Practicing letting go can take a number of forms, such as (1) letting go of anxiety by breathing deeply and allowing the body to relax; (2) turning over worries about money, health, and other issues to one's higher power; and (3) letting go of attempts to have a family member admit that he or she perpetrated abuse or was aware of abuse by another family member. Bit by bit, clients come to ask themselves whether a certain state or situation is in fact something they can control, and they begin to learn that they can tolerate and ultimately decrease the needless worry and anxiety that accompanies their frantic efforts to stay in charge of everything. Encouraging a here-and-now or one-day-at-a-time attitude is therapeutic for the broad range of survivor issues.

Step Four reads: "We made a searching and fearless moral inventory of ourselves." This step, which can be an overwhelming one for many survivors unless it is carefully modified, can often dredge up emotion-laden material that can be less than helpful in the early days of sobriety. In general and in accord with our recovery model, we recommend that a thorough Step Four be done as a part of the integration stage of recovery. A modified version can be done early as long as all the contingencies for safety are met. This modified version either focuses on current issues, with no reference to a historical review, or simply limits the discussion to issues associated with chemical use. In addition, the modified version makes certain to identify character strengths as well as character defects.

Step Four offers clients an opportunity to review in a comprehensive and in-depth way long-standing patterns of behavior to see which ones are helpful and which ones it may be appropriate to change. Some of these patterns of behavior may reveal previous self-sabotaging attempts to attain sobriety—as well as general well-being and happiness. This step is not meant to be an exercise in self-abuse for anyone, and therapists must ensure that it does not deteriorate into such an exercise for their clients, especially for the already shame-filled and acting-in survivor. Depressed and anxious survivors can already tell their therapist ad nauseam about all their poor choices, bad breaks, and situations gone awry. We are trying to offer survivors an accounting of their strengths as well as their liabilities. This process, if implemented in a positive manner, can further help survivor clients fight anxious and depressive thinking and find a grain of hope or consolation on a beach of fear and sorrow.

Readers will find examples of step work for depression and for anxiety in the appendix.

THE ANGRY SURVIVOR

The wounded survivor sometimes utilizes a protective strategy not of getting sad but of getting mad. At some level, all survivors have feelings of rage, and for some survivors this rage can be pervasive. The wounded part of all survivors is angry at not having been protected and nurtured and at the violation of trust that is at the core of most abuse experiences. The protector part of some survivors also settles on anger as a defense. Staying angry helps to ward off more painful feelings, such as depression and shame, and upsetting symptoms, such as flooding with hurtful memories or behavioral disorganization due to high levels of anxiety. In fact, as we have seen in Chapter 3, there is some research evidence to suggest that being angry leads to better survival outcomes for abused children than being placating or attempting to distance oneself through dissociation.

Most survivors have to get angry at some point if their treatment is to be successful. Being angry is the missing experience for many survivors. It provides the energy for moving away from placating others and passivity into more active stances toward their past and present experience. The therapeutic task for survivors is to safely have this anger, channel it productively, and integrate it as part of the working through of their trauma and grieving. We have worked with many survivors who at some point in their treatment experience homicidal fantasies. We are usually not overly disturbed by this and, in fact, generally see this as a sign of progress (provided clients appear able to contain their impulses). If there is any hint that a client might act on such impulses, we stress the notion of keeping safe and employ appropriate tactics based on our general recovery model. Working with spouses and others to help them avoid overreacting to the survivor in this angry phase is also part of our approach. However, persistent and volatile levels of anger and a routine, character-based use of this strategy for protection ultimately lead to a variety of problems later on. Being angry all the time is exhausting and alienates the individual from others, including treatment professionals as well as significant others. High levels of anger short-circuit productive thinking and impulse control and make reactive, shortsighted responding more likely. In some cases survivors with this kind of rage batter others and face legal charges for assault.

Chemical use exacerbates the situation, since intoxication reduces impulse control, and anger as a way of life makes problems with chemical use worse in a variety of ways. Anger-based character defenses make for double denial, intensifying tendencies toward projection and rationalization. Even when survivors are abstinent, these same defenses often impede their ability to stay sober and to develop healthy relationships in recovery. A common clinical occurrence, for example, is the relapse that involves drinking "at" someone when angry. The survivor uses anger and resentment as an excuse to drink or use drugs. This allows them to blame someone else for their relapse. "He made me so mad I had to get high," is an example of this thinking. The ingrained and reflexive use of chemicals to make things right and the tendency that accompanies anger to blame others and to make excuses are the antithesis of the principle of taking responsibility for the self to be in recovery—a mainstay of a recovery program for substance use disorders and, ultimately, for trauma.

To make matters even more complicated and challenging, anger-based defenses sometimes come bundled with other components that contribute to the difficulties survivors have in their lives and in their treatment. Authority is commonly a trigger for anger in survivors, and an antiauthority stance prevails. Thinking that is characterized by the attitude behind statements like "Don't tell me what to do" and "We'll do it my way or no way" and the power struggles associated with this thinking cause problems not only with bosses, spouses, and legal authorities but with therapists as well. (Professionals are automatically perceived as authority figures, and, of course, they are always telling clients what to do to get into and remain in recovery.) Also common is a strong need in survivors to look good and maintain a certain kind of image, a need that subverts honesty and leads to acting out when challenged by significant others and therapists. A sense of entitlement and a self-centered stance toward others are frequent accompaniments to anger-based defenses. "I deserve what I deserve" and "They're the ones with the problem" are oft-heard phrases that capture the flavor of this issue. At times these clients are often quite manipulative, taking the control issues of the survivor to new levels of dishonesty and adopting an unconcerned attitude toward the impact of their behavior on others.

The single-diagnosis *practicing* alcoholic/addict typically exhibits many of these same defenses. Prospective studies, however, have clearly demonstrated that no unique preexisting combination of personality traits or disorders characterizes the single-diagnosis alcoholic/addict; instead, the processes let loose by the chemical use and resulting substance dependence appear to promote these sorts of defenses (14). There are several differences between merely difficult chemically dependent individuals and those chemically dependent individuals who have these anger-based defenses as part of their character. For the angry survivor, these defenses tended to be present from an early age *prior* to any significant chemical use; second, the angry survivor demonstrates very intense levels of anger and even rage; and, third—and most importantly and tellingly—abstinent single-diagnosis alcoholics/addicts in early recovery quickly show little evidence of these traits (they are, instead, relatively anxious, depressed, and guilty) and recover quickly. The angry survivor, however, not only tends to demonstrate continued and significant difficulties in this area but occasionally these difficulties even intensify. More than once we have spoken with teachers, for example, who have noted an increase in a student's acting-out behavior at school once the student is not stoned on a daily basis.

Treatment for Anger-Based Personality Disorders

In this section we discuss treatment strategies and tactics, which complement our general recovery model, for survivors with personality disorders that present with anger-based defenses and the other accompanying issues discussed in the preceding paragraphs. The more a client exhibits aspects of these characteristics, the more we mix the approaches described in the following paragraphs into our model. These three personality disorders are antisocial disorder, narcissistic disorder, and borderline disorder.

We pay particular attention to exploring the worldview of individuals with a given personality disorder. Understanding their worldview, which is typically not that of most counselors, helps us to counsel these clients more effectively because we can use our appreciation of our differences in motivation and style to motivate clients and engage them in treatment.

Antisocial Personality

According to the DSM-IV, antisocial personality disorder is a pervasive pattern of disregard for and violation of the rights of others that begins in early childhood or early adolescence and continues into adulthood (2). Indications of antisocial personality disorder include at least three of the following: (1) failure to conform with social norms regarding what behaviors are lawful, (2) deceitfulness, (3) impulsivity and failure to plan ahead, (4) irritability and aggressiveness, (5) reckless disregard for the safety of self and others, (6) consistent irresponsibility, and (7) lack of remorse. Childhood indicators include aggression toward people and animals, destruction of property, deceitfulness or theft, and serious violations of rules.

The exact origin of antisocial personality disorder is unknown. There may be a genetic component that predisposes an individual at risk for this disorder not only to sensation seeking, anger, and impulsiveness but also to dependence on alcohol and other substances (15). The MacAndrews Scale for Alcoholism of the MMPI appears to tap some of these characteristics (12). Some research suggests that a childhood history of neglect and physical abuse may be a factor (16). Individuals with antisocial features often are persons who were very hurt in childhood and simply decided to get even in response. In many of these cases our experience has been that helping the client achieve sobriety and work through the antisocial defenses results in a depressed and anxious survivor. In some cases, however, the antisocial client is a so-called core sociopath: an individual (probably 10% of all those with antisocial personality disorder) who seems to be born bad and who is completely unable or unwilling to change (17). These individuals often present with a view of themselves as the victim, reporting a history of being abused as a child and of always getting the short end of the stick. After obtaining good collateral data, however, we find that the client is playing the role of victim as a way to avoid responsibility and manipulate others. Such clients might certainly have been spanked by an angry parent—after it is discovered that they have set the dog on fire! Psychological testing and the gradual establishment of a therapy relationship in which the client seems to care about, rather than tolerate, the counselor helps to sort out these two different subgroups.

While the majority of individuals endorse such values as altruism and self-actualization, antisocial persons have a different value system (17). Their core value is maintaining their image, that is, looking good and being Mr. Cool or Ms. Hot, no matter what. Another feature of the individual with an antisocial personality disorder, which supports the need to look good and be cool, is a strong need to have power and control; having power and being in charge feeds the ego of antisocial persons. A win–lose mindset is also a feature of this disorder; we have heard many antisocial people say, "Life is a game, and you are either the winner or the loser." Naturally, antisocial people almost always prefer to be the winner and view the hardworking person as a "schmuck" and a "loser." "What a fool! That guy works 60 hours a week for just $800. I can make that much in 2 hours by dealing drugs or robbing a convenience store!" is a comment that conveys a flavor of this winner–loser thinking. Another feature of the antisocial person is the very high value he or she places on having or getting plenty of money and sex; these symbolize success for the antisocial individual and serve to maintain and inflate his or her image. Antisocial persons exhibit yet another characteristic that is important to take into account when understanding this disorder: They have a strong need for immediate satisfaction of their needs. This distorts their sense of time, and waiting is not what they do best. For them, instant gratification takes too long, to quote a saying common in 12-step meetings. Antisocial persons are also often in conflict with authority; they resent the control and power over them that the authority figure can have. If, finally, we had to choose one word to best describe the antisocial person we would use the term *entitlement*. Antisocial persons feel entitled to everything that comes their way without having to pay for it or earn it; for example, they feel they should be given a high-paying job with great prestige without having to earn the position. And they would feel insulted to discover that they are expected to work once they obtain the position!

We have noticed that antisocial behavior, like addiction, appears to be progressive. Take the story of Bill. During a counseling session Bill told us that when he first started "doing break-ins," he would break into a house when the people were not home, take what he wanted, and then leave. Soon this became "boring" and did not offer Bill the "rush" that it once did, so he began sneaking into houses when people were home to commit his burglaries. Soon this too became "boring," and Bill then began knocking on doors and robbing people at gunpoint. This soon lost its luster. Finally, Bill started to rob people at gunpoint, to rape any women in the home while forcing family members to watch, and to then pistol-whip one or more of the family members.

Adding addiction to all this is like lighting a match to gasoline. In addition to the effects of the chemicals themselves, a life-style with the ups and downs of heavy chemical involvement fits in well with the dynamics of the antisocial. Substance dependence can, for example, lead to obtaining money through criminal means. Illegal drug trafficking and other aspects of criminal activity are perfect for generating excitement and for providing the opportunity to be Mr. or Ms. Cool; for those with antisocial personality disorder, evading the police, carrying weapons, and scamming others is very heady stuff.

As our discussion and Bill's story indicate, counseling individuals with both antisocial and addiction issues is challenging. We have found certain approaches helpful for this difficult counseling situation. We like to remember the three Cs when working with the antisocial client: corral, confront, and consequences. Unless antisocial persons face a firm external structure to corral them, they are likely to have little motivation to change. With their externalizing defenses they typically feel little internal distress and do not see themselves as having a problem. Examples of external structuring include having to report to a probation officer or being on a last-chance agreement with a spouse who has finally had enough. A firm treatment contract is another example of corralling; it is specific and detailed and requires the client's signature. The second C refers to the need to reinforce such clients' cooperation with treatment by confronting both their worldview and their need to look good. Respectfully confronting their thinking errors (to be discussed shortly) helps to modify their distorted worldview, and framing interventions with statements like, "A smart person like you can see that . . ." illustrates a way of intervening that uses their self-image to avoid resistance. The third C is for consequences. We never want to get in the way of a consequence for antisocial clients. If they have violated their probation and we are supposed to report this, we do so. This may make antisocial clients angry, but they will lose respect for you if they begin to think that you can be easily manipulated.

Their respect for the counselor is a main source of motivation for antisocial clients (other than the obvious ones like fear of going to jail). While these clients resent authority figures, they often respect the position and seek out people whom they see as powerful or important. As professionals, we counselors are authority figures, and this is especially true if the court has mandated treatment—as is often the case since most individuals with antisocial features do not feel they have a problem. Try as they might to subvert our authority, the antisocial person has a certain admiration for our power as they see it. Using this admiration for our power to get the antisocial person's respect is very important. The therapist who tries to be a "friend" to an antisocial client is making a strategic error; this behavior puts therapist and client at the level of peers and makes the therapist vulnerable to special requests and manipulation. At the same time, appearing to be harsh, judgmental, or eager to "catch" the antisocial client inevitably provokes an unproductive power struggle.

Earning these clients' respect is crucial, and there are several tactics therapists can use to promote this respect. Demonstrate a straightforward and businesslike attitude by expressing clearly to the client that your job is being a counselor and by letting the client know that regardless of whether he or she cooperates, you still get paid. Join with the *client's* motivation for recovery to create a mutual understanding of the goals of treatment and of the reasons the two of you are working together; that is, if the client's goal is, for example, to stay out of jail, you can build your treatment plan around strategies that will help accomplish this goal. These will most likely include (1) staying clean and sober; (2) attending 12-step meetings; (3) showing up for all counseling appointments; (4) submitting to random drug testing; and (5) fulfilling other treatment requirements, such as completing valid psychological testing and attending any other group meetings. If the client balks at any of the treatment strategies, either at the time of formulating the treatment plan or later in treatment, several moves to "corral" the client exist. Calmly remind him or her of the original goal. This is usually enough to get treatment back on track. In a few instances, however, this does not work. Without sarcasm, engage the client in picking a new goal, such as learning to survive jail or life without a spouse. Once again, this usually dissolves the resistance.

We use the thinking error work developed by Samenow and Yokelson and detailed in Chapter 4 to challenge the worldview of our antisocial clients (18). Thinking errors refer to the cognitive distortions that such clients inevitably evidence. One way to think about thinking errors is to consider them as specific examples of denial, rationalization, and projection. Challenging the worldview of clients with antisocial personality by pointing out their cognitive distortions is the core of our approach for dual recovery. We point out to our antisocial clients that they are making a lot of "mistakes" and that this is the reason they are in trouble. We present ourselves as experts who can, by means of our treatment contract, help the antisocial person eliminate all these mistakes and thus stay out of trouble. We also express confidence that the client is quite capable of quickly learning to spot these mistakes. We then give clients a copy of the thinking error material and ask them to give examples of their own thinking errors. Clients agree to focus on a few of these thinking errors as a way of getting on top of their own mistakes in thinking. Gradually over time our approach helps clients learn more and more to recognize automatically the mistakes in their thinking. We consider that we are making progress if after we lift an eyebrow at a particular comment, clients say something like, "I know, you're probably thinking that I'm making excuses." If they suddenly have a return of denial and fail to recognize their errors in thinking regarding a given situation or behavior, we express genuine surprise that someone with their intelligence, insight, progress in recovery, and so on, would not see their mistake. Remember that antisocial persons see themselves as good, bright, successful, and so forth. By working with antisocial clients' needs to feel important and set goals they want, such as staying out of jail, we can continue to corral these clients and work with their resistance instead of against it.

Besides not enabling antisocial clients, for example, by not helping them escape the consequences of their behavior, it is important for therapists to keep in mind that these individuals respond best to consequences that are immediate, concrete, and exciting, or that make them look good. They really do not care if they are hurting the feelings of their parents, for example, or that their behavior ultimately hurts their chances for a successful career. On the other hand, they might care if compliance means that they get a weekend pass, they get their license back, or their probation time is shortened. In a few instances we have even defined the goal or reward as no longer having to see us! Success is more likely if the therapist constantly and consistently presents to these clients equations involving basic concepts, if, for example, the therapist equates chemicals and antisocial thinking with jail or sobriety and honest, responsible thinking with the absence of a parole officer. Many antisocial clients are very visual, and having them imagine themselves as a film director with the script for their life or as the creator of a videotape of various scenarios of their past, present, and future sometimes helps them visualize the consequences of various behaviors.

The traditions of 12-step programs prohibit any one person from being in charge of the organization. The founders knew that the self-centeredness common to most alcoholics and addicts would make them want to be the top person. The politics of 12-step groups would rival that of the most corrupt governments if running for the president of AA were possible. Fortunately, no one gets to be president. In fact, the traditions of AA and related programs state: "Our leaders are but trusted servants; they do not govern" (19). Newly recovering alcoholics/addicts who, like people with antisocial personality disorder, have issues with authority find this organizational structure helpful. No one really tells them what to do. Other members simply share what has worked for them. Because of this process, antisocial survivors benefit greatly from attending 12-step meetings and will often continue to attend because meeting a great many people and speaking up at meetings makes them feel important.

The question of relapse for the antisocial survivor really is not a matter of if they will relapse but when. The ego inflation of antisocial persons inevitably leads them to think that they can maintain abstinence on their own, discarding the support groups and the tools of recovery that assisted them to get clean and sober in the first place. The humility required to work an active recovery program can be elusive for these individuals. Predicting early in treatment that a relapse is likely to occur and then assisting the antisocial survivor in identifying potential triggers for relapse is helpful. The fail-safe planning discussed in the last chapter is one way to approach this task.

A time of high risk for relapse occurs if and when these clients hit a so-called zero-state depression, which occurs when they experience an abrupt deflation of their image and feel that they have utterly failed. Often this condition precedes a jailhouse suicide and can precede a relapse to chemical use. Usually, however, these clients do not stay in this condition for long. They regroup quickly, using rationalization and projection to reinflate their ego. While never rescuing these clients from the consequences of their behavior, we try to avoid totally trapping and completely crushing their self-image in order to avoid a zero-state crisis; we always try to allow them to save face in at least some small way.

The step work found in the appendix illustrates and extends all these concepts. Remember to make written step work part of a signed treatment plan and in discussions of step-work-type issues to watch out for slippery, vague, and other thinking-error-laden responses. Work on surrender but always within the framework of the antisocial person's own goals and reasons; watch out for imposing your own values. A core issue to emphasize throughout step work counseling is the need for honesty. This is crucial. Honesty is the foundation of recovery for anyone but most especially for the antisocial client. Honesty encompasses truthfulness both with others and with one's self. Antisocial clients will relapse into dishonesty, just as they will relapse into chemical use. Set realistic goals for yourself in counseling these clients. Are they drinking and using less often now than before? Are they less dishonest? If so, they are demonstrating that the goal of 12-step programs is "progress, not perfection," as discussed in the Big Book of AA (19).

As mentioned earlier, many so-called antisocial clients become merely standard survivors once their antisocial defenses are dissolved. In these cases, the general recovery model presented in the last chapter guides our additional therapy efforts. Many times, however, antisocial clients remain antisocial in orientation, and our emphasis remains simply on assisting them to keep their antisocial behavior in check and avoid relapse.

The Narcissistic Survivor

Narcissistic personality disorder, as defined by the DSM-IV (2), is a pervasive pattern of grandiosity, need for admiration, and lack of empathy. Five or more of the following suggest this personality disorder: (1) grandiose sense of self-importance; (2) preoccupation with fantasies of unlimited success, power, beauty, brilliance, or ideal love; (3) believes he or she is unique or special and can only be understood by, or in association with, other special or high status people or institutions; (4) requires excessive admiration; (5) has a strong sense of entitlement; (6) exploits others; (7) lacks empathy; (8) envious of others or believes others are envious of him or her; (9) demonstrates arrogant, haughty attitudes.

Many similarities exist between the antisocial and the narcissistic individual. Both are extremely self-centered and demanding and feel entitled to whatever it is they desire. Both need to look good and maintain their image. And both exploit others for their own ends. There are some differences, however. The narcissistic person is less likely to be impulsive and focuses less on material gain and more on the promotion of feelings of being special and unique. We have worked with several narcissistic clients who satisfied these needs through charity work, although a careful consideration of what they actually did in the philanthropic organization revealed a taking-all-the-credit attitude that was not supported by significant work on their part. Narcissistic individuals are also very critical of themselves and have an underlying chronic low-grade level of anxiety, although this is not immediately obvious to observers.

Narcissistic behavior is difficult to empathize with or even tolerate. Nonetheless, our clinical experience treating narcissistic clients has led us to believe that they are wounded persons who became angry and feel entitled as a way to survive. This also matches our discussion in Chapter 3 of such issues as the avoidant attachment style. The histories of our clients contain certain common themes revolving primarily around abandonment. Narcissists almost always have a childhood history of serious emotional neglect within a "look good" family situation. Very often the parents of narcissists were also very critical and judgmental, the likely source of their hypersensitivity and their critical attitude toward themselves and others. Similarly, the emphasis in their families was on looking good at any price, if not through actual achievement then through any means necessary—and, off course, any accomplishments were never good enough. In addition, these individuals sometimes experienced some sort of physical or sexual abuse and had an inadequate parent (usually, but not always, the mother) who failed to protect and nurture them. Narcissists feel that there is no one who can help and support them and that they must therefore do it themselves. This leads to the development of a highly controlling personality style oriented not toward receiving but toward taking from others. Neediness becomes demandingness, and a substantial part of the narcissistic person's self remains stuck in childhood, with all the urgency and tantrums of a young child.

Whenever they feel slighted, criticized, or unappreciated, the pain of this narcissistic wound is triggered. The reaction of most narcissists to this perceived abandonment is intense rage. Anyone who has been the target of this rage, including counselors who had to cope with intense anger in their family of origin, can testify to its frightening and overwhelming nature.

Understandably, narcissists are at high risk for drug or alcohol use and dependency. Like all survivors, they have a strong wounded part that seeks relief from the pain. Chemicals offer needy narcissists a quick fix for this pain, one that is under their control and that they do not have to rely on others to bestow. Parental alcoholism and addiction provide a fertile breeding ground for narcissism in children and, through genetic and modeling influences, for their own subsequent chemical dependence. Several writers have commented on the narcissist's use of chemicals to combat fragmentation and to provide self-nurturing (20).

As with antisocial clients, we think of a trio of letters to remind us of the main issues when treating narcissistic clients, in this case three A's, which stand for acknowledge, align, and aware. *Acknowledge* refers to the need for the therapist to recognize the hypersensitivity of narcissistic clients and even to let them know that he or she recognizes how special they are and how they must feel that they do not get the appreciation from others they feel they deserve. This stance permits the therapist to join with the narcissist's hypersensitivity and also gives these clients a "missing experience" that counteracts the internal critic planted in their childhood. The second A is similar to the challenging of thinking errors discussed in the preceding section on antisocial clients. However, it is essential that therapists *align* themselves with narcissistic clients to try to help them succeed; thus, any confrontation or challenging of their thinking is done to help them win. The third A refers to the therapist's attempts to encourage narcissistic clients to become *aware* of their internal neediness and to discover that they can give to themselves and allow others to give them nurturing when they are tired, frightened, or alone.

The hypersensitivity of narcissists is both an impediment and an asset for engaging and maintaining them in treatment. We find that we must first join with the sensitive part of narcissists prior to challenging and confronting them. Gently joining with these clients by acknowledging the original wound and how hard it must be for them to always have to handle things without support or appreciation promotes the therapeutic alliance. Including ample praise and admiration for good qualities and initial achievements in therapy also helps. Talking to the hurt part of the narcissist invariably—and in most cases dramatically—produces regression to an earlier state, one that benefits from having the "missing experience" of a benevolent parental figure. This builds up a reservoir of goodwill, which increases the chance that the therapy relationship will last through challenges to the client's worldview and through any angry tirades that occur.

Challenging the narcissist's worldview can then proceed, but again caution is important. Referring to parts of the self allows therapists to give feedback to these clients in a way they are more likely to hear and absorb. Framing their less likable behaviors as a component of the protector part of the self permits therapists to describe these narcissistic clients to themselves by using expressions such as "that part of you that protects you by not seeing the needs of others." This is more palatable to them than discussing their self-centeredness. Or suppose a narcissistic client remains irate that the therapist has begun the therapy session 15 minutes late even after being told that an emergency phone call needed attention; having already introduced the notion of the wounded, hypersensitive part in an earlier session, the therapist could then explain that the client's hypersensitive part was feeling ignored or slighted despite the fact that the therapist very much wanted to be on time for the client and could also explain that the client's protective part was angry for the hurt part as a way for the self to feel safe. This strategy almost always defuses this sort of situation. The thinking error work that we discussed earlier in this chapter is also quite effective with the narcissist if a great deal of preliminary joining has taken place. Of particular importance is the need to challenge the victim-stance thinking that narcissists almost inevitably demonstrate.

The final part of the strategy for treating narcissists is to constantly acknowledge and give permission to their neediness while encouraging increased reliance on more effective ways of getting these needs met. The goal is to assist these clients to connect in a more nurturing fashion to themselves and to others. They need to learn more appropriate responses when they react to triggers and begin to act and feel like angry 4-year-olds. For example, we might first discuss with these clients how their protector part makes mistakes in thinking that actually make others pull away from them. We then might point out that this results in the repeated abandonment of their wounded part, and we might suggest a more assertive response as an alternative.

Assisting narcissistic clients to find a 12-step group that is right for them and whose meetings they will continue to attend requires some thought. Stressing that a group has unique qualities suitable for the client's unique needs is helpful. Once our narcissistic clients join a group, they usually enjoy getting close to those whom they see as having much "clean time" or some other perceived status in the group. Predictably, these members will eventually lose their status in the eyes of the narcissist and will no longer receive the admiration previously accorded them. This scenario re-creates one of the family-of-origin experiences typical of persons with a narcissistic personality disorder, namely, the experience of being ultimately let down by an authority figure. A similar process is likely to take place in treatment as the counselor or staff are no longer perfect and capable of meeting the idealizations of these clients. The challenge for therapists is to see this as excellent time to help narcissistic clients work through such issues as abandonment, idealization, and devaluation.

The time of highest risk for relapse for narcissistic clients is when they encounter an abandonment trigger and feel let down, slighted, or even abused by another person. Very often the reality of the situation does not merit such a strong response, but the triggered psychic wound distorts the client's perception. The risk is that using drugs or drinking alcohol can appear to the client to be the only option for managing this pain. Framing the relapse as a learning experience is important. Narcissistic survivors typically relapse or intensify their defenses if they feel their therapist is being very critical. Like antisocial clients, narcissistic clients can reach a zero state where they feel they have totally failed and there is no purpose in continuing to live. When in this state, they are at high risk for suicide, and therapists should implement all precautions and plans previously designed for helping survivor clients stay safe.

Skills building for narcissistic clients almost always has to focus on self-care and on assertion, especially assertively asking for what they need even if this makes them look bad. Ironically, as these individuals learn to allow nurturing of themselves through their own self-care efforts and the efforts of others, they become more nurturant of others.

We use the same step work with narcissistic clients that we use with those who have borderline personality disorder. Both types of clients represent very fragmented and wounded people whose protective parts, no matter how disagreeable at times, serve the function of trying to keep them safe.

The Borderline Survivor

The DSM-IV describes the cardinal characteristic of the borderline personality as a pervasive pattern of instability of affects, interpersonal relationships, and self-image as well as marked impulsivity (2). Other features of this disorder include the following: (1) demanding, hostile–dependent relationships; (2) affective instability; (3) angry outbursts and recurrent suicidal or self-mutilating behavior; (4) identity disturbance and poor self-esteem; (5) chronic feelings of emptiness and depression; and (6) strong triggering by abandonment, whether real or perceived (21). Additional disorders frequently associated with this disorder are mood disorders, eating disorders, posttraumatic stress disorder, attention-deficit/hyperactivity disorder, and, of course, substance-related disorders (2). Borderline clients also tend to have multiple and shifting symptoms and are notorious among treatment professionals for being difficult to treat.

Borderline clients often have substance use patterns that differ from those of other dual diagnosis clients. Borderline patterns include polysubstance use, a great deal of switching among chemicals of choice, and sometimes periods of abstinence (when, e.g., the borderline client is in a relationship with someone who is recovering or who is otherwise against drinking or drug use).

Whether these periods of abstinence mean that these individuals are just abusing the chemical or are variably but truly substance dependent, the argument for regarding abstinence as a goal for borderline individuals still applies. In our earlier days we spent much time engaged in lively debates with our dual disorder borderline clients on whether or not they were true alcoholics. While this may have sharpened our persuasive communication skills, it did little to encourage the insight of these clients or our enthusiasm for dual diagnosis work. What we have found more helpful for both ourselves and our clients is to remember the definition of substance abuse problems: What causes problems is a problem. Persons with this disorder who use substances are at the very least abusing chemicals, and this abuse almost always accelerates their other symptoms and problems, including suicide attempts.

Besides being angry, persons with borderline personality disorder sometimes evidence periods of psychotic-type symptoms. This appears to be particularly true in three sets of circumstances: (1) in response, not surprisingly, to hallucinogen or cannabis use (whether this is a unique biochemical sensitivity to these particular chemicals, an upsurge of severe anxiety in response to an extreme loss of control and hypervigilance, or some other process is unclear); (2) in response to specific triggers allied to experiences of severe abuse; and (3) in response to the more general trigger of abandonment. Distinguishing between psychosis and flashbacks with flooding can be very difficult, and we have sometimes struggled with whether a client has severe PTSD, incipient schizophrenia, or both. This occurs particularly when we discover (often some time into treatment) that there is a family history of schizophrenia.

Some general guidelines help to distinguish between PTSD and psychosis, with PTSD being diagnosed when the following conditions or symptoms exist: (1) predominance of visual over auditory illusions; (2) hallucinations experienced as internal rather than external; (3) short duration of the psychotic episode (several days or weeks) followed by a return to baseline functioning; (4) lack of formal thought disorder, such as thought blocking, and demonstrating appropriate affect; (5) psychosis congruent with the abuse event; (6) seeking out relationships rather than social avoidance; and (7) family genetic history negative for psychotic conditions. Sometimes we simply state that we do not know the psychiatric diagnosis, make a functional one instead, and obtain a medication evaluation to determine if neuroleptic or other medication is appropriate.

Borderline disorder was originally seen as a condition that represented a borderline state between neurosis and psychosis. Later formulations emphasized the affective instability that persons with this disorder demonstrate and tended to regard the disorder as a possible atypical affective disorder (22). One recent view sees the core issue as one of impulse control deficits (21). Consistent with our own long-held stance that persons with borderline personality disorder are survivors, more and more studies are finding that individuals suffering from this disorder typically have a history of serious childhood abuse, including a chaotic and/or dangerous family of origin, a childhood characterized by early parental loss and neglect, parents who suffer from chemical dependency and other severe psychiatric disorders, and substantial physical and sexual abuse (21, 23, 24).

In fact, the general survivor recovery model presented in the last chapter originally began with our work with clients who evidenced a borderline personality disorder. We characterized our initial formulation as the three S's: safety, skills, survivor. We gradually refined and expanded the model as we began to work with other survivors who in a crisis appeared borderline but whose diagnosis later resolved, after further observation and psychological testing, into other clinical pictures. We also found the 3-S model useful in dealing with other survivor syndromes.

Finally, we became increasingly sensitive to the negative connotations the term *borderline* had for us and other professionals and found it more therapeutically effective to consider borderline clients as survivors and not as horrendously difficult clients to treat. However, while our general recovery model is applicable to individuals with a borderline personality disorder, these individuals do present several treatment issues that warrant additional discussion.

Unlike the more uniform response of survivors with classic PTSD, some borderline survivors become significantly worse when taking antidepressant medication. Most notably, some patients show an increase in impulsive, assaultive, and suicidal behavior (25). Some research demonstrates a decrease of impulsive acting out in response to Tegretol and, most interestingly, a decrease in symptoms of depression in response to Haldol, an antipsychotic medication (26, 27). This latter research suggests that low doses of neuroleptic medication for short periods are likely to help borderline individuals through an acute crisis. As a group, persons with borderline personality disorder seem to be more unpredictable in their response to medication, as well as in terms of other aspects of their disorder. Consequently, standard medication practice with this group of clients often focuses on the symptom rather than the syndrome. The positive side to this approach is its empirical quality, its take-this-and-see strategy. The drawback is a tendency to prescribe multiple medications for borderline survivors to the point where sorting out which medication might be doing what becomes very difficult. Our experience, in fact, has been that a history of mixed or poor clinical response to multiple medication is an indicator of a possible borderline syndrome. Careful trials with close monitoring are our answer.

Treatment professionals tend to have strong, mixed feelings toward those with this disorder. Borderline clients are clearly in deep emotional pain, and we want to help. On the other hand, their acting-out defenses can prompt a desire in us to act out as well. Borderline individuals feel intense ambivalence toward parents and authority figures, toward others in relationships that are intimate, and toward life itself. The individual suffering from a borderline disorder experienced the ultimate double bind (see our discussion about attachment in Chapter 3) with the message "I love you; come here so I can abuse you." Having tried various strategies and experienced failure with them all, these persons play out the same double-bind dynamics with others, including treatment providers.

Managing transference and countertransference is critical when working with borderline survivors. This is especially true because of the acute hypersensitivity of these clients to others. They will know, even before the counselor does, what he or she feels about them. In addition, many of the borderline survivors we have treated have a specific trigger for being accused: The abuse scenario for these clients involved their having been specifically and repeatedly blamed for their own abuse. Any perception on their part that they are being accused, whether they surmise this from outright exasperated confrontation behaviors in others or from more subtle cues indicating critical frustration, typically escalates their acting-out defenses. An equally potent trigger is any behavior resembling abandonment. Frustrated with such clients for backsliding in treatment, we may, for example, give them a subtle (or perhaps not so subtle) critical message like "I am disappointed to see that you drank again so close to your 1-year sobriety birthday." Feeling criticized and/or abandoned, the borderline client's frustration may then escalate into a rage to punish us or descend in a spiral of self-hatred and self-harm for letting us down.

We have found a number of strategies and tactics useful for decreasing the chances of this happening and for managing acting-out defenses. We keep firmly and constantly in mind that this individual is not a "bad borderline" but a survivor of serious abuse. We even go so far as to avoid using the term *borderline* in our thinking and our conversations with clients and other providers, preferring instead such terms as *atypical PTSD* or *severe survivor syndrome*. We do discuss the meaning of the term *borderline* with clients when they are aware that other providers have given them this diagnosis, but we attempt to reframe this diagnosis as a survivor syndrome and always present our recovery model. As an extension of this approach, we also reframe the acting-out behavior for our clients (and ourselves) as being an understandable, if not always helpful, survivor strategy. Again, the notion that the behavior is a normal response to an abnormal situation captures the essence of this reinterpretation. Understanding that borderline clients simultaneously want our attention and approval and fear the power that this gives us also helps us keep a reasonable perspective when they do something to try to sabotage the relationship.

"Safety first!" is our guiding slogan for managing and treating the chemical use and the self-harm behaviors so frequently found in borderline clients. Understanding self-mutilation as a survivor strategy helps us avoid feeling manipulated or recoiling in fear or disgust. Although clinical lore sees self-mutilation as an attempt by borderline clients to manipulate others to reengage with them, we prefer a less judgmental interpretation; when we ask borderline clients why they cut themselves, the answer almost inevitably includes the idea of obtaining some sort of relief from "the pain." Furthermore, borderline clients are more likely to hide their cuts and wounds and to show shame at their behavior than to display them for public view or to consider them as some sort of badge of honor. We believe that self-mutilation is primarily a form of emotional management.

The somatic sensations produced by self-mutilation serve to disrupt dissociation and flooding and bring these clients back to the here and now rather than the there-and-then world of the flashback or the not-here-at-all sensation of strong dissociation. Some persons with a borderline personality disorder do appear to gradually learn that self-mutilation has certain reliable effects on others, and using this symptom to control others begins to become more central. Yet even in these cases we are more likely to view the issue as a social skills deficit than as manipulation and to intervene by validating the client's need for nurturing and protection and by encouraging the practice of "safer" ways to get this need satisfied.

Similar considerations hold for suicidal gestures and threats, which are often chronic. Some of the literature on this topic takes a very judgmental stance, with one writer, for example, referring to the "malignant narcissism" of parasuicidal behavior (28). Certainly the manipulative or attention-seeking quality of the suicide gestures of many borderline clients supports this contention. However, we believe that interpreting such behavior as manipulative, either to ourselves or to our clients, is not helpful. Through hard experience we have learned that this approach sometimes escalates the situation, and on more than one such occasion we felt uneasy about what a client might do after leaving a session. And whether it is because of impaired judgment due to intoxication, bad timing, bad luck, or legitimate despair, borderline clients do kill themselves. Therefore, we immediately take all suicidal thinking seriously, interpreting it as an indication that clients are not feeling safe, and implement safety precautions. Besides allowing us to sleep better at night, we have found that this policy and approach, consistently followed, is more likely to decrease any unsafe behavior over time.

Borderline clients are quite dissociative. Close observation of borderline clients who report feeling unsafe, act out, or are otherwise symptomatic reveals that they very often exhibit all the signs of dissociation and age regression (see next section for more detail). If they are acting as if they are 4 years old, chances are they are really operating at that age level. In our own experience and in supervising students and staff, we have found that it is a mistake, though commonly made, to continue to try to manage any outbursts or needy urgency by expecting clients who are age-regressed to respond to adult-to-adult explanations, rationales, and instructions. This is not likely to work. Instead, an intervention matching the presenting age is more likely to be effective. A client in a 3- or 4-year-old's state of rage needs kind, soothing, simple, and firm directives to contain the behavior and break the trance state: "I know you're angry, but you are out of control and unsafe. Breathe, relax, look around. You're safe here." These words, said again and again in a calm voice, exemplify such an intervention. Readers who are parents have an advantage here in being able to identify the age and in thus selecting an age-appropriate intervention.

Seductive behavior is one way the borderline survivor may try to stay safe and feel in control. Counselors who find that their client has fallen in love with them face a potentially explosive situation. Abundantly hypersensitive borderline clients may feel too embarrassed about their feelings to discuss this issue and may drop out of therapy. Counselors must be alert to these romantic feelings and must carefully raise the issue and set appropriate boundaries. A discussion with the client about the natural process of transference can provide an "intellectual" excuse and a graceful out for clients. Of course, therapists should NEVER engage in a romantic or sexual relationship with a person who is either a current or a former client. The therapeutic relationship bestows enormous power on the therapist, and these sorts of relationships are a repeat of clients' earlier violations of trust.

We assess and treat substance dependence from the standpoint that drug and alcohol use are unsafe behaviors for borderline clients. This allows us to sidestep any intellectual debate with borderline clients around whether they really are addicts. By not engaging in this initial power struggle with borderline clients over the exact nature of their chemical use, we have found that it is much easier to get a more accurate chemical use history as well as clients' agreement to initial treatment for chemical dependency.

As with other clients, we strongly promote participation in a 12-step program for borderline clients. Often this requires some preliminary work, however, to help clients feel safe in meetings. Feelings containment and assertion work provide a good foundation. Starting clients in our outpatient groups first and then bridging to outside groups is another way to get around their resistance to attending meetings. We suggest that borderline survivors begin their recovery at AA or NA meetings (or Overeaters Anonymous if food is their primary substance). Attending the often highly emotionally charged meetings of other self-help groups, such as ACOA (Adult Children of Alcoholics) or AMAC (Adults Molested As Children), can lead to a relapse and, in our experience, is best saved for the education stage of recovery.

We recommend same-sex sponsors, as well as therapists, to avoid confusing spiritual love with romantic love. We discourage our borderline clients from dating anyone from their 12-step group. The meeting is a place for honest and open sharing. A room full of potential or former dating partners can make honest and open sharing very difficult. Same-sex 12-step groups can keep things in appropriate perspective and offer the borderline client good role models for recovery.

We have found that making several modifications in our approach to doing step work with borderline clients avoids certain pitfalls and increases the effectiveness of this aspect of our counseling. In Step One we need to be sure that we have not overemphasized the concept of powerlessness. Power and control are two of the key ways borderlines have used to survive. We instead emphasize the unmanageablity of drug/alcohol use and how unsafe chemical use is in the client's life. We do gradually help borderline clients see that they are empowered when they accept their powerlessness over things they cannot control. However, understanding, accepting, and applying this highly spiritual–philosophical concept takes time for anyone, but particularly the survivor of severe abuse. Our approach is to go slowly with borderline clients who are addicted and to encourage them to incorporate this principle only gradually into their lives.

Step Two presents problems because it introduces both the concept of a higher power and the need for faith. Faith does not come easily to the survivor, and it can be a very elusive concept for borderline clients. Sometimes borderline clients already have some sort of spiritual belief system that counselors can utilize—although they sometimes develop attachments to satanism or other less than helpful spiritual systems or cults. Constantly demonstrating to these clients any improvements at all in their status helps to instill faith and hope. They learn to reach out for help from therapy groups or through the therapeutic alliance with the counselors, which shows that someone can help them. Step Three provides the opportunity for clients to learn how to let go instead of to hold on, and it helps to work with borderline clients on the "controlling part" of the self, as described earlier. We find that Step Four, if done at all in early recovery, needs to focus on here-and-now issues related to chemical use and other problems in daily living. Sexual inventories or questions about childhood are likely to be too much too soon unless borderline clients have achieved at least the education stage. The appendix contains examples of specialized step work for borderline clients (and, as stated earlier, is suitable for narcissists as well).

Working with alcoholic/addicted clients with borderline personality disorder means having to expect and respond therapeutically to relapses in both their psychiatric and their substance abuse disorders (29). Abandonment triggers are the most potent source of relapse. These clients benefit from early, frequent, and extensive fail-safe planning, all from the orientation of helping the client stay safe. While relapses will still occur, such fail-safe planning will help clients land safely, that is, without the need to return to a hospital and without a suicide attempt. The appendix contains a relapse exercise we use with borderline clients (which readers may find useful with other angry survivors).

Later integration work with borderline clients often involves working through memories of many years of abuse, especially abandonment. Quite often the "black hole" feelings experienced by borderline clients and other survivors, which clients often struggle to try to communicate in words, reflect their lack of nurturing. Because these feelings are often difficult to put into words and are often in the form of pictures and sensations, having clients use drawing and other art forms to express themselves is helpful. Supplying the missing nurturing experience is often difficult in the real world, but it helps to encourage these clients to be their own parent in their imagination or in real life (e.g., by using a rocking chair as a safe place).

Often, the cognitive distortions in the borderline survivor are quite global and sometimes take the form of such mental phenomena as massive mistrust of all people (owing to very early experiences in which all family members proved themselves to be unsafe). Chipping away at these beliefs is slow work, but it can be done. We have successfully treated numerous addicted borderline clients who have remained clean and sober and are reasonably functional in their daily lives.

THE DISSOCIATIVE SURVIVOR

The DSM-IV defines the essential feature of dissociative disorders "a disturbance in the usually integrated functions of consciousness, memory, identity, or perception of the environment. The disturbance may be sudden or gradual, transient or chronic."

Dissociative amnesia refers to an inability to recall important personal information that is substantially more extensive than that caused by ordinary forgetfulness. Dissociative fugue describes a condition where the person engages in "unexpected travel away from home or one's customary place of work, accompanied by an inability to recall one's past." It also includes "confusion about personal identity or the assumption of a new identity." DID (formerly known as multiple personality disorder) refers to "the presence of two or more distinct identities or personality states that recurrently take control of the individual's behavior" as well as evidence of dissociative amnesia. Depersonalization disorder is the "persistent or recurrent feeling of being detached from one's mental processes or body that is accompanied by intact reality testing" (2).

As we discussed in Chapter 3, traumatic events generally induce and produce dissociative states. In some ways, any and all trauma resolution work involves working with dissociation, and the more counselors know about dissociation, the more effective they are likely to be when treating survivors. In addition, the clinical presentation of some dual diagnosis clients, particularly those with DID, so strongly involves dissociative phenomena that the professional must maintain a strong focus on managing and treating dissociative symptoms from the start. Consequently, we have two aims for this section. The first is to present additional material on dissociation to help readers become more adept at assessing and identifying dissociative symptoms and syndromes. The second aim is to discuss some therapeutic strategies and tactics that we have employed in treating clients who suffer from both chemical dependence and a dissociative disorder.

Persons who have DID represent the most dramatic and fascinating form of dissociative disorder. Professionals for many years ignored or discounted DID, but recently a veritable explosion of interest and investigation has taken place. The experience of watching adults completely age-regress into a fetal position right before our eyes, of seeing the same person show dramatic changes in blood pressure and need for prescription eyeglasses, and of assisting in containing a meek, mild 98-pound female patient who was suddenly speaking in a gruff, almost male voice and who had just thrown a conference table weighing several hundred pounds across the room has made us believers. Such experiences have also given us a profound respect for the powers of the mind.

Describing and defining DID, especially the notion of personality, is difficult and tricky. Kluft, probably the leading expert on this subject, prefers the term "multiple reality disorder" in an attempt to get away from the idea that different entities occupy the individual and to emphasize that the DID-phenomena represent "configurations" of the same person's presentation (30). To combat the conclusion that everyone is a multiple personality because everyone experiences many states of mind, Kluft also makes several distinctions between normal variability and the DID variability (31). Compared to normal experience, DID experience involves (1) a complete change of identity and no sense of continuity, (2) a complete change (including physical) in the sense of self and the representation of self, (3) loss of continuity of memory, and (4) loss of the sense of ownership of what one does. The felt sense of awareness and continuity is the core issue for strongly dissociative survivors. Progress in treatment occurs as more and more of the personalities are aware of each other (a transition that is known as attaining "co-consciousness" among the "alters" or alternative personalities) and become more and more cooperative with each other. The ultimate goal of treatment (one not always achieved) is integration of the separate personalities into a unity (31, 32).

Individuals with DID generally appear to differ from other survivors of trauma not in kind but in degree. Individuals with DID may be more hypnotizable because of genetic influences, but research indicates that the experience of both severe (and even bizarre) childhood abuse (such as incest, frequent close exposure to death, and ritual abuse) and a failure to receive nurturing, soothing, and support is an essential part of the recipe for producing DID (31, 32). Braun's BASK model and his continuum of dissociation (discussed in Chapter 3) is a framework that argues for the continuity of DID with other dissociative and survivor syndromes and also seems to fit our clinical experience with survivors. And most descriptions of the components of treatment emphasize the importance of safety, skills building, education, and integration work (31, 32).

Not surprisingly, assessing and achieving a differential diagnosis for someone with a dissociative disorder is quite complicated, especially for individuals with DID. As with other survivors, persons with dissociative disorders are highly likely to evidence symptoms of depression and mood swings, somatoform symptoms, and various anxiety disorders (31). Classic symptoms of PTSD are very common, as are symptoms of borderline personality disorder and even symptoms consistent with schizophrenia. And, of course, this population has a high rate of chemical dependency. In addition to inquiring about PTSD symptoms, history of trauma, and substance abuse, we use a number of additional intake questions that have been suggested by experts for use in probing for dissociative symptoms (33). The most important question revolves around the experience of lost periods of time when the client is *not* under the influence of chemicals.

Sorting out the contributions of chemical-induced versus dissociation-based symptoms often requires detailed questioning and assumes that clients can accurately report these issues. A blackout, an alcohol-induced state of amnesia (34) and a common symptom of alcohol dependence, can mimic dissociative symptoms. In a blackout, the drinker continues to walk and talk as usual even though he or she is quite inebriated; however, the person is unable to remember what occurred during the blackout period. Some people have a total blackout and cannot remember anything at all; others have more of a "brownout," remembering some details sketchily. Some blackouts last only minutes, others last hours or even days. The amount of alcohol necessary to cause a blackout varies from person to person, and there seems to be a genetically based propensity for blackouts (35). Consequently, some especially vulnerable individuals may suffer a blackout every time they drink even if they have consumed only small amounts of alcohol. Others may experience blackouts intermittently, never knowing if or when a blackout has occurred (36); it usually takes large amounts of alcohol for these individuals to experience a blackout. And many alcoholics never experience a single blackout during the course of their drinking. Blackouts are, however, a symptom of alcoholism; thus, if someone experiences blackouts when drinking, he or she is most likely genetically predisposed to alcoholism.

Other drugs also can cause memory loss or other dissociative difficulties. Marijuana, for instance, can cause memory loss, both for the period of intoxication itself and, after sustained use, as a more prolonged impairment (37). Use of other chemicals enhances state-dependent learning, with details of complex information learned or experienced when intoxicated being difficult for the person to access when not intoxicated. There is generally some continuity of awareness, however, for global details of the situation. Asking careful and detailed questions about the time frame between using chemicals and the period of time lost to memory and about other suspicious symptoms is often helpful in differentiating the basis for the reported symptoms.

Both because of the complicating role of chemical use in producing such symptoms as personality change and blackouts and because of denial and dissociation, we find that observations of clients in session are likely to be helpful in establishing the existence of strong dissociative symptoms.

Signs of dissociation and perhaps even of switching to another personality include the following: prolonged lack of eye contact (usually with eyes focused up and away but sometimes looking down and to the side); frequent eye closure and/or bursts of blinking; eyelid fluttering; subtle twitching of the muscles around the eyes; and, most tellingly and dramatically, eyes rolling strongly upward (32). Distinct and coordinated shifts in facial and body posture or voice tone, inflection and phrasing that appear to be those of a younger or different person, and involuntary movements that the client has difficulty controlling are also diagnostic. In some cases clients with DID may even come to sessions with completely different mannerisms, styles of dress, preference for beverages offered in our waiting area, and so forth. We have also learned to observe ourselves in these sessions; if we start to feel spaced out, forgetful, etc. (and we are not sick and are not having our own problems), we begin to wonder if dissociation is occurring.

A few scales or tests are available that are designed specifically to assess for dissociative disorders, including one brief scale (the Dissociative Experiences Scale) that appears suitable for screening and another, more extensive, interview instrument (the Dissociative Disorders Interview Schedule) that apparently has good test characteristics (33, 38). We do not routinely use these devices because of the structure of our clinic, but we have found reviewing them helpful in fine-tuning our interviewing.

Our experience has been that patterns of drug and alcohol use among strongly dissociative survivors are as variable as their presentation in other areas. Clear-cut progression is also sometimes difficult to establish, mainly because of difficulties in using self-report as a source of data.

However, a general pattern of using more chemicals and of things getting generally worse is usually clear. As with all survivors, strongly dissociated survivors are at high risk for substance use disorders, and the interaction of their two disorders is synergistic. The use of chemicals not only mimics but also promotes further dissociation; it intensifies the customary use of "checking out" in order to cope for those survivors who effectively disengage from reality via dissociation. In other words, if survivors are using psychic numbing to detach from their feelings, alcohol and other drugs can aid them in their effort to numb the pain.

Chemicals, however, are unpredictable friends. While on one occasion they may help push away negative feelings, on another occasion they may enhance these feelings and trigger flooding. Chemical use can cause additional psychiatric difficulties as well. The survivor who uses hallucinogens increases the chance of a psychotic break. We have worked with many adolescent survivors who enjoyed the use of hallucinogens. Often, at some point they experience a "bad trip," which resembles a paranoid, psychotic experience. Following their use of drugs such as LSD their mental status and results of psychological testing resemble those of a person with schizophrenia. We have spent years working with strongly dissociative survivor clients who have encapsulated "mini-psychotic" symptoms revolving around flashbacks of their "bad trip," these symptoms being associated with explanations for their existence that sometimes drift off into delusional thinking, often with a religious component.

Differentiating between severe dissociation and schizophrenia, rapid cycling bipolar disorder, and even partial seizures is sometimes difficult. Auditory illusions and other flashback phenomena, incoherence and confusion, and autistic-style thinking are common among survivors with high levels of dissociation. Some guidelines do help with this process. Compared to persons suffering from schizophrenia or other psychotic conditions, strongly dissociative individuals are much more likely to hear voices coming from inside their heads rather than outside, to have more focal episodes with discrete triggers, to not demonstrate looseness of associations and consistently blunted affect, to not show gross deterioration of social functioning, and to have the ability to carry out activities of daily living. Compared to rapid cycling mood disorders, strongly dissociative persons are more likely to report and demonstrate the mood shifts in a matter of minutes and even seconds. And compared to those with a seizure disorder, they are more likely to show sustained and complex behavior as opposed to the simple automatisms seen with seizures. Once again, however, we sometimes are simply not sure of the diagnosis and have to treat the symptoms while maintaining a provisional diagnosis, to be revised over time, in our heads.

We have also worked with a number of survivors who at some point in their treatment reveal that they have different names for different aspects of themselves. One client, for example, referred to one aspect of herself as Judy, the tough one, and to another aspect as Mary, the sweet one, and saw herself as being organized like a diamond with many facets. Careful questioning and observations indicated that this client was co-conscious of all these parts, was aware when a different "part" was operating, was able to maintain a sense of control, and showed no obvious signs of switching during therapy sessions. We finally decided that this particular client was using metaphorical language as a way to describe and organize various aspects of an essentially unified self.

We did an evaluation on a young man (whom we will call Ralph) who presented with a severe depression, a very recent suicide attempt, and an alcohol intake of a fifth a day. Ralph referred to his family as being "strange" but had difficulty elaborating on this. He also let us know that he had been recently charged with molesting several nieces and nephews, and with great shame and distress he admitted that the charges were true. Several times during the intake interview Ralph stopped, his head was pulled back, and his eyes rolled upward. Afterward, he "came back" and continued the interview. Questioning him about dissociative symptoms revealed that he was positive for many of them, even during the periods when he had tried to stop drinking. We gave him a diagnosis not only of major depression, pedophilia, and alcohol dependence but also of disso-ciative disorder not otherwise specified, and ruled out DID. After a brief hospitalization for detoxification and to forestall another suicide attempt, Ralph gradually revealed in his work with us a history of terrible sexual abuse and an elaborate interior world populated by 12 personalities, including one, named Ivan, who did both the drinking and the molesting.

Linda was a client who did not have DID but who was strongly dissociative. Her case also illustrates the dangers of attempting to prema-turely work through traumatic material. Linda was referred to us for dual diagnosis treatment. She had attained over a year of sobriety at the time she sought help, but she continued to experience urges to use and strong dissociative symptoms. Linda attended AA meetings and had accepted the fact that she was an alcoholic. She had also been in counseling for childhood sexual abuse with another therapist for over a year.

Linda presented as highly dissociative. During the first session she came in and compliantly sat down and began slowly and deliberately relating details of her childhood sexual abuse by her brother. Linda stared off into space as she discussed these details, very slowly reciting each word and pausing for long periods of time. Her account was so slow and rhythmic that it had a lulling quality to it. Katie (Evans) found herself having to shake her head to try to stay alert and she felt as if she were being hypnotized. For several weeks the therapy proceeded the same way:

Linda would come into the office to discuss her trauma in a highly dissociated state, sit in the same chair, and then literally look and feel very young in age.

Psychological testing revealed severe depression with a highly elevated score on the schizophrenia scale of the MMPI. We referred Linda for a medication consultation with our psychiatric consultant. He prescribed a medication with both antidepressant and antipsychotic properties, which Linda took for several months and then rejected because she felt it was not helping her. (Katie could see that the medication made no difference.)

Highly dissociative survivors are highly suggestible. Ironically, Linda's previous therapist had not only tried to deal with her dissociation but apparently promoted it by encouraging her to practice dissociating traumatic material. Linda needed to learn some different ways to stay emotionally safe other than dissociation before she could do her integration work. We decided not only that she was highly dissociative but that she was also in a therapy-induced trance, trying to work through her trauma but in such a dissociated way that her work would never become integrated. Instead of hypnotizing Linda, we decided that she needed to be dehypnotized and to have her trance broken. In the next session Katie explained to her that she was stuck in a trance state. Katie then began to wave her hand in Linda's face and say her name loudly whenever she appeared to be going into a trance state, an intervention that interrupted her dissociated monologue about her abuse. Katie also suggested to Linda that she say her name to herself each and every time she felt herself drifting off in this way. This felt strange for both Katie and the client at first. All of our previous therapy training (and all of Linda's experience in therapy) involved a prohibition against distracting clients from their process. Intentionally and consistently interrupting a client seemed like some sort of therapeutic blasphemy. Nonetheless, it worked. Linda very quickly learned to stay in the here and now, both in sessions and outside of them.

Consistent with our recovery treatment model, Katie then spent the next several weeks encouraging Linda to learn safety skills. She had an extremely difficult time being assertive and was also fearful of rejection from almost everyone. She focused on finding her own boundaries and figuring out who she was and what she wanted to do in her life. She quit trying to please everyone and began learning how to respect and take care of all parts of her self. Linda's urges to drink disappeared, and over the next year she worked through her abuse issues in an integrated way.

When overly stressed, Linda still occasionally starts to dissociate again. She makes an appointment, comes in for a "checkup," and is then able to get back in control of her dissociation. She does complain from time to time that therapy has wrecked her ability to get lost "in space." She acknowledges that she can still dissociate, however, and she accepts that dissociating consciously and with awareness is better than dissociating automatically.

Linda's feelings about losing her facility to dissociate typify a reaction sometimes found among highly dissociative survivors. Whether it is because of fear of a new way of living or because of the deep (but ultimately transient) pain of working through the trauma, the grief, or, as one writer put it, the narcissistic investment in the old parts (33), some survivors do not want to let go of their old self. Once again, persons with DID most dramatically illustrate this issue. Some achieve co-consciousness and a high degree of internal cooperation among their parts/personalities. Equipped with new skills and a recovering identity, they no longer need their various personalities to cope. Nonetheless, they choose to retain their personalities and to forgo fusion of their different parts.

Our philosophy is that clients are always the ones to choose their treatment goals. We do make this distinction, however. We agree that dissociation is a valuable tool and one that clients should always keep in their tool kit. We further emphasize, however, that having many tools is important for living the most satisfying life possible and that until they are free to refrain from dissociating, they are not truly free to dissociate. We stress that a key aim of treatment is "conscious unconsciousness" rather than uncontrollable, automatic reactivity. Our goal, in collaboration with the client, is to disable the dissociation defense as an automatic response. We want survivors to be able to dissociate, if they find it helpful, but we want them to be able to do it mindfully and deliberately.

Much of the discussion about the use of medications for survivors with borderline personality disorder applies to strongly dissociative survivors as well. In our experience there is no "magic bullet" medication for these clients, and their response is highly variable even when their presenting symptoms seem to indicate that a certain medication might be helpful. We have sometimes tried antipsychotic medication with these clients when they suffer from a psychosis that appears to be a result of their chemical use. These antipsychotic medications are sometimes effective for the acute psychotic symptoms, such as hallucinations and paranoid thinking, that are part of this condition. These same medications, taken at a low dosage for a brief period of time, are sometimes helpful for strongly dissociative clients who are suffering from traumatic flashbacks and nightmares. We have observed two major drawbacks to the use of neuroleptics: (1) negative side effects, such as muscle stiffness and thick tongue, which are uncomfortable and cause clients to become very reluctant to take the medication, and (2) an effect of sedation that interferes with some survivors' hypervigilance ("jams their radar"), lead-ing them to feel less alert and therefore unsafe. For clients with dissocia-tive disorder we use the step work for borderline personality disorder provided in the appendix.

We find our general treatment model applicable to persons with DID who also have a substance use disorder. For example, we use the same step work with DID clients that we use for clients with borderline personality disorder. The difference is that we may need to do these steps with several different personalities depending on "who" drinks or does drugs. We also find, however, that we have to apply the model creatively at times. We offer the following discussion of issues, strategies, and tactics as a work in progress. We have not treated enough of this sort of client to have the same degree of certainty we have with other groups of clients.

In many ways we find ourselves thinking of the multiple personalities of each client as constituting a family and working with them as we would with any family. Consistent with this, we help each of the personalities with strong survivor issues through each of the stages of our model. While the literature suggests that the modal number of personalities, or alters, is 13–15, typically half a dozen or fewer alters appear to spend the most time "out" (32). We start by engaging as many of these important personalities as we can in the therapy process and by assessing, in a preliminary way, their general level of denial and insight, their availability and cooperativeness, and their role in the client's presenting problems and in the internal family structure. We are careful to keep good notes in this preliminary survey of the system because things can get quite complicated and because we do not want to insult any of the personalities by forgetting their name and so forth. We add to these notes as more information becomes available, and they become the basis for more extensive mapping in the later stages of treatment. Assessing which alter is the alcoholic/addict can be complicated. Sometimes only one person-ality is the culprit, as was the case with Ralph. Sometimes there is one personality who uses one chemical, another personality who uses a different drug, and yet another personality who is an abstainer.

Within the general orientation of honoring all the parts of the self, we try to establish the best possible therapeutic alliance with all "family members." Just as in family therapy, sometimes the younger "children" are best left at home until later and sometimes certain members are in denial or are not interested in working with us.

Sometimes some of the personalities have the characteristics of various personality disorders that we discussed in the last section. We consequently keep in mind our various strategies and tactics for these disorders when trying to engage these personalities, for example, being careful to join with the hurt and initially protect the image of a narcissistic part. Sometimes some of the personalities do not want to attend a session; in that case we announce, "All of you who need to know what's going on and who can safely participate are invited to listen," which sometimes engages parts that appear to have been "no shows" and reduces the amount of repetition of necessary material.

We then introduce to the engaged members of a client's internal system our reframing of both the survivor issues and the substance use in terms of safety. We attempt to obtain an agreement to the terms of our standard safety agreement with respect to abstinence, self-harm, attendance, and so forth with the appropriate "parts" who engage in the unsafe behaviors. We also try to intervene with any enabling alters. In one case we even organized an intervention with cooperative parts to get the chemically dependent one into treatment. We have used some of the tactics of network therapy (39) (see Chapter 9 for a more detailed discussion), prompting the addicted alter to identify helpful parts that would support its efforts to stay abstinent and that would share with us and the substance-using alter (or part) their impressions of the alter's progress, signs of relapse, or actual relapse.

We work with the protector part or parts to not only help the other parts stay clean and sober but also to get them to attend 12-step meetings. We have found it important to clarify which part will show up at those meetings and to ensure that the part or parts most needing the information will attend and listen. Checking whether this happens is also important. This proved important in Ralph's case. He was attending AA meetings, but Ivan, the alter who was doing the drinking, never deigned to show up. Ivan, who was very antisocial, did finally agree to go after we corralled him (as per our approach with antisocial clients) by working with the lawyer Ralph had retained to defend himself against the molestation charges. Ivan was not very keen on going to jail, and pointing out that the molestations always occurred when Ivan was drinking helped us identify sobriety as a way to stay out of jail.

We also work to build additional safety skills for protection and nurturing to enhance the abilities of the protector and nurturer parts to more effectively do their jobs. For example, we have borrowed a tactic from a colleague to implement the notion of a safe place. We suggest that clients create a house with many safe rooms for various parts to go to where they can feel safe, rest, and find refuge when they are scared, a house that also has special places in which to contain dangerous parts so that they can "chill out" and not bother the others (40). Clients find this helpful in containing their acting-out parts, in keeping safe the vulnerable personalities, and in simply quieting things in their mind when many alters are competing for "air time" and things get confusing. Sometimes clients already have the appropriately skilled part but have blocks to using that part. One female client had a strong protector, for example, but this part was female and, because of the client's history, strong women triggered her. Her wounded-child part generally refused to ask for the protector's help. We tried several different ways to overcome this block but without success. We finally suggested that the client would figure out a way to do this herself by the following week, and, sure enough, the client came in announcing that she had "converted" the protector to an older brother figure and that this worked for her. Instances like this reveal the creativity of survivors, especially those with DID.

Attention to nurturing skills is always important. Inevitably, the nurturing parts are at best underdeveloped and at worst almost nonexistent. We also try to keep in mind the developmental age of a part and adjust our expectations of the skills that part can learn accordingly. For example, we might work with a 6-year-old alter on learning to ask for help from an older alter who, in turn, is learning to be more assertive in the standard sense of the word.

In the education phase we are careful to do elaborate mapping of the internal structure and to identify the age, main characteristics, and, most importantly, the function of each personality. Understanding this function is crucial. Perhaps the personality's main job or function is to take the abuse, or maybe there is a "smart personality" whose job is to do well in school. We take care to include the response of each part to the use of mood-altering chemicals, and we work with that part accordingly. We give each personality the opportunity to tell his or her story and correct cognitive distortions as they arise. We also attempt to foster communication and mutual self-help between personalities when this seems possible.

We begin the work on fusing and merging the different personalities during the integration stage of the recovery process. Often, some of the personalities have spontaneously merged by then. Sometimes they still exist but in closer harmony. The abreacting of painful memories and the merging of personalities are therapeutic interventions that require a highly trained expert in DID. We still consider ourselves apprentices in this area and request outside supervision from an expert on DID when we do this work. We refer readers to the resources listed in the notes for this chapter for additional material on the treatment of DID.

REFERENCES

1. Kranzler, H. R., & Liebowitz, N. R. (1988). Anxiety and depression in substance abuse: Clinical implications. *Medical Clinics of North America*, 72(4), 867–885.

2. American Psychiatric Association. (1987). *Diagnostic and statistical manual of mental disorders* (4th ed.). Washington, DC: Author.
3. Friedman, M. J. (1990). Interrelationships between biological mechanisms and pharmacotherapy of posttraumatic stress disorder. In M. E. Wolf & A. D. Mosnaim (Eds.), *Posttraumatic stress disorder: Etiology, phenomenology and treatment.* Washington, DC: American Psychiatric Press.
4. Koss, M. P. (1993). Rape: Scope, impact, interventions and public policy responses. *American Psychologist, 48*(10), 1062–1069.
5. Ross, C. C., & Anderson, G. (1988). Phenomenological overlap of multiple personality disorder and obsessive-compulsive disorder. *Journal of Nervous and Mental Diseases, 176,* 295–299.
6. Southwick, S. M., Yehuda, R., & Giller, E. L. (1991). Characterization of depression in war-related posttraumatic stress disorder. *American Journal of Psychiatry, 148*(2), 179–183.
7. Hamilton, M. (1960). A rating scale for depression. *Journal of Neurology, Neurosurgery, and Psychiatry, 28,* 56–62.
8. Kofoed, L., Friedman, M. J., & Peck, R. (1993). Alcoholism and drug abuse in patients with PTSD. *Psychiatric Quarterly, 64*(2), 151–171.
9. Coie, J. D., Watt, N. F., West, S. G., et al. (1993). The science of prevention: A conceptual framework and some directions for a national research program. *American Psychologist, 48*(10), 1013–1022.
10. Liepman, M. R. Nirenberg, T. D., Forgers, R. E., et al. (1987). Depression associated with substance abuse. In O. G. Cameron (Ed.), *Presentations of depression.* New York: Wiley.
11. Beattie, M. (1987). *Codependent no more.* New York: Harper/Hazelden.
12. Greene, R. L. (1991). *The MMPI-2/MMPI: An interpretative manual.* Needham Heights, MA: Bacon/Simon & Schuster.
13. Kosten, T. R., & Krystal, J. (1988). Biological mechanisms in posttraumatic stress disorder: Relevance for alcohol abuse. *Recent Developments in Alcoholism, 6,* 49–68.
14. Kammeier, M. L., Hoffman, M., & Loper, R. G. (1973). Personality characteristics of alcoholics as college freshman and at the time of treatment. *Quarterly Journal of Studies on Alcohol, 34,* 309–399.
15. Cloninger, C. R. (1987). Neurogenetic adaptive mechanisms in alcoholism. *Science, 236,* 410–416.
16. Zanarini, M. C., & Gunderson, J. B. (1987). Childhood abuse common in borderline personality disorder. *Clinical Psychiatry News, 6,* 1–2.
17. Samenow, S. (1987). *Inside the criminal mind.* New York: Times Books/Random House.
18. Yokelson, S., & Samenow, S. (1976). *The criminal personality: Vol. 4. The drug abuser.* New York: Jason Aronson.
19. Alcoholics Anonymous World Services. (1976). *Alcoholics Anonymous.* New York: Author.
20. Kohut, H. (1971). *The analysis of self.* New York: International Universities Press.
21. Gunderson, J. G., & Phillips, K. A. (1991). A current view of the interface

between borderline personality disorder and depression. *American Journal of Psychiatry, 148*(8), 967–975.

22. Gunderson, J. G., & Elliott, G. R. (1985). The interface between borderline personality and affective disorder. *American Journal of Psychiatry, 142*, 277–288.

23. Akiskal, H. S., Chen, S. E., Davis, G. C., et al. (1985). Borderline: An adjective in search of a noun. *Journal of Clinical Psychiatry, 46*, 41–48.

24. Ogata, S. N., Slik, K. R., Goodrich, S., et al. (1990). Childhood sexual and physical abuse in adult patients with borderline personality disorder. *American Journal of Psychiatry, 147*, 1008–1013.

25. Soloff, P. H., George, S., Nathan, R. S., et al. (1986). Paradoxical effects of amitriptyline on borderline patients. *American Journal of Psychiatry, 143*, 1603–1605.

26. Gardner, D. L., & Cowdry, D. I. (1989). Pharmacotherapy of borderline personality disorder. *Psychopharmacology Bulletin, 25*, 515–523.

27. Soloff, P. P. H., George, A., Nathan, R. S., et al. (1989). Amitriptyline versus haloperidol in borderlines: Final outcomes and predictors of response. *Journal of Clinical Psychopharmacology, 9*, 238–246.

28. Kernberg, O. (1975). *Borderline conditions and pathological narcissism.* New York: Aronson.

29. Nace, E. P. (1987). *The treatment of alcoholism.* New York: Brunner/Mazel.

30. Kluft, R. P. (1991). Personal communication.

31. Kluft, R. P. (1991). Multiple personality disorder. In A. Tasman & S. M. Goldfinger (Eds.), *Review of psychiatry* (Vol. 10). Washington, DC: American Psychiatric Press.

32. Putnam, F. W. (1989). *The diagnosis and treatment of multiple personality disorder.* New York: Guilford Press.

33. Loewenstein, R. J. (1991). An office mental status examination for complex chronic dissociative symptoms and multiple personality disorder. *Psychiatric Clinics of North America, 14*(3), 567–603.

34. Valliant, G. (1983). *The natural history of alcoholism.* Cambridge, MA: Harvard University Press.

35. Milam, J. R., & Ketchem, K. (1981). *Under the influence.* New York: Bantam Books.

36. Schukit, M. A. (1986). Genetic and clinical implications of alcoholism and affective disorders. *American Journal of Psychiatry, 143*(2), 140–147.

37. Blum, K. (1984). *Handbook of abusable drugs.* New York: Gardner Press.

38. Ross, C. A., Heber, S., Norton, G. R., et al. (1989). Differences between multiple personality disorder and other diagnostic groups on structured interview. *Journal of Nervous and Mental Disease, 177*, 487–491.

39. Galanter, M. (1993). *Network therapy for alcohol and drug abuse: A new approach in practice.* New York: Basic Books.

40. Seutter, S. (1989). Personal communication.

The Addicted Adolescent Survivor

✧

Ditto (written about a teen survivors recovery group)

You are the only ones who can understand how I feel,
I consider you all my friends,
and I'll stand by you 'till the end.
When you need a shoulder or a listening ear,
I am someone who won't disappear.
I am on your side when you need somewhere to hide,
I'll be here, you need not fear.

—GINA, age 15

Our goal in this chapter is to explore some of the special issues that arise when treating alcoholic/addicted survivors who are adolescents. While our general approach is the same for our addicted adolescent survivors as for adults, adolescent clients wrestling with both survivor and chemical use difficulties present several unique issues that providers need to take into account to increase the chance of treatment being more effective.

ADOLESCENCE: A DISEASE OR A DEVELOPMENTAL STAGE?

Mark Twain stated very well the adolescent worldview in his famous quote: "When I was a boy of fourteen, my father was so ignorant I could hardly stand it" (1). Many adults and some treatment professionals exhibit a profound prejudice toward adolescents. Professionals tend to be more subtle in their biases, usually choosing to avoid treating adolescents. Members of the public tend to be more obvious, reacting in a hostile way to adolescents in their stores, recreation centers, and other public areas even when teenagers' behavior is well within acceptable limits. We have even had to move our own clinic operations in response to complaints from area tenants about "those kids constantly hanging around causing trouble," when, in fact, our teen clients have generally been orderly, polite, and in the area for only 15 minutes before and after group meetings a few times a week.

These issues are likely to be even more evident when working with addicted/alcoholic adolescent survivors. As our discussions in earlier chapters have made abundantly clear, the majority of individuals with both survivor syndromes and chemical dependence are likely to have family members who are troubled by chemical dependence, other psychiatric difficulties, divorce, and joblessness; moreover, these families are likely to live in a neighborhood that is characterized by violence, guns, and general chaos. Denial, stress, and lack of resources are all likely to contribute to a family's dismissal of their adolescent's difficulties, to their tendency to see their adolescent as the basic problem, and to their being unwilling or unable to participate actively in the young person's treatment.

Recent research and our own experience have painted a more complex picture of adolescents' issues. Some individuals begin a downward spiral in early adolescence at the time of the transition to junior high school. The majority of adolescents, especially females, show some decrease in academic performance at this time and exhibit behaviors that lead to an increase in family conflicts, especially in the areas of autonomy and control (2, 3). Reports in the media on the tremendous increase in teen suicide, homicide, and pregnancy have been widespread in recent years. Epidemiological estimates are that one in five adolescents has a diagnosable mental disorder (4); poor peer relationships in adolescence are among the strongest predictors of adult disorder (5).

On the other hand, the majority of adolescents of both genders get through the second decade of life quite successfully (6). Evidence suggests that the problems are not due to adolescence per se but to other factors that interact with adolescent issues. For example, findings indicate that the standard bureaucratic structure of most junior high schools fails to meet the needs of students for emotional support (7). Other findings indicate that weak bonding to families and strong bonding to deviant peers and a great deal of unsupervised time predict future chemical use problems and delinquency (8, 9). Adolescence, then, is a time of transition, but it is not in and of itself a problem.

DEVELOPMENTAL ISSUES, TRAUMA, AND CHEMICAL USE

Authorities universally see adolescence as a time of rapid developmental change and as a period with its own unique developmental tasks. In his classic formulation Erikson saw the main task of adolescence as the development of an integrated identity, with successful achievement of this task resulting in a state he termed "devotion and fidelity" and failure resulting in role confusion (10). As we saw in Chapter 3, Cole and Putnam identified issues of abstract thought, intimacy, identity, sexuality, and boundaries as the key developmental issues of adolescence (11). Havighurst offers another description of the developmental tasks of adolescence (12). Table 8.1 outlines these tasks.

Details of developmental models may differ, but it is clear that adolescents must face and master critical developmental tasks. Even normal adolescents find these issues a challenge. Individuals who have a history of trauma and who are chemically dependent are massively challenged. Plagued by PTSD symptoms and by the failure to negotiate earlier developmental phases and develop life skills, survivors of childhood trauma, especially severe and/or ongoing trauma, face adolescence ill prepared. Chemical use also interferes with accomplishing these tasks. A common clinical finding in working with individuals who are chemically dependent is that they stopped developing (at least partially) at about the time of onset of heavy use. We often hear individuals in recovery whose chemical use started in their teen years wrestle with adolescent issues. When trauma and chemical use are combined, successful negotiation of adolescence becomes a very chancy proposition.

Adolescence is ripe with opportunities to trigger and play out survivor issues perhaps even more intensely than in earlier years. Chemical use, like gasoline poured on a fire, exacerbates these difficulties. The most common pattern we see at intake with adolescent survivors is the presence of preexisting difficulties (mainly of the acting-in type) in the early years. These difficulties begin to escalate in junior high school, and

TABLE 8.1. Havighurst's Developmental Tasks of Adolescence

1. Achieve new and more mature relations with age-mates of both sexes.

2. Achieve a masculine or feminine identity.

3. Accept one's physique and view the use of one's body as being effective.

4. Achieve emotional independence from parents and other adults.

5. Prepare for marriage and family life.

6. Prepare for economic career.

7. Develop values as a guide to behavior.

8. Achieve socially responsible behavior.

when behavior often converts to a more acting-out pattern. Chemical use exacerbates these problems.

THE ADDICTED TEEN SURVIVOR'S WORLDVIEW

Addicted adolescent survivors, even more so than their less troubled peers, show peculiarities in their thinking. Their extremely black-and-white thinking typically serves as a barrier to change. These teens hold strongly to their own positions and have a difficult time seeing that options and other ways of looking at things exist. Their thinking also tends to be concrete. Abstract concepts like letting go and being a survivor are difficult enough for adults, never mind adolescent survivors whose brains are affected by toxic chemicals. A related phenomenon is the tendency of adolescents to take the short view of things; that is, they often fail to take into account the long-term effects of their actions. Having a long-term perspective requires a belief that there is a future that matters and the capacity to envision it. Teen survivors have little hope in the future, little belief that they are in control of their destiny, and difficulty making the abstract leap from the present to the future. Frustrated parents may turn to their 15-year-old and say, "Don't you see that if you don't get good grades you will never get into college?" The teen is likely to meet this statement with a blank look and to respond with a comment like "Whatever. Besides, that is really a long time off, and I have plenty of time to pull it together later."

During a recent drug and alcohol evaluation, we asked a teenage boy when he last smoked marijuana. He responded, "A really long time ago." Further questioning revealed that this was 4 days prior to the interview. We adults consider the '60s a long time ago, not last week. Time distortion also affects adolescents' perception of their new "good behavior." We often hear the complaint, "I've been clean and sober for 3 whole weeks, and my mother still doesn't trust me!" These youth are unable to see that after 2 years of failing grades, truancy, and drug abuse all is not forgotten and forgiven just because they have been in a recovery program for "a whole month."

A corollary issue in the treatment of adolescents is their strong need for excitement and their difficulty in delaying gratification. Being patient is not what the majority of adolescents do best, and boredom is the bane of adolescent existence. A humorous but pointed saying commonly heard in 12-step meetings is "Instant gratification takes too long!" This is doubly true of the addicted survivor teen. Chemicals promote an "I want it now" attitude, which combines with the adolescent future-denying tendency and natural adrenaline and hormonal drive to counteract the numbing and depersonalization that is typically part of PTSD-type syndromes. Pushing serenity as part of recovery is not likely to impress adolescents. Even suggesting that they will die if they continue chemical abuse—a statement commonly made to adults facing Step One issues—is likely to be met with a statement such as, "I'll probably die anyway but not for a while, and, besides, I can do a lot of partying before that."

A common mistake we see parents make is using such disciplinary techniques as grounding for a month or longer. This is too long and almost inevitably results in some sort of flare-up, including running away from home. Their distorted sense of time makes a "whole month" seem like the rest of their life to teens and can often lead to their ignoring and disregarding the wishes of their parents and not complying with the grounding when the parents are not home. As parents we also realize that grounding an adolescent for as long as a month is a penalty to both parent and child alike. Most of us give up or give in long before the month is over when we are trapped in our homes with an angry or petulant teen!

Ironically, once adolescent clients accept recovery, their black-and-white thinking makes them militant about it, and the task is to slow them down a bit. Until this happens, however, asking questions, making distinctions, and soliciting input from other adolescents in a group helps to combat their global all-or-none thinking. For example, a common statement made by teens in early recovery is, "Everyone at my school uses drugs!" As the group's facilitator we may ask other group members, "Do you think that it is possible that all 2000 teens attending school with Mary are *all* using drugs?" This usually results in input from group members concerning the black-and-white thinking that leads to the conclusion that one's stoned peer group makes up the entire student body of one's school. It is also common in group to hear a teen state, "No one can understand what it feels like to be out of all the cliques at school." Again, the group of peers can confront this thinking. Other group members, for example, may admit that they too often feel they do not fit in with the other teens at school, and they may share ways they handle this.

Pointing out to the teens we see the fact that going to school this week means that their parents are more likely to increase their allowance and let them use the car is a more effective approach than discussing the impact of their current behavior on their retirement options. We also use the principle of immediate reward and punishment in consulting with parents about disciplinary issues; we advise them to save the lectures and let their consequences do the talking. Frequently, parents have a set of lectures they fall into automatically, and as the parent pontificates, the glassy-eyed youth is clearly not listening but is, instead, looking into space, watching the clock, or in some other way "not present" for the lecture.

We usually politely interrupt the parent and point out that while it is a fine lecture indeed, it appears that the audience is not attending. We have found it much more helpful to remind parents (and ourselves) that it is to the here and now that the teen relates and that actions, not words, are more likely to get the teen's attention.

As part of helping our adolescent survivor clients take the long view, we are careful to make all the intermediate steps clear. Prompting them for input in a step-by-step review of what is likely to happen next as they imagine a scenario helps teens begin to adopt a longer-range time frame. Creating an imaginary videotape of the past, present, and future is one exercise that sometimes helps more visually oriented survivors; this technique allows them to step back and take a look at their behavior in small, digestible bites and in a way that is less personal. One of our standard interventions in family sessions is to point out again and again the impact of the adolescent's behavior on the parents and to show how this furthers or hinders his or her immediate goals. The narcissistic view of these teens prevents them from seeing things from their parents' point of view. They usually view their parents as being in their way and blocking them from many desirable freedoms. Examining in small sequential steps what will happen if they show up for school or follow family rules and tying the consequences directly to their goals help adolescents transcend their concrete thinking and time-distorted worldviews.

Helping these adolescents find alternative ways to get some healthful intensity in their lives is also important. Sometimes we can encourage our teen survivor to get involved with sports, such as downhill skiing, that provide a rush. Going to dances sponsored by local Alano clubs gives these teens a party environment that is more likely to be protective of their recovery. Because these clients are still going to attend the parties of their age-mates, we are also careful to rehearse "saying no" strategies and to do fail-safe planning around this issue. We even construct a scenario of the day after a party, with our clients knowing everything that went on at the party and taking the one-up position instead of being the target of gossip about what they did in a blackout. With client and parental permission, we have even promoted our clients' telling their stories of recovery from drugs and alcohol to local organizations and in the local media. Being a celebrity is one way to create some prorecovery excitement, and correlating success and status with duration of abstinence and commitment to working the steps facilitates a prorecovery identity. Even with these sorts of interventions, the best 12-step group and the dances it sponsors do not hold the same excitement as taking 20 hits of LSD and playing "dodge the car" on the local interstate. Drug-dependent teen survivors have a distorted sense of what excitement is and will need to readjust their definition of a good time if they are to be successful in their dual recovery programs.

ADOLESCENT NARCISSISM

Intense preoccupation with self is a hallmark of adolescence; in some cases it takes the form of blatant narcissism. Underneath the narcissism lurks the fear of not being good enough, a fear that can emerge if the narcissistic bubble bursts. This is especially true of hypersensitive teen survivors, who have an enormous sense of shame. A 17-year-old girl who was recently in our office for counseling told Katie (Evans) how important the therapeutic relationship was for her. "You are the only one I can talk to!" she insisted. "I have a lot of friends, but all they want to do is talk about their own problems. No one ever wants to listen to my problems!" The same young woman asked, "Will I always have to have a counselor in order to have someone to listen to me?" Katie replied, "I think you will find that as you get older your friends will become better listeners." Whether this young woman's friends were really so preoccupied with themselves or whether this perception of them was merely her own self-centered response, her comments are a classic example of the egocentricity of the adolescent.

The self-centeredness of adolescents tends to distort their sense of how important their own thoughts, feelings, and needs are (13). There is also an element of grandiosity in this self-centeredness (14). Adolescents are more likely to shout at their parents, "You're not listening to me!" than to ask, "Won't you talk to me and tell me what you think is best for me?" A young girl recently talked on and on about her (uneventful) week in a group therapy session, totally oblivious to the needs of the other group members, including one who had made a suicide attempt. When this was pointed out to her, she was highly indignant. Her lengthy, tedious account of her week seemed more important to her than the needs of the rest of the group, even with one member in crisis.

This self-centeredness also can take on a very negative tone. For example, youths who are depressed may feel it is a sign that their therapist does not like them if they are kept waiting for 5 minutes beyond the scheduled start of their therapy session; yet they would have no qualms about extending their own therapy session if they were having a crisis. Often survivors assume the worst: If their mother says, "I need to talk to you," they are flooded with fear and anxiety over why they are in trouble when perhaps the parent only wanted to coordinate transportation plans. This often leads teens to blow up at the parent unexpectedly. Teens may be so worried about getting into trouble that when a parent finally does talk to them, they are so stressed and anxious that they erupt before the parent has finished the first sentence!

Addicted teen survivors are also characterized by grandiosity, which often leads to haphazard and unrealistic planning and contributes to the difficulties they have in being realistic about the consequences of behavior (15). When a young man who was in treatment at our clinic for a serious drug problem was confronted with the potentially life-threatening consequences of his behavior, he replied, "If I die, it won't be from drugs!" Note that in his mind the issue was not *when* but *if*. This thinking can sometimes interfere with young people's willingness to participate in 12-step programs for recovery. They often believe that they can do it on their own, and this prevents them from getting support for their sobriety, which is essential for adolescent recovery from addiction.

Challenging this stance directly is an invitation to a blowup or a depressive collapse. Most of the strategies discussed in the previous chapter on narcissistic personality disorder are relevant here. We also use this preoccupation with self to motivate therapeutic progress. We encourage our teen survivors to write poetry or paint pictures, and we take the time to familiarize ourselves with these productions as a way to promote positive transference. Framing interventions in terms of self-interest is another way to work with, rather than against, this current. We might ask, for example, "How do you think it's going to look to the other members of your recovery group if you keep going out with people who are not kind to you?" If this appeal to peer review does not elicit the desired reaction, we might use a more paradoxical approach and state, "I am surprised that you want to give all your power away to your mother by staying angry. You're the one who loses when you blow up, not your mother."

Notions of powerlessness engender resistance for all kinds of reasons among these clients. Using the aforementioned paradoxical approach or framing the issue as one of safety are ways of dealing with this. Step One paradoxically teaches that you get control by admitting that you have no control. Continually pairing the notion of getting out of control with the idea of losing power, not gaining it, is one strategy for doing Step One work with these teens.

PEER ORIENTATION

Ironically, intense preoccupation with peers accompanies intense preoccupation with self. "Where do I belong and what do they think?" are questions that adolescents constantly ask themselves. This is part of mastering such tasks as establishing the boundary between self and others and formulating an integrated identity. Identifying with a given peer group is a way to accomplish the transition from adolescence to young adulthood and independence from the family. Serving as a temporary bridge and a second family providing interim support and a stage on which to try out a new identity and practice friendship and intimacy skills, the peer group is the essence of gangs and other groups that adults see as antisocial. The family attraction to your "homies" (fellow gang members) can be a very strong draw.

Feeling ashamed a great deal of the time and often lacking advanced social skills, adolescent teen survivors struggle with finding an appropriate balance between themselves and others. The failure of their own families to often provide worthy role models or conditions promoting bonding also leads to either a lack of counterbalance between family and peers or even to overidentification with adults. This fixation on not separating from family is sometimes not immediately obvious in the case of adolescent teen survivors who have a more acting-in stance. At first glance they appear anything but overinvolved with their peers inasmuch as they report few friends, spend enormous amounts of time in their room, and pursue only solitary hobbies (if any). However, even a few quick questions or a few minutes letting them talk about their concerns reveals a massive preoccupation with what others think of them, intense feelings of resentment (and abandonment) at not being part of a group, and a constant judgment of self based on what they think others think of them. These teens are always looking over their shoulders, even if at a distance. In contrast, those teens who are more prone to act out are clearly and dramatically involved with others and tend to hand over more parts of themselves to peers than is safe or wise, often to their detriment.

The acting-out mode of expressing anger through violence to self and others coupled with a desire for a family beyond their biological one also propels the addicted survivor into the maw of gangs either as a fully "jumped-in member" or as someone who uses one "color" or "set" as her dating pool. (Color and set are gang terms that refer to the gang's identity, for example, the "East Side Bloods" is a set and their color is red. All of their gang members wear red to demonstrate unity.)

Gangs and youth violence in this country are currently grave problems. Many of us wonder what could be fueling the violence and gangster behavior among an alarming number of youth. There are many opinions. Some argue that it is the lack of employment for young people today, others that it is the breakdown of the family. Some say it is drugs, easy access to firearms, or an educational system that no longer works. We think all of these theories hold a part of the truth. Clearly, teens join gangs for self-protection, as a way to feel safe should opposing gang members threaten them; but we also believe, on the basis of our clinical experience, that there are other factors that lead gang life to have a strong appeal for the addicted teen survivor.

Many of the addicted teen survivors we see are affiliated with gangs. Being part of a gang appears to offer these youth critical ingredients, such as feelings of safety, support, and validation, they have not received elsewhere. The excitement of delinquent activity, in addition, is very addictive. Gangs offer a highly seductive way to obtain these missing experiences and to relieve emotional numbness and pain. A gang-affiliated client will often say, "My gang is more like a family than my real family." These teens tell us that the loyalty their gang membership provides helps them feel that someone is really there for them, and this "even to death" loyalty provides a heady sense of protection and nurturing.

Gangs serve other purposes for the teen survivor. Violence, a core ingredient of the gang experience, begins when the new member is "jumped in" or initiated into the gang by being beat up for a number of seconds or minutes by gang members. The violence, of course, extends to conflict with rival gangs. Teen survivors' trauma-induced anger finds a channel for expression in these conflicts, where it becomes a source of status, power, and even legitimacy. Moreover, adoption of gang values solves the identity problem and gang affiliation provides a promising opportunity for men and women alike to use the psychological defense of projection. Many girls in our acting-out survivor group hold a lot of rage toward the perpetrator of their early childhood abuse. Instead of keeping a journal or writing colorful poetry to express their anger, they will instead look for an opportunity to "kick the shit" out of a stranger who has slighted them or another gang member. The same tearful, suicidal girl in our office on Tuesday will pull a knife on another girl in a gang fight at school on Wednesday. This fragmentaion, classic to all survivors, can be even more dramatically played out in the addicted teen survivor.

Amy's story illustrates some of these issues. Her parents, both of whom were alcoholics, divorced when she was only 5 years old. Amy was left alone for long periods of time while her mother, who had custody, sought support and companionship in the local tavern. Amy's older brother, a key figure in her life, often served as a substitute parent when no adults were available. When Amy turned 11, her mother remarried; her second husband was also an alcoholic, but Amy was happy to have a dad. Along with her new dad came a stepbrother, her own brother's age. Amy was desperate for attention and acceptance from this stepbrother; at the same time, she also felt she was losing her brother to him because the two 15-year-old boys were doing more and more things together. One night Amy's brother and stepbrother were drinking beer, and Amy, in an attempt to fit in, joined them in their drinking. When Amy's brother passed out, her stepbrother began undressing her. Amy says she "went along with it" in order to please him, and her stepbrother had intercourse with her. The next day at school, shaken and guilty, Amy told the school counselor about the incident. Her stepbrother was charged with "Rape 1," but since he was a juvenile the charges were deferred provided the family participated in therapy. Amy's stepfather blamed both Amy and his son for "letting this legal stuff happen!" He definitely did not see it as rape despite the fact that his son was 4 years older than Amy. Amy's father and even her mother also blamed her for what happened. Amy soon began hanging around gang members and finally joined the gang. Her initiation involved, among other things, having sex with the male gang members. When we explored the reasons for her gang membership, Amy revealed the following themes: a feeling of finally belonging, a delight in the rush of beating others up, and a sense of being a sex object as the price of belonging.

Establishing healthy peer relationships is difficult for teen survivors. They do not have a strong sense of who they are, and they do not like what they think they are. "I am too emotional," one teen survivor told us. "And sometimes I feel like I am just crazy! There is no one my age that I can relate to. I just feel like I am the only person in the whole world who feels the way I do!" This statement illustrates the common dilemma of adolescent survivors who want to be a part of a wholesome teen group but feel they do not fit in. The trauma experience and its effect on trust and self-esteem make the development of healthy peer relations extremely difficult for teen survivors. Not knowing whom they can trust and feeling unsafe with others, these adolescent survivors experience the development of a friendship as a traumatic experience in and of itself. For girls, same-sex peers may represent the mother who failed to protect them from their abuse—or, even more damaging, who blamed them for the abuse once it was discovered.

Even under normal circumstances, the peer group in many instances becomes a second family, since adolescents often feel that their parents do not understand them but that their peers do. The phone company has undoubtedly made significant profits from the installation of a second telephone line in many homes. The use of the telephone is probably second only to school performance as the most debated subject at our clinic. The telephone is an adolescent's lifeline to other teens, especially in the years before independent transportation is available. Lengthy nightly phone calls in which daily conversations with peers are processed are a hallmark of adolescence. Hypersensitive and very needy teen survivors, however, may feel that their friends are not there for them. If the teen is not home when they call or forgets to return a call, survivors may perceive this as abandonment. Their intense need for support wears on most friendships.

Teenagers also constantly compare themselves with same-sex peers to see how they measure up. This process for the wounded teen is very painful; their shame-based thinking tells them they are never good enough. We have worked with many teen survivors who find the standard teenage ribbing and kidding so intolerable that they end up reacting too strongly, either by blowing up or falling to pieces, and then become a target for further and truly damaging insults.

Dealing with peer issues is absolutely critical for therapeutic success with teenage survivors. One common mistake is to immediately forbid all contact with any and all peers who exert an unwholesome influence on the client once his or her problems become apparent. For many teen survivors this is like asking them to cut out their hearts and is an invitation to rebellion. Weaning these teens away from peers who are a negative influence is a tricky process and requires time.

ESTABLISHING A NEW IDENTITY

Besides providing a high, relief from painful feelings, and a way to relate to peers, chemical use also provides a way to establish an identity. School authorities promote abstinence, and health classes teach the dangers of chemical use. The majority of parents—even if their words do not always match their actions—warn against drinking and drug use (although we have encountered several situations where parents used chemicals with their children to help them "learn how to handle it" or to be "buddies" with their children). Drinking and doing drugs provides a ready-made way to be different from parents and other authority figures. Chemical use also forms part of the identity of many peer subgroups, whether the subgroup is one of jocks who frequent keg parties, "stoners" who smoke pot, "alternatives" who do hallucinogens, or "gang bangers" who drink the gang's preferred brand of ale. Taking on the identity of the group typically means engaging in the chemical use rituals of the group as well as sharing the antisocial values characteristic of these subgroups. Teens who are increasingly dependent on chemicals will also increasingly spend more and more time with chemically dependent peers, finding support and justification for their accelerating use of substances. A very common comment we hear from substance-involved adolescents is, "Everyone is doing it; what's the big deal?" Quite often this is not offered merely as an excuse but reflects the fact that all the client's buddies are indeed heavily involved in substance use.

Identification with peer groups with a strong component of chemical use provides the opportunity and payoff for increasing involvement with chemicals. The influence works both ways: Using chemicals makes these groups "cool" and increasing dependence on chemicals makes seeking out these groups more imperative. Unfortunately, it is more and more common that female survivors who attend "gang banger parties" are raped by one or more gang members. Sometimes these "tough chicks" do not want to tell anyone about the rape, since they see it as a weakness on their part that they could not "kick their ass." Other times the survivor feels she deserved it because she was drunk and flirting. There is also the issue of loyalty to the gang or "set": If the survivor and the rapist are both members of the same gang, she may not want to get a "family member" into trouble by talking about him to other people or, most importantly, to authority figures.

Encouraging the formation of a "recovering addicted survivor" identity is an essential component of treatment for these teens. We use all the strategies and tactics described in previous chapters to accomplish this. This view is not, however, without its opponents. Some professionals express particular concern about labeling adolescents, addicts, or alcoholics. These professionals feel that the identity of "recovering addicted survivor" is a negative one—with its emphasis on once a survivor/addict, always a survivor/addict—that dooms these teens for the rest of their lives.

We answer these concerned critics by making several points: First, the label empowers adolescents through honest validation of their experience and points the way to how they can heal. It reinforces the conclusion that they are not bad but are suffering from a disease over which they have no control. Second, through the experience of working the steps of a recovery program they find that this new identity bestows previously missing protection and nurturing experiences and makes it possible for them to learn skills that will ultimately promote their chances of leading a more satisfying and productive life. Third, the recovering identity promotes honesty; the notion of sharing with and helping others; a realistic understanding of control; and other prosocial values. Finally, successful work in the integration stage frees these adolescents to move beyond being a recovering addict/survivor. Many suffer serious "victim stance" thinking, which if uninterrupted can follow them well into adulthood. Seeing oneself as a *survivor* and not a *victim* may appear to be a subtle shift in worldview, but it is a strongly empowering one indeed!

We also acknowledge the importance of taking into account the special needs of adolescents and not expecting them to respond as adults do in working a 12-step program. Individual counseling offers the youth the chance to learn how to manage painful affects in ways other than drug/alcohol use.

Creating bonds to a substitute peer group is the number one task

with addicted adolescent survivors. Strongly promoting a 12-step program is part of this process. Many locales have teen-oriented 12-step
groups that can facilitate addicted teen survivors' acceptance of meetings
as part of the recovery process and help them deal with the standard teen
perception that "those meetings are full of old people carrying on about
the Big Book." In the face of such complaints, challenging teens to listen
for what they have in common with other people in the meeting is another
way to deal with this complaint. We also strive to provide an alternative
peer group by making our recovery groups at the clinic cohesive ones.
Our efforts range from ensuring that the group atmosphere is supportive
but also has the norm of confronting unsafe behavior and thinking to
handing out coins and providing a cake to celebrate significant milestones
of group members. Sometimes schools provide support groups as well,
although our teen clients sometimes resist attending such groups out of
fear of what their peers might think. A charismatic counselor with a gentle
touch who can define the group as "cool" is helpful here. It is also helpful
when attendance at group meetings translates into school credit, even if
it does mean missing that history class.

It is also important to refrain from assuming that addicted teen
survivors have the social skills necessary to relate successfully to peers.
For example, sometimes "I won't" is really "I can't." Engaging in successful and healthy social interaction (including attending 12-step meetings)
means that one can start conversations, listen to others without interrupting, speak up about feelings and concerns, learn to set boundaries with
others, and communicate needs. For all the reasons discussed throughout
this book, teen survivors are not likely to have high levels of these skills.
Therefore, therapy sessions must provide opportunities for them to
endlessly practice social skills and for therapists to give them feedback
about boundaries, respect for self and others, and related issues.

BODY IMAGE AND SEXUALITY

Accepting one's physique, developing a healthy body image, and being
able to set good sexual boundaries are often difficult tasks even for the
average teen. Youths with a history of childhood sexual abuse have even
more difficulty in these areas and may try to hide their sexuality by
wearing heavy or baggy clothing and plain hairstyles or through obesity.

Audrey was only 4 years old when a cousin 10 years older molested
her. Initially, he fondled her, but this gradually led to sexual intercourse.
Unable to keep herself physically safe and very frightened, Audrey began
the use of dissociation to mentally leave her body during the abuse. A
series of sexually abusive baby-sitters only confirmed her belief that the

world was not a safe place. In adolescence Audrey became a beautiful young woman, slender and willowy. Her beauty did not go unnoticed. Male passersby would whistle and call out to her such remarks as "Hey baby, you can keep me warm tonight!" This behavior massively increased Audrey's fear that "all men are unsafe." Audrey then deliberately gained over 75 pounds in a single year so that "those men would stop."

Some teen survivors believe the only way they can get love and approval is through sex. Sometimes this is an attempt to get some nurturing, no matter how false or brief. Some survivors, including some males who prostitute, use their sexuality as a way to feel powerful; we have had many of these adolescents marvel at how sex gives them power over men. Young women who were previously frightened and exploited by men now notice how males will say or do almost anything in order to have sex. Sometimes young women attempt to gain a sense of personal power and self-esteem through their promiscuity. They want to see how many men they can have sex with, and each name on the list adds to their sense of power. Unfortunately, in spite of the glee the protector part of the young woman feels over each new "conquest," the wounded part experiences each encounter as yet another episode of abuse by someone who cares nothing for her as a person and only wants her body for sex. This reinforces her fragmentation, for she must then push the feelings of being unsafe and hurt further and further away.

Many teen survivors who are promiscuous have difficulty consistently having safe sex. They often find it difficult to ask an ardent partner to use a condom, or they are uncomfortable having to set the boundary, or they are too impulsive to slow down and get protection. Unwanted pregnancy is a serious problem in this population. It is sad indeed to see how the wounded child part of the survivor teen believes that having a baby will fill that hole inside of her that longs for unconditional love. The romanticized view of motherhood is quickly shattered by colicky babies, absent fathers, and the public welfare system.

Often, sexual abuse survivors have had sexuality linked to self-esteem as part of the abuse scenario. For example, the father who tells his daughter that she is a very "special little girl" when he molests her causes her to link sexuality, self-esteem, and body image (16). This promotes a dynamic whereby the survivor sees herself as only having worth as a sexual object and feels unworthy because she has been the object of sexual abuse. The messages she receives from the abuse scenario create a double bind for her; she learns both that her only worth is as a sexual person and that sex is unsafe. As discussed in Chapter 3, these sorts of double-bind messages lead to classic PTSD-type symptomatology.

This abuse cycle associated with sex often leads the survivor to choose sexual partners who are not terribly loyal or who can be emotionally, physically, or sexually abusive. Trying to convince a starry-eyed 15-year-old that she is being deceived when she believes it is love is a challenge indeed. This is where a therapy group of same-sex peers can give feedback that is more easily accepted than that of parents or other authority figures.

The conflict over losing versus maintaining virginity is an issue for most adolescents (17), but survivors of sexual abuse approach this conflict with many unresolved issues; for example, they often feel like "damaged goods." As one 15-year-old survivor put it: "My dad had already done so much worse to me than my boyfriend wanted to do; what was the point in trying to say no? It's like saying no is a lie or something." Survivors who lost their virginity at the hands of a sexual offender are very confused about what normal sexual relations are. A 17-year-old survivor, who was in recovery from addiction and who identified with traditional Christian values, told us that she now considered herself a virgin, having become "re-virginized" when she became a Christian. She was adamant about wanting to marry a man who was also a virgin, explaining to us, after some discussion, that his virginity would ensure that he would be unable to tell what her father had done to her. The young woman shared with us and the members of her all-female addicted survivors group the fact that her father had taught her a variety of sexual techniques, particularly those involving oral sex. She reported that her father always ejaculated in her mouth and admitted that she felt dirty all the time and felt that a man's penis was dirty as well. She believed that if she married a virgin, he would be clean.

Sexual identity confusion is common for most survivors of sexual as well as other types of abuse. For the male sexual abuse survivor who was abused by a same-sex partner, there is an even greater sense of confusion. Adolescent males are often quite homophobic, their pervasive bias and tendency to taunt revealing their fear of being a "queer" or "faggot"; it is as if they need to firmly disclaim what they are not before they can identify what they are. An adolescent male who has been sexually abused very often wrestles with whether he is homosexual. He may also feel that his body betrayed him if any sexual response was generated to the abuse. As with female survivors, sexuality for abused males also becomes contaminated with distorted notions of power and control.

OTHER IDENTITY ISSUES

Achieving a sense of who one is and an integrated identity is a core developmental task facing teenagers. For adolescent survivors of trauma this task is a tremendous challenge. Those who adopted the "placating others" strategy have for years practiced being what they thought others wanted them to be. Many continue with this strategy and never go through the identity crisis necessary to discover who they are. Unfortunately, after a lifelong experience without a sense of self they sometimes hit a delayed identity crisis later on in their life following some sort of major life event such as marriage or childbirth.

Other individuals reach adolescence and adopt a stance in which they completely reject all values espoused by various authority figures. Some children have been angry and difficult for many years; for them, adolescence merely provides the opportunity for more of the same. Teen survivors who are heavily dissociated lack unimpeded access to their own experience. Either they do not know what they think, feel, and sense and therefore remain lost, or their different self parts trigger in contradictory ways that are difficult to coordinate in a coherent fashion. For example, there is the "nice guy" or "good girl" teen who periodically explodes in an assaultive rage over trivial matters, leading both the teen and those around him or her fearful and confused. The trauma experienced by teen survivors has contaminated such personality features as their trust in and connections with others, the way they see issues of power and control, and their sense of self-efficacy and competence. These contaminations distort their ability to explore identity issues, leading them to be overly accepting of things as they are, compulsively rejecting of certain possibilities, or frozen between the two extremes. Teen survivors' enormous legacy of shame and self-loathing greatly interferes with their ability to answer the "Who am I?" question.

The difficulty with identity issues plays out in many ways. In some cases survivors, having seen the abusive parent as having power and therefore as being worthy of emulation, identify with the aggressor and turn tough. Males may adopt a macho pose, and females, viewing their own sexuality and femininity as what made them vulnerable, may begin to dress in a more masculine fashion, may get into physical fights, may gain prowess in being tough, and may attempt to deny their feminine selves. Angry survivors, as we have seen in our discussion of gangs, find an antisocial identity appealing.

POWER STRUGGLES AND THE NEED FOR AUTONOMY

Adolescents, at least in our culture, begin to press for more autonomy and control when they enter junior high as part of their move to define themselves. The transition to junior high school leads to a dramatic increase in exposure to new peers and other families and in time spent in peer relationships, where power and control are more symmetrical. Discovering and experiencing new and different values and ways to relate, together with the development of increased abstract thinking, may contribute to the adolescent's tendency to question parental rules and the rules of other authorities (18). Whatever the reasons for its existence, our society acknowledges this phenomenon with the term "teen rebellion," and some level of it is an accepted rite of passage for adolescents in Western cultures.

Numerous books, the frequency of questions to advice columns, and periodic special coverage in the media indicate the intense salience in our culture of the question of how parents, teachers, and others responsible for teenagers can best handle this phenomenon. An increasing amount of research provides some general guidelines in this area. Again and again, high levels of parental support and moderate levels of control appear to be associated with fewer problems in school and with adolescent substance use; weaker orientation to negative peers; and less delinquency, depression, and other difficulties (19). A high level of parental support includes praising, encouraging, and giving physical affection to the child. An optimum level of parental control over the adolescent involves the maintenance of moderate levels of monitoring and supervision, and some reasonable type of punishment, and the consistent enforcement of clear and explicit rules; unclear expectations, inconsistent discipline, and harsh mentally and physically abusive consequences appear to have particularly damaging consequences. Research also suggests that a similar pattern holds true in junior high school settings, with low levels of support and high levels of control by teachers being associated with a decrease in students' school performance, motivation, and identification with teachers as models (7). Even well-functioning parents and teachers wrestle with maintaining the proper balance of support and control with adolescents. A friend of ours, who has done a fine job of raising her own children and is an effective leader of the teen groups in her church, explained with good humor that her philosophy for dealing with teenagers starts with the assumption that she is automatically wrong in their eyes. Ironically, many well-meaning parents and teachers actually increase their control efforts and decrease their support of adolescents, out of fear, just at the time when adolescents need as much support as before, if not more, and reasonable levels of control.

Adolescent addicted survivors are ripe for teenage rebellion, which they usually express overtly but sometimes display covertly, in a passive aggressive manner. Since school is one arena in which these issues play themselves out, we commonly see these behaviors when teen survivors enter high school and encounter a structure that is simultaneously more formal and authoritarian and less supportive than that of grade school and junior high school. Some adolescent survivors have difficulty handling the increased need for independent work, because they have never learned to structure time and tasks for themselves, or they have difficulty asking for help if they are falling behind. Others trigger strongly to teachers and administrators who are likely to be less understanding and supportive of individual students because of time constraints and a heavier work load. These same school authority figures are also more likely to expect that students will follow the rules and be accepting of the consequences. Whether they are triggered by anger at the control exercised by these authorities or by the lack of warmth and support, adolescent survivors often act out in a host of ways in the school setting. Add in chemicals, and the stage is set for their complete disengagement from school, either by sitting quietly intoxicated in class or by skipping school altogether to get high with drug-using friends. A drop in grades or school suspensions for truancy or attitude problems are often the problems that lead a frustrated parent to reach out to the mental health community for help for their child. Some readers may recall fondly the special times of junior high and high school. For the wounded teen with a fragile commitment to a recovery program, a lack of self-esteem, and a weak sense of identity, school is a very painful experience. For many survivors it is a fear of peer rejection and a sense of alienation that gets in the way of their school attendance.

An alternative school that can offer a more therapeutic environment is often helpful; a special group for recovering drug-free teens is a safe harbor for at least one period a day. Many school districts across the country have excellent student support services for recovering youth. Sadly, funding cuts in many parts of the country are leading to the dismantling of some of these fine programs, which are thought of by some as unimportant. If safety is the core issue for all survivors and if it is the basis upon which all steps for recovery are built, then providing safety in schools is ultimately far more basic and fundamental to learning than any other part of the educational system.

Adolescents are sometimes still in the families where the trauma occurred. By definition, abusive families are low on support and are undercontrolling and neglectful or overcontrolling and intrusive, or they are highly inconsistent on these dimensions. Sometimes abuse is still occurring but the adolescent has an increasing awareness of the injustice of it and/or an increased sense of power and support from peers. The adolescent then rebels, and the abuse stops. We see this a great deal of the time in cases of physical abuse when adolescents come into their own in terms of size and strength. In other cases the abuse stopped some time before, but in either instance the issues are unresolved and the atmosphere in the family is heavy with this. Sometimes the spouse has divorced the perpetrator but the adolescent survivor begins to explode with rage toward the "abandoning" parent. We often see this with adolescent girls who finally explode at their mothers for failing to protect them when they were younger. This rage often accompanies a profound fear of separation and abandonment, and this anxious/ambivalent attachment (as discussed in Chapter 3) keeps the parent and adolescent angrily enmeshed. These adolescents feel that if they pull away from the family they will no longer be wanted or loved. At the same time, they resent the control of the authorities in their life and often act out their anger toward their parents with a sense of being helplessly trapped.

Carefully assessing the roots and dynamics of these adolescents' rebellion is important. Acting-out behaviors can have many roots, and different etiologies call for different treatment approaches. And although parents or school officials sometimes seek an evaluation for a teen because of their concerns about severe anxiety or depression, particularly where the question of suicide potential is an issue, it is usually, as the saying goes, the squeaky wheel that gets the grease. The more common presenting problems are outbursts of anger and a negative attitude toward authorities, being caught at school by a teacher or in the park by the police in possession of chemicals, declining grades and truancy, and running away from home or defiance of family rules. Sometimes our evaluation, which includes interviewing adolescents, parents, and school officials; administering psychological testing; and ordering urinalysis to test for drug use, demonstrates not only the existence of a substance use disorder but a conduct or oppositional defiant disorder. Consequently, our treatment will put more emphasis on corralling and containing the adolescent and on appropriately challenging the acting-out defenses.

More often than not, however, we are likely to find one of two other clinical pictures. The first is what a colleague of ours calls "tootsie pop kids," referring to the hard exterior that covers the soft wound inside (20). This term describes those adolescents who typically were anxious and placating as children. They often have histories of at least adequate achievement, separation difficulties, and extended thumb sucking and bed wetting as children. In other instances, they have a long history of acting-out difficulties, which have recently accelerated. When these individuals hit adolescence, they switch to an angrier stance, one fueled by their chemical use. Psychological test results typically demonstrate both the acting-out exterior and the underlying mistrust, confusion, and anxious depression of the survivor. These adolescents are in some ways the most difficult to treat because they require a balance between corralling and supporting that can be difficult for counselors, parents, and school officials to maintain. A combination of the strategies for managing and treating the narcissistic and borderline personality disorders (described in the last chapter) is likely to be more effective than simply supporting disruptive and inappropriate behavior. When they are abstinent from chemicals and able to experience safety under conditions of simultaneous containing and support, these adolescents typically quickly decrease their acting-out behaviors.

Tom illustrates this type of teen. When he was 15 years old, school officials referred him to our clinic for a drug and alcohol evaluation. Tom, who enjoyed a reputation for being "a hard ass," had been caught selling LSD at school. He had a history of fighting with peers that went back to the first grade. We took a social history from Tom and discovered that between the ages of 4 and 8 he had been molested by an uncle. Tom disclosed this information without emotion, but when we commented that it sounded like he did not feel very safe when he was a child, he noticeably softened. And when we commented on how sad it was that he needed to learn to protect himself at such an early age because the adults in his life did not, Tom burst into tears and sobbed off and on for the rest of the session.

The second common clinical picture is one in which the adolescent acts out to a relatively limited degree and in response to discrete triggers, typically either PTSD symptoms or anger at parents. Evaluation generally shows sporadic chemical use and continued good performance at school and in other areas. Often, we also see a "social worker" mentality in these adolescents: They are constantly trying to rescue friends even if this means skipping classes to console a friend who just found out she is pregnant or hiding a runaway friend in their bedroom after the friend tried to stop his stepfather from once again beating up his mother in an intoxicated rage. These adolescents often go through a phase of using chemicals and are at high risk for continuing the progression of use; at evaluation they may or may not be chemically dependent and experiencing a loss of control over chemicals as well as other aspects of their lives. Abstinence, together with individual and group therapy coupled with family therapy, typically results in quick improvement in their behavior.

Although we discuss issues regarding family treatment in more depth in the next chapter, certain issues involving adolescents and their families arise often enough to merit some discussion here. For example, we work very hard to involve parents from the very start of treatment and to keep them engaged in the treatment process. We do this in a number of ways: We strongly insist that at least one parent—and if it is not a single-parent family, then both parents—accompany the adolescent to the intake interview. Our first move is to interview the parents to identify their concerns and to obtain information from them about their child. The parent or parents (or, in some cases, the legal guardian) often know more about the history of the extended family and about the adolescent's early developmental history. We do inquire about any difficulties the parents themselves may be having in terms of issues such as depression and stress, and we also seek information on how other children in the family are doing and about the state of the parents' marital relationship. Moreover, we are careful to join with the parents in their concern for the child. Standard tactics include praising them for caring enough to bring their child in for an assessment and framing all questions and interventions as being "for the sake of the child." For example, we might start our exploration of the parents' marital relationship by stating that having a child in trouble is stressful for everyone and that this stress sometimes makes even loving spouses irritable. We also ask parents to take an MMPI and a SASSI (Substance Abuse Subtle Screening Inventory) (if there is suggestion of parental chemical use), and we urge them to return to discuss the results of their child's psychological testing as well as their own.

We believe that joining with the parents is crucial, a belief that is sorely tested in several situations. In some cases, the adolescent discloses that active and acute physical or sexual abuse is still occurring. We then speak directly with the parents and in a matter-of-fact manner tell them that state laws require that we report this situation. Whenever possible, we try to get the parents—or, in some cases, the child—to make the report. This serves to counteract the teen's perception that the parent has abandoned them or to empower the teen. Obviously, this approach is likely to be difficult for the parent or the adolescent; it is often the case that they cannot make the report or that issues of immediate safety do not permit the time to work on this in therapy. Parents have all kinds of reactions to our informing them of the requirement to report, ranging from relief to disbelief to rage, all of which we are prepared to handle. Using the safety reframe, as always, seems to decrease negative reactions.

A more common dilemma occurs when the assessment process reveals that one or both parents are using chemicals or have some other serious but not acknowledged mental or emotional difficulty. We have found that discounting the parents' perception that the child is the problem and instead focusing exclusively on them is a strategic mistake for several reasons: Sometimes a parent with acting-in problems such as depression is quite amenable to going for help. However, even in this situation, the teen typically still has serious difficulties that require treatment. Parents with more acting-out difficulties, ranging from being highly critical, angry, and controlling to chemical dependence, are likely to blow up and pull the teen out of treatment. We take a middle road in these cases. Having psychological testing to validate our conclusions is helpful because people see this as less "opinionated." We also continue to frame the need for parental work as being for the sake of the child; we might say, for example, "We must clear this matter up and give your child one less excuse to avoid his [or her] own issues." Referring a parent to an outside source for an independent evaluation is another tactic we use to establish a boundary between the parent's reactions or issues and the teen's. This also communicates the message to adolescents that as unfair as it may be they are going to have to give up their futile "codependent" wish to control, save, or dominate the parent and keep the focus on their own recovery. We refer to this process as "psychological emancipation," and this is often the only course left open if parents refuse to acknowledge and deal with their own issues.

Trust is an enormous issue for adolescent survivors. Clear and firm boundaries in the counseling relationship are essential for success. The balancing act for counselors is between respecting the adolescent's need for a safe place to process issues and not enabling the keeping of secrets about the family. There is also the issue of the parents' right to know what is going on in treatment and their need to know in order to keep them engaged in the process. We handle this by establishing the following at the time of intake: the purposes of the evaluation, who is going to receive information about the results of the evaluation, the standard requirement for all adolescents to take a urine drug screen if there is any question at all of chemical use (including our policy that we consider a refusal as the equivalent of a "dirty result"), our legal and ethical responsibility to inform parents of risky behaviors on the part of their child, and our policy of keeping parents informed of the adolescent's general issues. We also establish an agreement with adolescent clients that if they tell us something they do not want their parents or the school to know, we might need to discuss the issue further. We do let the adolescent know that the details of what they tell us, with the exception of matters that threaten their safety and health, will be kept confidential. If a safety issue is involved, we will need to inform parents and school counselors. If the adolescent relapses (which is particularly likely to happen with either renewed use of chemicals or a return of self-harm impulses) during treatment, our standard approach is to hold him or her accountable for telling the parents. We tell the teen that we are willing to negotiate a reasonable time frame for this (e.g., 3 days) and that if he or she still cannot comply, we will tell the parents. We then handle as a counseling issue whatever resistances, fears, or concerns arise. Generally speaking, we frame the issue as one of "honesty in recovery" and also point out to teens the likely advantages of having the parents receive the information about relapse from them rather than from us. Finally, we tell the adolescent about all phone conversations, letters, and hallway and other meetings between us and the parents unless there is some very good reason not to do this, and we prefer to hold all parental meetings with the teen in the room. We usually find that once trust has been established in our relationship, our adolescent clients prefer that we speak with their parents without them in the room, since they wish to avoid being in such close quarters with their concerned or angry parent.

Owing to issues related both to trust and good boundaries (not to mention transference), we usually have different counselors for individual and family therapy, and it is imperative that the two therapists work as a team. This approach defuses some of the problems that often arise when a single therapist attempts both roles. The few times early in our practice that we attempted to assume both roles the therapy ended in disaster. This is particularly likely because the majority of the adolescents we treat need both corralling and supporting. For individual counseling with addicted adolescent survivors in early recovery to work, some form of positive transference based on support for the counseling is required. Family work is more likely to focus on helping corral these adolescents, who have very strong negative reactions if the counselor they have for individual therapy is supportive (but not enabling) in one session but firmly (but not unkindly) backs the parents to maintain a reasonable level of control in the next. These teens are very black and white in their thinking, and splitting is a common defense; they have a difficult time not feeling abandoned by the individual counselor who is also the family therapist. We use a family counselor either in our agency or in the community, being very careful to maintain constant communication with that therapist in order to exchange information and develop a clear picture of what is going on with the adolescent and the family. It is also common for the sensitive teen survivor to interpret the neutral stance of the family therapist as indicative of abandonment or of being on the parents' side. The individual counselor, however, can go on to smooth the way for successful family meetings and can begin to chip away at the black-and-white thinking of the adolescent as part of the individual therapy sessions. To keep the boundaries as clear as possible, we also arrange for parents who require a great deal of support and who call frequently with minicrises to contact the family therapist and not the individual counselor.

MEDICATIONS

Many parents express strong reservations about the use of medication. We also tend to be conservative about recommending a medication evaluation with adolescents and do so only when there are strong indications from our evaluation and/or ongoing observations that medication is likely to be an issue. Depression that interferes with the ability of the adolescent to attend school or retain information, anxiety that is so high that he or she cannot even attend to therapy, or mood swings so severe that sessions are a constant stream of crisis management are all signs that medication is indicated and can be helpful. It sometimes reassures parents when we take the time to carefully review with them the basis for our recommendations and/or decide by mutual agreement on a certain point in time by which we expect to see improvement and beyond which, if improvement is not evident, we will get a medication evaluation.

Other issues around medication sometimes come up. A few parents, whether because they are stressed out or passive aggressive, forget to fill prescriptions or just never seem to get around to making the necessary appointments; a kind but insistent phone call from us, particularly after a minicrisis, is often enough to do the trick. Sometimes adolescents refuse to take their prescribed medication. Questioning often reveals that this is due to their intolerance of side effects, and working with the consulting physician to come up with alternatives resolves this issue. Occasionally, adolescents refuse to take their medication either because they want to win in a power struggle or because they are planning to use chemicals again and fear a bad reaction. We advise parents not to get into the position of forcing pills down their adolescent's throat. We encourage them to continue to apply reasonable consequences for misbehavior and to allow their son or daughter's therapist to help the adolescent make the connection between taking medication (and thus following the behavior contract previously agreed to) and, say, the increased likelihood of having the car for the weekend.

OTHER THERAPY STRATEGIES WITH ADDICTED TEEN SURVIVORS

This would not be a very practical model for treating the adolescent survivor if we did not address the issue of the therapeutic alliance. In all therapeutic relationships it is the job of the clinician to facilitate a helpful alliance that can lead to therapeutic change. It is essential that those of us who work with teens understand their point of view yet also demonstrate ourselves to be competent and trustworthy authority figures. Some counselors try too hard to be youthful and "cool"; while adolescents may enjoy the chat, it is unlikely that they will be able to take the counselor's advice seriously. Other counselors are too parental, and this approach is also unsuccessful.

Counselors have a unique opportunity to offer teens a safe and helpful relationship with an authority figure. In order to develop this key relationship there are some things that need to take place: To begin with, counselors need to *join* with their adolescent client, that is, to understand through reflective listening what the *teen* sees as the problem; it is important to the teen survivor to feel heard. Next, counselors need to convey the fact that they have information or skills that might help improve the teen's current problem or situation and that they are an *expert* in this area. Counselors must be prepared to prove that they can be *consistently caring* about adolescent clients and their situation without enabling them. Survivors are highly intuitive; if they sense that a counselor does not care or is not being honest, they will not be able to develop trust in the relationship. In sharing who they are as a real person counselors assist the teen survivor in seeing them as more than a well-read observer and as someone who has had problems and has overcome them. Clearly, boundaries about appropriate personal disclosure apply here; nevertheless, when counselors share some of their true self, it is easier for adolescents to share those wounded parts of themselves.

Most of the recovery suggestions discussed for survivors in Chapter 4 are helpful for teens as well. It is important not only that all individual therapy be geared to the client's learning the symptoms of PTSD and understanding issues of safety but that the chemical dependency recovery be integrated into treatment. We constantly refer to the need to work a *dual* recovery program. An excellent example of this is our conclusion that modifications in doing step work are necessary with adolescents, especially those who are survivors. For example, even more than other survivors, adolescent survivors have difficulty with Step One's notion of powerlessness. Surrender is often the last thing these teens want to do. The notion of a higher power is also especially difficult for these teens. They often see themselves as their own higher power and dislike the idea that they should have to ask for help from any other person or entity. God is, of course, the ultimate authority figure. Youth who have issues with authority find that giving their power and life to God is difficult. Our orientation toward safety is the way we deal with issues of powerlessness. We also work very slowly with teens to help them find some form of a higher power they can feel safe with and toward which they can develop a reasonable relationship. Many youth choose their own unique higher power, such as "the universe" or "karma" or "special energy." Allowing them to tailor their concept of a higher power to their own needs gives these adolescents more ownership in the process and avoids power struggles.

As a preview of parts of the next chapter, we use the same recovery model for families as we do for individuals. We work to establish safety in the home, setting up no-harm agreements and fail-safe plans to handle acute issues. We develop a home behavior contract to handle issues of behavior and discipline and use the negotiation of this contract as an opportunity to educate parents about appropriate levels of control and to teach negotiation skills to all parties.

We have watched many sensitive mothers attempt mother–daughter counseling with a hypersensitive, hypervigilant survivor daughter. The mothers find that there is no way they can say anything right. The daughters may complain that a detached mother is abandoning them, or they may complain that the attentive mother is "too nosy" and "bugs" them all the time. Many tired and frustrated parents are no longer sure how to behave in their child's presence. We often use a home behavior contract to provide for some structure and consistency in the home. These contracts may be simplistic target behaviors or more elaborate systems.

We encourage parents to attend support groups such as Al-Anon; to begin to take their own medication, when appropriate; and to begin their own therapy, as needed. We run a three-session education program for parents that covers material about both chemical dependence and PTSD, and we give parents tips for handling difficult situations that commonly arise, including incidents of self-harm, chemical use relapse, and outbursts of anger. As the home situation settles down, we pinpoint trigger sequences of various family members and work to anchor new skills into these situations. And if all goes well, we arrange for family clarification sessions as part of integration work. Often, parents end up in their own therapy groups working on their own issues of learning more helpful coping skills and how to set firm boundaries on their child while keeping an eye toward safety for themselves as well as their child.

REFERENCES

1. Harnsberger, C. T. (Ed.). (1948). *Mark Twain at your fingertips*. New York: Beechhurst Press.
2. Eccles, J. S., Midgley, C., & Adler, T. (1984). Grade-related changes in the school environment: Effects on achievement motivation. In J. G. Nicholls (Ed.), *The development of achievement motivation* (pp. 283–331). Greenwich, CT: JAI Press.
3. Buchanan, C. M., Eccles, J. S., & Becker, J. B. (1992). Are adolescents the victims of raging hormones? Evidence for the activational effects of hormones on moods and behavior in adolescence. *Psychological Bulletin, 111*, 62–107.
4. U.S. Congress/Office of Technology Assessment. (1991). *Adolescent health: Vol. 2. Background and the effectiveness of selected prevention and treatment services* (OTA-H-465). Washington, DC: U.S. Government Printing Office.
5. Sroufe, A., & Rutter, M. (1984). The domain of developmental psychopathology. *Journal of Child Development, 55*, 17–29.

6. Powers, S. I., Hauser, S. T., & Kilner, L. A. (1989). Adolescent mental health. *American Psychologist, 44,* 200–208.

7. Eddles, J. S., Midgley, C., Wigfield, A., et al. (1993). Development during adolescence: The impact of stage–environment fit on young adolescents' experiences in schools and in families. *American Psychologist, 48*(2), 90–101.

8. Elliott, D. D., Huizinga, D., & Ageton, S. S. (1985). *Multiple problem youth: Delinquency, substance abuse and mental health problems.* Beverly Hills, CA: Sage.

9. Richardson, J. L., Dwyer, K., McQuigan, K., et al. (1989). Substance use among eighth-grade students who take care of themselves after school. *Pediatrics, 84,* 556–566.

10. Erikson, E. H. (1963). *Childhood and society* (2nd ed.). New York: Norton.

11. Cole, P. M., & Putnam, F. W. (1992). Effect of incest on self and social functioning: A developmental psychopathological perspective. *Journal of Consulting and Clinical Psychology, 60*(2), 174–182.

12. Havighurst, R. J. (1972). *Developmental tasks and education* (3rd ed.). New York: McKay.

13. Elkind, D. (1967). Egocentrism in adolescence. *Child Development, 38,* 1025–1037.

14. Enright, R. D., Shulka, D. G., & Lapsey, D. K. (1980). Adolescent egocentrism-sociocentrism and self-consciousness. *Journal of Youth and Adolescence, 9,* 101–109.

15. Keating, D. P. (1980). Thinking processes in adolescence. In J. Adelson (Ed.), *Handbook of adolescent psychology.* New York: Wiley.

16. Black-Grubman, S. D. (1990). *Broken boys: Mending men.* New York: Ivy Books.

17. Grotevant, H. D. (1984). The contribution of the family to the facilitation of identity in early adolescence. *Journal of Early Adolescence, 2,* 28–35.

18. Higgings, E. T., & Parsons, J. E. (1983). Social cognition and the social life of the child: Stages as subcultures. In E. T. Higgings, D. W. Ruble, & W. W. Hartup (Eds.), *Social cognition and social behavior: Developmental issues* (pp. 15–62). Cambridge: Cambridge University Press.

19. Barnes, G. G., Farrell, M. P., & Cairns, A. L. (1986). Parental socialization factors and adolescent drinking behaviors. *Journal of Marriage and the Family, 48,* 27–36.

20. Meyers, J. D. (1986). Personal communication.

Addicted Survivors in Their Families, at Work, and in Therapy Groups

✧

Memorabilia: A Journal Entry

"I've been spending more time alone in my room lately. I'm usually just thinking, thinking of all the questions I have about my future. But I suppose this behavior is not uncommon for a 20-year-old. The age of 20 feels so isolated, as though all other 20-year-olds are stranded together on an island, not wanting to be teenagers, yet not allowed to be adults.

"Yesterday while examining these thoughts in my room, I began picking through my good-luck charm box. It's a small wooden box, about 2 inches by 3 inches. The inside of the box is lined with velvet, and the box itself is only an inch deep. Inside this small space I keep trinkets that mean much more than the space they demand. In the box there are five miniature antique dice which I always won craps with when the game was in fashion among my friends; a small handful of quartz crystals that were given to me at a Grateful Dead concert; and a penny from 1977. I felt the year 1977 to be a lucky one because the Portland Trailblazers brought home the world championship that year. As I flipped the tarnishing coin between my fingers, my mind rolled back to the year that I had believed to be so lucky. . . . I could almost see the images perfectly in my mind; the particular day I remember from 1977 was the day that I, as a 5-year-old child, was separated from my innocence and hope for a painless future.

"I was a tiny thing, only about 3 feet tall at the age of 5. I sat in one of my mother's antique school desks, and I practiced writing my name. My angel-white hair hung before my eyes as I formed a large and unproportioned 'M' with my pencil. The pencil seemed so long and fat that my little fingers could barely control it. Suddenly I realized that I could spell my name no further than 'Ma.' I was so frustrated. I knew that my mother had just showed me yesterday how to spell my first and last name; why couldn't I remember? At that moment my oldest of two brothers came into the room. He was 15. I knew that I could trust him to give me the proper spelling, so I asked him, 'How do I spell my name? Mom told me and I forgot.'

"He sat beside me on the desk bench, and he spelled out my name as I fumbled to get the letters out legibly; this was very important to a 5-year-old who was entering kindergarten. He explained that I could write better if he put his hand over mine and helped me form the letters. I was excited about the idea. I couldn't wait until I was 15 and could come up with such smart ideas!

"He put one arm over my left shoulder and hovered over me as he guided my right hand with his. My writing was much better, I was very pleased, and I was eager to write even more when he pulled the pencil from my grasp and asked me to sit on the couch. I had been holding my small baby doll in my left hand, which I carried with me to the couch. He sat down beside me and told me to lie down; I obeyed. He then proceeded to lie down beside me and covered us both with an orange blanket. I didn't know why I had to lie down; I figured it must be nap time. I pulled my baby doll close to my chest to hug while I slept. When my brother saw the doll, he tore it from my hands and threw it across the room, explaining that I wouldn't be needing her. I looked at him curiously. He asked me, 'Do you remember those magazines that we looked at in the tree house?' 'Yes,' I said. 'Do you remember what those people were doing in those pictures?' 'Yes,' I said, remembering the nude men and women and the strange positions, playing with each other's pee-pees. 'Well, we are going to do those things, because they are fun, and you can't tell anyone because we will get into trouble.' I learned quickly that it was not fun. He touched my body in places that only my mother had touched with a washcloth in the bathtub. He tried to put his fingers in the place that I thought that pee-pee came from. After a while he began to use his tongue to examine the area rather than his fingers. My whole body tensed up, this was so foreign, so strange. He told me to do the same to him, and he told me just how to do it. He told me that big girls like to do this. Being big was very important to a 5-year-old.

"That day in 1977 set the pattern for the next 5 years. Each time that I was left alone with my older brother, these things would occur. I would stuff each occurrence into the back of my mind, where they would stew until 1990.

"Sometimes it feels like no one really believes me because no one in my family really wants to. I know that none of them really understands the severity of my abuse, none but my eldest brother. When I confronted my parents with the reality in 1990, they were put into a state of numbness where I believe that they have remained, unable to give me the emotional support that I needed and still need. My sister grieved briefly but has put the situation to the back of her mind. I told my other brother this year in 1993. He said that he is 'here for me' but isn't 'ready' to hear the details or to face the depths of my abuse. Today the tarnished penny dated 1977 is gone. It has been replaced by a shiny 1990 edition— 1990 was the year I began regaining my self-worth and hope; those things are important to everyone."

—MAUREEN, age 20

Maureen's story illustrates how the trauma of sexual abuse reverberates throughout the family. Even trauma that is "external," such as rape or abuse perpetrated by someone outside the family, has an impact on families. Both trauma and chemical dependency (simply living with a practicing alcoholic/addict is very likely to be traumatic) are family "dis-eases." Since these diseases are embedded in a family context, affecting parents, siblings, spouses, and children of addicted survivors, no discussion of dual recovery for addicted survivors would be complete without exploring family issues.

Although our main focus in this chapter is on families, we also briefly explore issues that arise for addicted survivors in work settings and in treatment groups, both those that are professionally run and self-help ones. These groups often resemble second families for members and are settings where addicted survivors are likely to encounter triggers that can prompt the re-creation of family-of-origin dynamics.

FAMILY LIFE, PAST AND PRESENT

Addicted survivors bring with them into their current lives a family legacy that operates at many different levels and in many different ways, a legacy that treatment must take into account. This is immediately obvious in treating addicted survivors who are adolescents or who are young adults still living at home. However, even clients who have separated from home and whose grandparents and parents may be long dead bring "ghosts" with them into their current relationships, including therapy.

The literature on the impact of growing up in an alcoholic home provides important insights into family issues, insights that clients can often easily recognize as applicable to themselves. Many addicted survivors are children of alcoholics regardless of who their abusers were. Growing up in a family where parents are emotionally unavailable owing to their preoccupation with alcohol or with the alcoholic family member is often enough, in and of itself, to cause traumatic damage. Much of this damage revolves around intense feelings of emotional abandonment. Cermak, who has written about adult children of alcoholics, has been a forceful proponent of the need to consider not only what happened to these individuals but also what did not happen (1). If parents are unavailable emotionally or are inconsistent or untrustworthy because of their addiction or "coaddiction" (dependent relationship with an addict), the child develops intense survivor issues even when no overt physical or sexual abuse occurs. We worked with one man, for example, who described his father as the "12-hour dad." Warm, nurturing, and supportive when sober, this father became distant and critical as the evening cocktail time progressed. Many COAs (children of alcoholics) grow up scared and have an "empty hole" inside. COAs may seek to fill this hole, this sense of being empty inside, through chemicals, sexual acting out, food compulsions, relationship addiction, or other external fixes.

The following is a philosophy statement, taken from the ACOA (Adult Children of Alcoholics) group in our area, that illustrates these issues and points toward a solution:

The Problem
Many of us find that we have several characteristics in common as a result of being brought up in a alcoholic household. We came to feel isolated, uneasy with other people, especially authority figures. To protect ourselves, we became people-pleasers even though we lost our identities in the process. Personal criticism is perceived as a threat. We either become alcoholics ourselves or marry them, or both. Failing that we find another compulsive personality such as a workaholic to fulfill our sick need for abandonment. We live life from the standpoint of being victims. We have an overdeveloped sense of responsibility and prefer to be concerned with others rather than ourselves. We somehow get guilt feelings if we stand up for ourselves rather than giving in to others. Thus, we become reactors rather than actors, letting others take the initiative. We are dependent personalities who are terrified of abandonment, who will do almost anything to hold onto a relationship in order not to be abandoned emotionally. Yet we keep choosing insecure relationships because they match our childhood relationship with our alcoholic parents. Thus, alcoholism can be seen as a family disease and we can be seen as coalcoholics, those who take on the

characteristics of the disease without necessarily ever taking a drink. We learned to stuff our feelings in childhood and keep them buried as adults through that conditioning. In consequence, we confuse love and pity and tend to love those that we can rescue. Even more self-defeating, we become addicted to excitement in all of our affairs, preferring constant upsets to workable relationships.

This is a description not an indictment!

The Solution

By attending Al-Anon meetings on a regular basis, we learn that we can work our lives in a meaningful manner. We learn to change our attitudes and habits and find serenity and even happiness! We accept alcoholism as a threefold disease—mental, physical, and spiritual. We came to see our parents as victims of this disease that if not arrested ends in insanity or death. We see ourselves as covictims who must forgive ourselves and other victims, especially our parents. We learn the three Cs of alcoholism: We didn't Cause it, we can't Control it, we can't Cure it. We learned to detach with love and how to practice tough love—the love that allows everyone concerned to exchange role-playing for reality. We use the Al-Anon slogans. We learn to feel our feelings and express them. We apply the serenity prayer to our daily lives and use the telephone to share experiences, strength, and hope on a regular basis.

Meanwhile we work the Al-Anon steps that allow us to accept the disease, realize that our lives have become unmanageable and that we are powerless over the disease and the alcoholic. This work gives us a chance to look at our defects and thinking in a nonjudgmental way—in a heal-thyself way that promotes healthy attitudes and actions. Through this work experience, we come to believe there is a solution other than ourselves . . . a spiritual solution that includes a power greater than ourselves in the group and in a Creative Spirit that many of us call God and others call "the Good." We learn, we act, we love. This is the program that we invite you to accept into your life—one day at a time (2).

COAs may also find it difficult to accept their own chemical dependence if they still have a lot of unresolved anger toward the alcoholic parent (3). Many COAs promised God and themselves that they would never grow up and be like the alcoholic parent. The realization that they too have become addicted to a chemical challenges this pledge as well as the belief that the alcoholic parent was weak-willed. Accepting that addiction is a disease means they not only have to forgive themselves for breaking their childhood pledge but also have to begin to see that their parents were sick, not bad. Counselors need to be alert to this as a possible source of denial and must be prepared to address this as part of the acceptance process. Attendance at group meetings for adult children of alcoholics during the education stage of dual recovery can be helpful to addicted survivors of alcoholic homes as part of working through these issues.

Claudia Brown has written about the three unspoken rules that characterize interactions in an alcoholic family: Don't talk, don't feel, and don't trust (4). These rules also apply to other unhealthy families. The "don't tell" rule describes the denial and secret keeping common to these families. Survivors receive the message to keep the secret in ways that range from subtle to gross. Sometimes the perpetrator makes direct threats designed to maintain secrecy, such as threats of killing the victim or a member of the family. Sometimes the abandoning parent accuses family members who speak up of lying or of wanting to break up the family. Sometimes family members minimize the abuse, change the topic when it arises, or express such obvious discomfort that survivors, ever hypervigilant, know that their truth is not welcome. Maureen's journal entry, with which this chapter begins, reflects this process. Dishonesty, in such forms as lying, minimizing, repressing, and keeping up appearances while actually in a lot of emotional pain on the inside, becomes a way of life. Survivors also automatically assume that they know what others are thinking, intending, and so forth, having had little experience with people who are likely to be honest and with the notion that open and explicit communication, problem solving, and negotiating are possible. The "don't feel" rule refers to the need to bury, stuff, deny, repress, and dissociate feelings. Expressions of genuine feelings are not welcome in these homes. Being hit even harder to "give you something to really cry about," being told to "respect your [abusive] parents, young lady," or being asked "Can't you see I'm sick [hung over]?" hardly encourages a person to have real feelings; going numb and dissociating is typically the only available option. The "don't trust" rule refers to the unpredictability and inconsistency of so many abusive and neglectful families as well as to the violation of basic trust that occurs with trauma. "I can't count on people" is the form of this lesson that so many survivors carry with them and that perpetuates their inclination to seek safety through disconnection.

Apart from their contribution to the various survivor syndromes, these rules serve to contribute to the maintenance of an addiction or coaddiction. Chemicals serve to either help numb feelings or induce artificial ones. Moreover, chemically dependent persons already have ready access to the dishonesty that supports denial about chemical use, having had years of practice in dishonesty in their family of origin. Firmly believing that this is how families function, survivors simply use the same denial strategies for coping with an addicted or otherwise seriously impaired family member and even with "normal" family life.

Several authors, though using somewhat different schemes, have

used the notion of roles to describe what happens in an alcoholic family
(4, 5). In this context a role refers to a set of standard behaviors and its
place in the family structure. We use the following role descriptions to
help clients identify their stereotypical roles and the changes they need
to make to relate to others in a healthier way. Readers should keep in mind
that while we identify some roles as being more commonly filled by
parents and others as being more commonly assumed by children, other
configurations are possible.

- *The Sick Person* (who is alcoholic/addicted, mentally ill, or emotionally unavailable). This person is the one whose illness, disorder, or condition is responsible for the family's need to compensate or cope. Other family members organize themselves around
  this individual, and dealing with that member's behavior is the
  preoccupation of all family members.
- *The Enabler or Coalcoholic.* This person spends all of his or her time
  and emotional energy trying to save or rescue the sick person. If
  the sick person is alcoholic, the enabler might be hiding the bottle
  or the car keys. The enabler often assumes the role of martyr,
  complaining, "I do so much for everyone else, and no one appre-
  ciates me!" The enabler's helpfulness, which is often done with the
  best of intentions and/or out of fear of the consequences of the
  sick person's problem behaviors, is very often, ironically, part of
  the problem, not the solution. The enabler's attempts to help
  actually maintain the problem by, for example, minimizing the
  consequences that would naturally follow from the sick person's
  behavior, thus making it easier for the alcoholic/addict to continue the substance use. Bailing the alcoholic/addict out of jail or
  calling in sick for this person when he or she is hung over are just
  two examples of this type of enabling. Enabling can reach insane
  proportions, as in, for example, cases where the mother helps her
  daughter "clean up" after the father has molested the child.
- *The Hero.* This person tries to be perfect and to avoid getting into
  trouble. He or she thinks, "If I can just be a good enough girl or
  boy, then maybe I will be able to get the love and attention I need."
  This is not likely to happen, however, because the parents' dysfunction leaves no room for the needs of the children, resulting in the
  hero being ignored or criticized no matter how well he or she does.
  The hero also allows family members to think they are doing
  something right to have such a good child. The oldest child is a
  natural for this role. Heroes are chronically hardworking and
  placating, but they are also lonely, depressed, anxious, and resentful.

- *The Scapegoat.* This person carries the blame for all the troubles of the rest of the family. "If little Bill didn't get into so much trouble all the time, then maybe we would all be happy and Dad [or Mom] wouldn't have to drink so much!" is an example of the dynamic of this role. And, in fact, the person taking on the scapegoat role is often acting out. It is the scapegoat who often comes to the attention of counselors and juvenile court officials when his or her anger outbursts, drug use, and/or delinquency gets him or her in trouble. At other times, the scapegoat's behavior is well within normal limits but he or she still gets targeted as the problem by family members. Either way, the scapegoat serves to keep the focus off some or all of the difficulties in the family.
- *The Lost Child.* This person "checks out" to escape what is going on in the family. Lost children often develop an active fantasy world or spend a great deal of time alone in their rooms reading or playing computer games. They are so good at not being noticed that they may find they are ignored in other social settings; they are easy to overlook in the classroom and even in therapy groups. Usually shy and withdrawn, lost children have little sense of self and of their feelings. As adults, these persons tend to disappear in their marriages and from their children.
- *The Mascot.* This person clowns around, tells jokes, or otherwise engages in behavior that distracts the family from upsetting conversations or situations. Like persons in the lost child role, mascots deny their own anger and depression and deflect all negative input with a funny one-liner or a distracting comment.

The Three Triggers

We have identified the issues of survivors in Chapter 3. These trauma related responses include focal, fear-based triggers; more generalized abandonment triggers; and shame triggers. Survivors carry all three sets of triggers into their current relationships. The classic example involves the sexual fears and dysfunction that survivors of sexual abuse carry into their relationships with boyfriends/girlfriends, spouses, and lovers. Quite often these difficulties are not evident early in the relationship but emerge later on. Whether because of the initial rush provided by the infatuation of early courtship and/or because of the insulation provided by intoxication, survivors and their partners often report at least an adequate sexual adjustment early in their relationship. However, the waning of infatuation and, most importantly for addicted survivors, attempts at sexual relations when the partners are sober reveal the underlying sexual fears. Another common fear trigger for survivors is the anger trigger, especially for survivors of physical abuse. Survivors with this fear trigger tend to overreact to anger in others, either by blowing up and raging all out of proportion to the situation or by completely going to pieces. We very commonly see this with mothers, themselves survivors, of angry survivor teens.

Abandonment triggers are more generalized and in some ways more devastating to family relationships because they are more pervasive. The chances are that survivors will, in fact, routinely reexperience abandonment in a vicious cycle of self-confirming and self-defeating behavior in their intimate relationships. We are constantly saying to clients in our therapy sessions "Ask for what you need; you might just get it," or "Don't guess; ask what your family member needs and wants from you right now." The third question in this intervention is to prompt the client to ask him- or herself, "What can I do to help myself feel safe and supported?" The goal with this intervention is to establish that the task is a mutual one and to abort any one-sided thinking that it is all up to the survivor or all up to a family member to provide all of the protection and support.

The final trigger that influences families is the one that involves shame. Whether it is the shame of the trauma or the shame of addiction, shame issues infiltrate and pollute family life. Shame leads to denial, to unrealistic needs to be perfect and look good, and/or to isolation from others out of a fear that if others knew about one's past and "real" self, they would be appalled. Shame interferes with the development of healthy intimacy, whether between spouses/partners or between parent and child. So much of the hypersensitivity of the survivor is a product of this "shame wound" and its self-centered quality, which constantly distorts the survivor's reactions to others and makes him or her see the moods and behaviors of family members as being totally in reaction to himself or herself. "He's mad at me, and I didn't do anything," is an example of this automatic thinking. This grandiosity, whether expressed narcissistically or codependently, contributes to enmeshment in the family. We encourage clients and their family members to ask and honestly answer the question "Is this my problem, their problem, or our problem?" to remedy this destructive distortion. We also constantly promote the themes of "sick, not bad" and "making a mistake does not make you a mistake" to combat shame-based reactions.

The classic situation that ignites both abandonment and shame issues for survivors is the response of others when they tell their story. Statements of outright denial or blaming of the survivor—"You're lying!" or "You caused it!"—are examples of responses that trigger feelings of shame and abandonment in survivors. More subtle but just as powerful are responses that imply denial but that may actually represent well-meaning but clumsy attempts of family members to cope with the trauma themselves. Examples of such responses include the following: "Why didn't you tell me?" "Why didn't you run away?" "Why were you walking down that street?" and even "How could you be alcoholic?" No matter what the intention and motivation of the family member, survivors inevitably hear such responses as confirmation of their worst fears, namely, that family members will blame them, will fail to understand them, will refuse to support them, or will not gratify their wish for the "missing experience." Helping survivor clients come to terms with family members who remain in denial is a crucial part of our treatment with them. We help clients facing this situation to understand that powerful forces are working in the family to maintain the "secret" and that family members are clinging to their statements of denial primarily to affirm their own truth and only secondarily to have others believe them. We also ask clients to explore the possibility that their family members' reactions are an unfortunate but understandable narcissistic response to their learning about what happened, not a statement about the client. We also work with willing family members to help them understand why the survivor is so touchy about this issue and to help them accept and integrate what happened.

The Two Axes

Many models of family functioning exist, but none have achieved universal acceptance. A colleague uses a model with two axes to summarize a great deal of the literature on family dysfunction and conceptualize some of the key clinical issues found in troubled families (6). The first axis has the endpoints of chaos and rigidity, and the second axis has the endpoints of enmeshment and disengagement. Putting together these two axes results in the following schema:

Families in general (and relationships between family members) fall somewhere on the rigid–chaotic and enmeshed–detached dimensions.

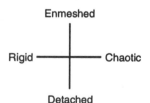

The further their position on these axes is from the center, the more unhealthy their functioning. Rigid families have inflexible, overly determined rules; they have a difficult time responding to exceptions or changes in circumstances and seem to have rules mainly for the sake of rules: "We only have dessert on Fridays, and, no matter what, all kids should be in bed at 7:00 P.M." Families that are chaotic are unpredictable and inconsistent in their behaviors, and rules (if made at all) are made to be broken; schedules are erratic, expectations are unclear or uncertain, and interactions vary widely from day to day. Enmeshed families have very weak boundaries and feel totally responsible for each other's feelings and problems; the members of such families are too connected to each other. The members of detached families are very distant from each other, communication is poor, and relationships are cool and distant. Members of detached and chaotic families have no idea what is going on with each other because of the disorganization and distance in the family. Enmeshed and chaotic families are disorganized and highly reactive to whatever crisis comes along. Rigid and detached families leave children feeling criticized and abandoned whereas enmeshed and rigid families monitor their family members with a vengeance.

The ideal is for a family to be as close to the middle of these axes as possible. The family therapist can help a family strive for emotional boundaries that allow its members to be both a part of the family and themselves and for rules that provide structure but do so flexibly.

FAMILIES AND THE GENERAL RECOVERY MODEL

The beauty and utility of our general recovery model is that it applies to work with families as well as with individuals (and even with the "internal family" of the client with DID). We use the five stages of crisis, skills building, education, integration, and maintenance to pinpoint the interventions necessary for a given family. We ask ourselves, "Is the family situation dangerous, very chaotic, abusive, or obviously unhealthy?" An affirmative answer suggests the implementation of crisis-type interventions, perhaps filing a report of abuse with children's protective services, getting clients and family members to agree to a contract for no physical or emotional abuse, or developing fail-safe plans such as calling 911 or other emergency numbers or staying with another relative or family if things begin to escalate. Affirmative answers to such questions as "Does the family appear to have difficulty discussing issues calmly and productively or to have difficulty observing their own process?" and "Are they lacking in support?" suggest the need for skills-level interventions, with an emphasis on communication and negotiation skills. Referrals to Al-Anon and/or to codependency groups also appear indicated. Do family members appear to be struggling with the implications of the diagnoses of chemical dependency and PTSD? If so, a referral to our parent and spouse education series appears indicated. These classes cover such topics as the signs and symptoms of these diagnoses, common problems that family members face and how to handle them, and the material presented earlier on dysfunctional families. Does the family know all the right things but still relapse on certain trigger issues? Do family members appear to have done their grieving? Integration sessions helping family members continue to work on acceptance of what happened and its impact and on busting old "trance loops" are likely to be helpful. Are families ready to proceed on their own? Developing a maintenance plan prior to discharge is likely to prevent relapses down the road.

TEEN SURVIVORS AND FAMILY THERAPY

Many of the survivor families we see often respond in a reactive fashion and are unable to form a balanced structure that would prevent constant crisis and overreactions. A written agreement provides an external structure that all parties can use in the heat of the moment or when everyone is tired and worn-out. We start by joining with adolescents around how helpful this contract is likely to be to them in getting more of what they want by getting their parents under control. We also let them know that although their parents have the final say, they have a chance to give input and that we will serve as a referee to make sure things are fair. We join with the parents by outlining the virtues of having a clear system for themselves and their child that ensures that they will respond fairly and that the adolescent will be under control. Readers will note the importance of finessing compliance with the details of the written agreement by presenting the control issue in positive terms to all parties and of having everyone commit to the agreement.

We use a standard contract that we modify to fit the individual family (7). The contract addresses such issues as curfews, school attendance, homework completion, chores, clothing and grooming, and other typical hot spots. It also contains items that prohibit chemical use by the client and verbal and physical abuse on the part of all family members; treatment requirements for the adolescent and the family; guidelines for handling requests by the adolescent and denials by the parents; and provisions for decreasing nagging and increasing praise and compliments by the parents. Items pertinent to the particular family are added to the contract. For example, if the adolescent has complained that he or she never gets to spend any time with the father, we negotiate with the family on the wording of an item addressing this issue.

Consequences come in the form of a system of levels in which all rewards come to the adolescent when he or she is on level three. Driving and dating privileges, later curfews, allowances, and all the freedom the family can tolerate are part of Level 3 privileges. An infraction of the behavior contract, such as skipping school or missing a curfew, leads to a drop to a lower level. Level 2 involves being grounded and doing a work task but with some privileges, such as phone use and time-limited visits by friends, still intact. Level 1 is restriction to one's room with nothing electrical in the room except a light bulb. The level drop per infraction is generally limited to 24 hours except in cases of violence, stealing, and chemical use, and adolescents work their way back up to Level 3 with 24 hours of compliance at each level.

The contract and the process of negotiating it allows us to intervene in several ways: By reinforcing appropriate family structures and levels of control the process allows us to correct the family's distorted notions of what constitutes an appropriate amount of control and freedom for an adolescent. By negotiating contract items in a reasonable fashion we actually model behaviors family members can use when they negotiate issues. And by exploring issues of safety, protection, and nurturing with families we attempt to shift the atmosphere in the family so that more of these ingredients can be provided.

SPECIAL ISSUES FOR SURVIVOR PARTNERS

Resuming or attempting sexual relations when sober reveals the survivor's underlying sexual fears. One of two scenarios then commences. The first is the complete cessation of all sexual activity or the beginning of dissociated once-a-month sex that is accompanied by a "maybe now I'll be left alone" attitude. The second scenario is the conducting of an affair, a solution that may feel familiar to the survivor since it mimics the dissociation of sex and true intimacy that was part of their early conditioning around sexual activity.

We worked with one couple whose sex life involved having sexual relations once a month. After redefining sex as "safe touch," we then explored specific touch triggers. In the therapy session we asked the couple to hug and "notice what happens." The survivor wife noticed that she felt "suffocated" if the hug lasted more than a few seconds. The husband noticed that his wife seemed to go "limp," a response he experienced as rejection; he noticed that he, in turn, wanted to withdraw in anger. Tracing the roots of this trigger for him revealed the fact that his parents were masters of qualified praise who always made a critical comment no matter what he did. Exploring the source of her sensation of suffocating, the wife disclosed that her perpetrator often held her down and put his hand over her mouth. She had learned to go limp and to dissociate in order to survive an overwhelming sense of helplessness and powerlessness. Both partners, hearing these revelations, were able to take the other's reactions less personally. Further investigation showed that the wife felt more comfortable with hugging if she and her husband were sitting side by side on the couch, if they negotiated specific rules about the contact, and if she could say "Stop" at any point. Incorporating these elements into exercises at home proved helpful in gradually increasing the frequency and contact of touching for the couple.

We work with many couples who have had extensive individual and couples counseling in the past but who still have difficulty applying what they know. "We have a fair-fight contract," one couple told us, "but it goes right out the window when we discuss the kids." We inevitably find that couples reach these "stuck" places when they mutually trigger and age-regress, that is, when suddenly they become a 5-year-old and a 7-year-old attempting to maintain a mature relationship. Clients respond very positively when the notion of trance is introduced. This corresponds exactly to their subjective sense of what happens, provides a nonjudgmental frame for their own and their partner's behavior, and gives them hope that something can change. Couples report that the following accomplishments are the most helpful consequences of counseling: learning to take responsibility for their own issues and process, getting out of the habit of blaming each other for problems, learning shuttling skills (as discussed in Chapter 6), and understanding the origins of their own and their partner's triggers.

OTHER COMMON CORE SURVIVOR ISSUES AND THEIR IMPACT ON THE FAMILY

Many addicted survivors are relentlessly critical and dissatisfied with themselves and others. A friend of ours who is a member of a 12-step program describes himself and other recovering alcoholics as "chronically malcontent." We think of this characteristic of survivors as being, at least partially, a component of the protector part of themselves. Being perfect is often a strategy for avoiding the criticism (or even worse actions) of others. Yet the survivor's internal critic also appears to be addicted to criticism. It seems that it just cannot get enough time or topics to satisfy its urgent need for finding fault. Addicted survivors can never be smart enough, fit enough, attractive enough, perfect enough, or far enough in recovery to satisfy their internal critic. This is a defense that has run amok. The resulting anxiety and depression that this internal critic produces contributes to a survivor's unhappiness in recovery and to relapses to chemical use or other unsafe or less than helpful behaviors.

Unfortunately, this perfectionism spills over onto those in the addicted survivor's inner circle. Lovers, spouses, children, and friends are also subject to this relentlessly critical part that so many of our clients exhibit. Therapy needs to address this perfectionism and its impact on clients themselves and on their intimate relationships. Children who get all A's and one B on their report card deserve congratulations on the A's and not an interrogation about the B. And clients need to learn not to be so critical of their spouses. When a survivor has a difficult time responding objectively to off-the-cuff comments, which he or she hears as massively critical, the spouse can help by learning how to give feedback in a gentle, measured way that reduces the likelihood of a major blowup. The spouse and family members also need to work on setting firm limits when they feel attacked or picked on by a hypercritical survivor. Helping clients and their family members understand that no one is perfect and that "easy does it" is a more appropriate attitude will make everyone's life more serene.

Hypersensitivity is a second characteristic we commonly see addicted survivors exhibit that contributes to problems with family members. Our clients' hypersensitivity leads them to be acutely aware of, and to take very personally, the feelings and actions of others. This hypersensitivity also has a self-centered quality in that the core belief is that everything others feel and do somehow always has something to do with the client.

While it might sound appealing to feel as if one is the center of the universe, the reality is far less glamorous. Hypersensitivity does not necessarily make one feel powerful; rather, one tends to have a sense of being buffeted and overwhelmed. When hypersensitive individuals see a scowl on the face of their mate, they may believe their mate is angry with them. To make matters worse, they may inadvertently solicit blame by asking, "Did I do something wrong? Are you mad at me?" If spouses (or angry teenagers) would rather blame others than take responsibility for their own feelings, they now have an opportunity to blame the solicitous survivor for deeds for which the survivor bears no responsibility. In addition, the self-centeredness that is a component of survivors' shame-based narcissistically wounded part can lead survivors to behave at times like a hurt child. This hurt child may be very demanding, wanting constant attention and viewing anything less as complete abandonment. This can lead to some very intense family and marital sessions in which survivors present a long list of their own unmet needs but are totally unaware of the needs of other family members.

If two survivors are in a committed relationship, they bring to it twice the hypersensitivity and its associated features. They each have their own list of expectations of the relationship, such as, "You should *always* be there for me no matter what." Two hyperalert, hypersensitive people sharing love and life together will predictably experience many intense emotional states. Some of these states will be love, adoration, and a spiritual connection never before known, with a feeling of almost merging. At other times, however, the states will include rage and intense feelings of emotional abandonment. Two people who take everything very personally will have a difficult time riding out the waves of daily interactions and talking productively about issues that arise. Helping hypersensitive family members learn to listen to each other objectively and find reasonable ways to respond to each other's triggered urgent sense of need is a necessary task for the counselor.

Projection bedevils addicted survivors' relationships with others, especially intimate ones, and leads to reenactments of old issues. We view projection as the automatic assumptions individuals make about others when unresolved issues become triggered. Projections often cause a self-fulfilling prophecy. Automatically assuming one knows what others are thinking or are likely to do and then acting on these assumptions without checking them out first may bring about the very reaction (often a negative one) that will confirm the assumption. For example, if survivors assume that their spouse is angry because of something the spouse thinks they did (e.g., rather than try to discover whether the spouse had a rough day at work) and if they then react to that unspoken, undeserved charge by getting angry and angrily questioning the spouse, the result may be that the spouse will indeed now feel angry.

The therapeutic task is to help addicted survivors, in both their individual and family sessions, slow down, learn to recognize these assumptions they make, question them on their own, confer with others whom they trust, and then take the risk of trying something different. We find that we have to walk a thin line here. Many times survivors do know how significant others will react and feel angry or ashamed if their judgment is questioned. We find a number of tactics useful in this case: One is to listen for the presentation of a childlike belief, suggesting old trance-based notions that need examining, rather than one that is a factual, adult one. Another is to look for a long-standing pattern of the same difficulties across numerous different relationships. A third is to be tentative and to invite the survivor to reflect on the basis for the belief and to consider some safe tests of it. Working with actual trance states, as described in Chapter 6, helps to dissolve old beliefs and to substitute more realistic ones. "Let's check out that assumption" is a constant refrain in our sessions with our clients. And the fact that survivors make these assumptions in our office during marital and family work provides wonderful opportunities for us to point out that they are doing so and encourage them to do the opposite. This often helps to create a much improved communication system and more reasonable boundaries (neither detached nor enmeshed).

The final issue that constantly causes difficulties in the relationships of addicted survivors is the issue of control. Almost without exception, we find that addicted survivors have strong control needs and that other family members are also likely to have a propensity for wanting excessive control. This oftentimes takes the form of countercontrol reactions.

Keeping things under control is a key survival strategy used by survivors, and substance dependence also encourages a "my way or no way" attitude. Whether this control is an obvious very demanding authoritarian style or a subtle, passive–aggressive manner, control issues make for conflicted and unhappy relationships. Power struggles abound, issues remain unresolved, and gridlock prevails. "He *must* hear what I'm saying about needing good grades to get into college," or, "Tell me what to do to *make* her do it" are comments that illustrate this dynamic. The use of words like *should* or *must*; expressions like "I'm right, and they're wrong"; and the rationale that one must apply still more energy to a tactic that is not working in a relationship with another suggest control issues at work.

Family members are often quite ready to acknowledge control issues when we bring these to their attention. Psychological testing, considered objective by clients, is also helpful here. We ask family members whether control has worked for them and explore the ways in which they try to excessively control interactions with other family members. We point out that the issue is not right or wrong but what is more or less helpful. We work to encourage our clients and their family members to accept limits to the control they have over others and to learn to recognize the signals (such as rage, high levels of frustration, focused intensity) that indicate they are in high "control mode." Encouraging clients to let go, to try something different, or to just wait and see what happens if they refrain from trying to impose control on a situation are ways of helping them experiment with control issues as part of the therapeutic process. When the need to impose control is reframed as a protective strategy and when clients attempt to come to terms with their underlying fear, new insights into what this need for control is all about for them often result. Clients who are increasingly grounded in 12-step attitudes can benefit from being encouraged to "do a Step One or a Step Three" on this issue.

GENERAL TREATMENT STRATEGIES AND ISSUES

Addicted survivors' families, past and present, have an important role to play in successful dual recovery. Assessing family history for at least three generations is important to provide the context for understanding a particular client. At intake we of course ask about a family history of chemical dependence, psychiatric disorders, and traumatic events, internal and external.

Involving the members of the immediate family, as we have already indicated, is essential. A client's significant others are an important source of information about his or her chemical use and survivor syndrome symptoms. Members of the immediate family can also help corral acting-out clients by providing accurate information about their chemical use and other behaviors and about leverage to motivate change (8). Clients who suddenly rescind or cancel their release-of-information agreement to contact family members are very likely relapsing into chemical use and/or other serious psychiatric symptoms or otherwise protecting some "secret."

A corollary to successful treatment is acceptance by clients of the importance of taking responsibility for their own recovery and their own contribution to their problems. So often, clients and their family members arrive at our office blaming each other for what has happened, with each person holding tightly to the belief that he or she can only be happy and healthy if the other person agrees to cooperate with his or her plans for correcting the situation. This inevitably leads to the adoption of a defensive stance by each family member and a control struggle that ends up in gridlock. Parents accuse their children of ruining their lives, and spouses accuse each other with charges of, "You're driving me to drink," or, "You don't love me." Many times the covert agenda of family members is to get the therapist to agree that the identified client is, in fact, the "bad" person and the cause of *all* the family's problems.

We begin our family counseling by developing a good rapport with all family members. We acknowledge them for caring enough to seek help for their "problem," whether this problem is their out-of-control adolescent or a wife that is threatening to leave. We are careful to avoid prematurely using labels such as *addict* or *perpetrator*. Instead, we keep the original statement of the problem simultaneously general and specific by speaking in such terms as "problems with pot use" or "anger issues"; similarly, we begin by referring to family sessions as "conferences" or "consultations." We accept the family's goals in a general sense as treatment objectives but begin to introduce the safety reframe of our general recovery model. Most families can immediately agree with a statement that the initial goal must be the immediate safety and health of all family members. We explain how treatment will benefit each member; for example, we might say to an angry father, "Part of the objective of treatment is to get your kid back in line and your life more manageable." We present ourselves as experts and, wherever possible, try to do something immediately that gives families reason to regard us as resources (e.g., calling the school to inform personnel there that an adolescent has completed an alcohol and drug assessment and can now return to classes). Having done this, we also send the message kindly but firmly that we expect family involvement.

Other postulates that we follow are the cardinal ones of always empowering clients and family members and of eliminating secrets, an issue that comes up repeatedly with respect to reporting abuse and relapses. For example, we work with clients and/or a parent to make the phone call to children's protective services if there is a question of current abuse, and we encourage them to do this right in the session; we are even comfortable spending a session or two encouraging such a phone call, if that is what is required, unless the issue is one of immediate safety and health. Another example of empowering a client is our attempt to encourage a relapsing client, especially an adolescent, to report the relapse directly to family members, as needed. We structure this by first explaining the importance of honesty and accountability for all family members in the matter of maintaining safety and health. We then state that we will wait several days before making the report ourselves but that we prefer that the responsible family member make the report. In the majority of instances clients and family members, although reluctant, do proceed with the necessary reporting.

Communications with family members also raise issues of empowerment and secrecy. We always let everyone know that we will respect client confidence but will not keep secrets, unless there are questions of immediate safety and health. When parents call us to let us know that they think their child has relapsed, we ask them if they have spoken to the child (and we explore the reasons for this with them if they have not) encourage them to confront the child, and tell them that we will tell their child that they have called us. If we have a conference with the spouse of a client, we carefully explore the client's feelings about this and also make sure that the client is in the session. Sometimes there is a question of whether clients should remain in a marriage. We have seen many therapists recommend quickly and without reservation that a client should immediately leave the spouse; these clients, often in early recovery and confused about what they want and need, then spend years feeling ambivalent about and regretful of their decision. We take a different stance. We do believe that clients should take immediate steps to protect themselves and keep themselves safe. However, our stance is that we do not decide for clients whether to stay or leave a marriage. Our policy is that we will help them get as clear as possible about their situation, their feelings, and their options and make as clean a decision as possible.

Trust Issues

Addicted survivors have enormous trust issues. Being clear on who is saying what to whom is crucial in maintaining this trust, avoiding triangulation, and refraining from enabling. The issue of trust influences our decisions about which therapist does what piece of the treatment. We seldom have the same therapist do individual therapy as well as marital or family therapy with the same client. At most, the counselor for individual therapy might have one conference at the beginning of treatment with involved family members, and he or she might maintain occasional phone contact with the parents of an adolescent client. We advise parents needing a great deal of support in coping with their adolescent to contact a family therapist first and to contact the individual therapist only if an emergency exists and they are unable to reach the family therapist. This is consistent with standard clinical practice and is a matter of maintaining good boundaries. However, sometimes addicted survivors, with their strong idealizations and positive transferences, come to believe that their individual therapist is the only therapist in the world who can do the job or that this therapist should be exclusively theirs. Processing these issues with clients, clarifying boundaries with all parties, and making appropriate referrals to other therapists are the necessary tasks in this situation. Obtaining releases to the other therapists helps to avoid triangulation.

False Memory Syndrome

A matter related to the issue of trust is the so-called false memory syndrome (9). Advocates of this phenomena (generally, parents accused of and, in some cases, sued in court by their adult children for alleged abuse) hold that therapists and support groups have sometimes persuaded and brainwashed clients into falsely believing that abuse occurred. According to the advocates, the scenario plays out in this way: A client enters therapy or joins a support group for any of a variety of symptoms and problems. Professionals and/or support group members quickly persuade the client that he or she was probably abused, despite the fact that the client has no memories of any such abuse. Consistent messages to this effect, checklists suggesting that every conceivable emotional and personal problem is an effect of abuse, and, most especially, the use of hypnosis and guided imagery to recapture "lost" memories convert and convince the client that abuse did take place and that a family member perpetrated the abuse. Research demonstrating that children can be convinced after repeated and leading questions by experimenters that they experienced highly unpleasant events that never happened supports the contention that a false memory syndrome exists.

The possibility of false memory syndrome poses tremendous clinical, legal, and ethical dilemmas for professionals. Therapeutic relationships presuppose a great deal of trust, and power adheres to the position of being a counselor and therapist. Clients are certainly suggestible, and a defensible position is that all therapy relies primarily on persuasion. Survivors, who may have had an abuse experience different from the one they end up remembering (i.e., involving a different form or perpetrator), appear to be particularly suggestible. There is no definitive survivor syndrome, and many symptoms associated with the experience of trauma (such as generalized anxiety disorder) can occur without any experience of trauma. False accusations and legal charges can cause tremendous wreckage in the lives of innocent individuals accused of perpetrating abuse. And therapists increasingly run the risk of being sued themselves in these cases. On the other hand, denial and dissociation characterize the memories, feelings, and actions of survivors of childhood abuse and their family members. Many clients do not enter therapy with memories of childhood abuse and only recover them later. This is particularly likely to be true for addicted survivors who enter sobriety; the chemicals no longer preoccupy them and no longer screen unpleasant memories and feelings. Many therapists view the notion of a false memory syndrome merely as a very sophisticated form of denial that inflicts further abuse on survivors. Hypersensitive survivors can detect even the slightest questioning of their position by others, which they experience as abandonment.

At the time of writing this chapter, the American Psychological Association had established a high-powered task force to study this issue and to formulate guidelines and recommendations for researchers and clinicians. Our guess is that its conclusions will be reasonable but qualified as needing more research. The results of court decisions will also begin to point the way to necessary safeguards and procedures for dealing with this issue. Meanwhile, practicing clinicians must make their own way as best they can.

We employ several procedures with our clients that we feel strike a reasonable balance on this issue and protect everyone's interests. Even when clients have memories, we are careful to document their reports and the basis for any clinical conclusions we make in their chart. We phrase our statements to clients who have no memories very carefully. For example, we state that having no memories or other signs and symptoms associated with an experience of childhood trauma might indicate that such trauma took place or might indicate other psychiatric conditions. We are careful to avoid leading questions such as, "Who do you think might have abused you?" or, "What abusive experience must you have had to account for these feelings?" Instead, we ask more neutral questions such as, "What was it like growing up in your home?" or, "I wonder if you can recall the first time you felt like that?" This neutrality is particularly important if the therapist uses hypnosis, guided imagery, or other techniques focused on memory reconstruction. We seek out clinical consultation with a colleague when doing this kind of work to review our procedures and get feedback about possible countertransference issues that might interfere with an objective, helpful stance. In instances of possible current abuse we have another therapist/supervisor listen to audiotapes or sit in on sessions. Finally, it is important for therapists to discuss with clients who are contemplating confronting perpetrators or launching lawsuits the risks as well as the benefits of these actions. Many clients have the fantasy that they will finally and most certainly get the validation they want from family members when, in fact, this is often not the case. Many clients also do not understand that there is a vast difference between psychotherapy, where the bias is to support and validate their subjective experience, and a court hearing, where the emphasis is on demonstrable facts and the path to those facts is an adversarial process. (Readers interested in a more extended discussion of this may find references 10 and 11 helpful.)

It is helpful for therapists and family members to remember that the family, *as a whole*, only progresses through the stages of recovery at the pace determined by the member whose progress is slowest. This is not to say that individual or even partial family recovery is not possible when one or more family members are stuck in the recovery process. What it does mean is that one or more family members are likely to be increasingly left behind by the rest of the family. A classic example of this is the couple composed of an addicted survivor in recovery and a practicing alcoholic/addict. To expect that marital therapy in this case is going to reach the integration stage is naive and counterproductive. We typically tell clients in this situation that marital work, while possibly addressing at least safety issues, is very likely to be a waste of time until both spouses are abstinent and working a program. We encourage spouses in recovery to continue in their own recovery program and to practice loving detachment in the Al-Anon fashion. Similarly, an adolescent with a formerly abusive and still simmering parent who is unwilling to take a look at his or her own issues is not likely to have the evolved relationship he or she might like with that parent. Quite often we recommend that other family members obtain their own individual treatment first before entering into any in-depth family work beyond the crisis stage.

THE WORKPLACE AS FAMILY

Several authors have written about the ways in which organizations can have dynamics resembling alcoholic or otherwise dysfunctional families (12). Whether cause or effect, projection or reality, addicted survivors often trigger in their workplace and reenact old patterns established in their families of origin. Survivors may see incompetent and/or abandoning authority figures right and left. They may cast coworkers in sibling roles such as scapegoat. They may get into triangular situations, speaking to this person about that one, situations that can set off reactive ripples that either reinforce unhealthy dynamics or create them to the point of negatively influencing other members of the work team.

We have found it helpful to assess our clients' work situations and their relationships with coworkers at intake and periodically throughout treatment. This is particularly important for two reasons: Sometimes survivors have no immediate relatives and those in their workplace constitute their family, meaning that a prime source of data about "family relationships" is, therefore, what happens at work. The second reason is that since clients, in our experience, may start to revert to old behaviors and relapse for no immediately apparent reason, asking what is going on at work can sometimes suggest the possible basis for the relapse. Perhaps clients work with individuals whose idea of promoting workplace bonding is getting drunk on Friday nights after work. Perhaps a new boss is on the scene and is very critical of employees. Perhaps management has promoted a coworker into a position the client thought was his or hers.

Assisting clients to resolve workplace issues can be an important part of their recovery. Workplace situations present the opportunity to work through not only important issues in reality but also important internal issues related to family dynamics. Clients may need to quit their job if the situation is realistically intolerable or unsafe. Difficulty in the workplace raises important and often unresolved issues of loyalty, fear, and self-care; it may also motivate the client to learn the difference between running away from family members (or coworkers), standing up to them and challenging their inappropriate behaviors, and detaching from them and moving on. Apart from issues of economic security, our general philosophy is to consider quitting a job as a last-resort option. We believe that clients are always better off working through the situation if this is at all possible; even if they eventually decide to leave, they are then able to do so cleanly and with a better understanding of themselves. A client's interactions with others in an organization raise other issues and provide opportunities for self-understanding that he or she can explore in therapy. For example, a client may be motivated to ask the following questions: Am I projecting old issues? How can I tell? Can I be assertive at work? Avoid being drawn into a triangle? Give up the wish for the perfect boss? Be honest about my alcoholism with coworkers without being ashamed? Accept the need to deal with my compulsive workaholism? Workplaces and families are often, psychologically speaking, the same, and both require some treatment attention.

GROUP WORK WITH ADDICTED SURVIVORS

Apart from their cost-effectiveness in these days of managed health care, groups also offer a uniquely therapeutic experience for addicted survivors. Groups provide a setting where family-of-origin issues are likely to exhibit themselves and where they can be readily identified and processed. Groups, in addition, can serve as a substitute family and can give clients many of the experiences of protection and nurturing they failed to receive when younger. There are a number of important considerations in utilizing groups therapeutically with addicted survivors. In our discussion of these we include both groups that are professionally run and self-help groups.

Crisis Stage Groups

The focus of the crisis stage of recovery is immediate safety and health. Consistent with our safety frame is the conviction that chemical use is not safe and that the focus of groups at this stage must be the identification of safety options that can reinforce abstinence and provide basic levels of protection and nurturing. Both AA and NA offer a structured, predictable, ritualized format that emphasizes the importance and benefits of managing "life on life's terms" without the use of drugs or alcohol. The atmosphere in a 12-step group is nonjudgmental, and the emphasis is on a shameless communication of one's own experience and on sharing strength and hope. We strongly encourage regular attendance (at least two to three times a week) at the meetings of a specific 12-step home group. We also encourage clients to acquire a sponsor for individual support as soon as possible. The support and unconditional love offered in this setting can provide a safe and readily available free haven for survivors both in the initial stages of their dual recovery and for the rest of their lives. These programs also provide opportunities for social activities that can help fight loneliness and introduce survivors to other clean and sober people who are trying to put their lives in order. We do explicitly advise clients against developing sexual and romantic relationships with members of their support groups. We emphasize that a 12-step program is not meant to be a dating service and that keeping clear boundaries in this area is important. A disastrous romance with a fellow group member can rob a client of an important source of support.

Many clients initially resist going to 12-step meetings. Occasionally this is simply denial and needs to be challenged. More often, however, our clients suffer from strong social phobias, and the prospect of, for example, having to raise their hand and let others know they are in the first 30 days of sobriety precipitates anxiety and shame. This is especially true if they keep relapsing and thus have to raise their hand again and again. We offer a same-sex dual diagnosis relapse prevention group to not only provide active treatment for clients but to serve as an interim holding environment to help them prepare for attending 12-step meetings. The key focus in this group is on relapse prevention, with a particular emphasis on learning ways to manage painful feelings and on speaking up and offering and receiving support. We screen clients prior to their entering the group to be sure that they are not actively drinking or using and are at least trying to stay clean and sober. These small groups (typically, there are five to seven members) offer a safe place for early recovery to blossom.

In most cases women and men stay in our relapse prevention groups for 8 to 12 months. Some stay longer if they appear to continue to need this additional support and/or if they have not established group support outside of treatment.

The Skills-Building Stage

Groups grounded in 12-step recovery and self-help philosophies are very helpful during the skills-building stage. Learning to share in meetings, accepting recovery slogans, and being comfortable calling a sponsor are skills that are therapeutic for survivors. In our relapse prevention groups we also focus on such topics as anger management and assertiveness. Clients not only learn about such skills in a conceptual way but also see other group members who are more advanced in these areas model these skills. Most importantly, clients have an opportunity to practice these skills with each other under the watchful eye of a therapist who can help ensure that this process is a safe one.

The Education Stage

In the education stage survivors continue to learn more about the process of recovery. Groups designed to support survivor recovery, such as AMAC groups (Adults Molested As Children), complement professional and other self-help groups. With supports and skills in place, clients are now in a better position to handle therapy groups that specifically target survivor issues; they now have a decreased chance of relapsing and an increased chance of truly benefiting from such groups (and not merely dissociating the experience).

The Integration Stage

In the integration stage survivors continue to make gains from attendance at meetings of a self-help group whose focus is not chemical use but family-of-origin issues. Groups such as Incest Anonymous or ACOA offer clients a place to continue to work on integrating all their parts into recovery. Survivors now have the ability to tolerate the intense emotions experienced and encountered in these groups (which are not professionally facilitated). Survivors can now also begin to benefit from groups with a more traditional (i.e., psychodynamic) emphasis on working through transference and projection among members. Continued attendance at 12-step groups to reinforce abstinence is important.

The Maintenance Stage

Addicted survivors benefit from lifetime involvement in a self-help program that anchors their recovery and continues to help them to "live life on life's terms." For survivors to consider themselves recovered rather than recovering from either addiction or one of the survivor syndromes is a potentially dangerous stance. Both conditions are chronic, and the potential for relapse, though less and less with time and treatment, always exists. Thinking "I'm recovered" can lead to thinking "I can now drink." Addiction is a disease of body, mind, and spirit; improved thinking and functioning does not magically confer bodily immunity to addiction. Survivors may also encounter triggers that require going back into treatment to finish up another unresolved issue.

The following sections discuss the key therapeutic ingredients we feel it is important for groups to provide to be effective for addicted survivors.

Abstinence

The norm for all therapy/recovery groups and the goal of each member should be one of abstinence from mood-altering chemicals (with the exception of nonaddictive medications prescribed by a physician). A relapse, while not excused or enabled, is not grounds for dismissal from the group if clients show a willingness to stick to the group norm and if they are honest about what happened. If a member of one of our groups relapses, we do not shame the person and kick him or her out of the group. Instead, we ask such members to discuss how their relapse was unsafe and to replay the steps leading up to the relapse in the group. Group members help by giving feedback about possible triggers for the relapse and suggestions about "safer" ways to manage these triggers.

The group also includes a review of other unsafe behavior in the category of relapse. Self-harm, sexually acting out, and bingeing or purging with food are all examples of other kinds of relapses.

The group norm is to provide a supportive but clear message that interprets relapses as "sick behaviors and symptoms of a lack of safety and good self-care." Many relapsing survivors grow to dislike groups like AA or NA because they perceive members of these self-help groups as being shaming and blaming in the face of a relapse. In fact, this does sometimes occur and is not just a projection. Shaming and blaming of addicted survivors by other group members is not the way to help them build a healthy foundation for their dual recovery program. On the other hand, enabling the relapse by minimizing, ignoring, or justifying it only leads to further relapses.

We have found that many survivors are reluctant to count their days of recovery, a practice that is common in 12-step programs. Our clients tend to see the group as waiting to catch them fail, or they resort to magical and distorted thinking and believe that the greater the number of days of abstinence, the greater the likelihood that they will eventually relapse. Nevertheless, we still encourage them to count their days of abstinence. We are careful in doing this to prompt clients to count the successful days rather than focus on the times they failed. We have noticed that survivors who refuse to count successful days tend to relapse more often; they appear to have less investment in abstinence if they do not count these days.

Honesty and Safety

Safety is the general anchor point for all our group discussions. Anyone who is unsafe or knows that another group member is unsafe has a contract with the group to discuss these behaviors. Violating this contract—or struggling to keep it—raises all sorts of issues around denial, triangles, enabling, and so forth that are a treasure trove of therapeutic opportunity.

We have found it important to take into account several key issues that distinguish group work with male survivors from group work with female survivors. The first issue is the differences in attitude toward painful feelings and emotions and in the generally accepted style of managing them. In Western society men are supposed to be macho, tough, and strong, and most males (despite several decades of liberation talk) still believe that acknowledging painful feelings is a sign of weakness. Because of these gender differences, our group work with female survivors focuses on "managing" the pain and work with male survivors deals with "honoring" the pain. The concept of "respecting your wounded part" seems to give male survivors greater permission to explore painful thoughts, feelings, and emotions in front of their peers. Another key issue that needs to be addressed with male clients is the vulnerability of the abuse victim. To openly discuss their vulnerability, whether past or present, is a very difficult task for most men and threatens their concept of "manliness." Clarifying that being a victim of abuse does not mean that one is homosexual or weak is very important. Male survivors who are also addicted to chemicals need dual support. Our male survivors relapse prevention group provides the opportunity, under the aegis of a group norm that "honors" the pain, for males to safely discuss such issues as feelings of shame and powerlessness and the role of chemicals in their lives.

The transference issues that arise in teen survivor groups are similar to those in the adult groups. The difference is that the teen is much more likely to be obvious. In some ways this makes treatment easier, and in other ways more difficult. If they plan to drink and use, adolescents will often tell you. They will make it clear if they dislike a group member and will often not pretend to be nice about it. Clients in our teen survivor groups often accord Katie (Evans), who runs these groups, the status of being "the good mom." These teens then think that Katie is capable of performing miracles with family members and outside parties. When she fails to deliver on the miracle, these clients are often hurt or disappointed and may relapse. Strong loyalty to other group members can lead to very negative reactions when they relapse. On the other hand, this loyalty and transference is often what keeps teen clients on the road to recovery. Most teen survivors have trouble achieving more than a year of clean and sober time—they tend to go on brief binges (usually under 2 weeks). However, they typically return to group, stricken with guilt over their relapse and ready to recommit to recovery. The ability to keep expectations clear and to understand the special issues of adolescent addicted survivors, a tolerance for intense affect, and a high energy level help therapists who do groups with these teens.

DEFINING THE NORMAL FAMILY

What is a normal family? We have no good models to represent this, and given the cultural diversity of our population, elevating any one model is fraught with the dangers of prejudice and bias. However, we have evolved one standard for helping clients decide if an experience was normal or abusive. We ask them to notice what their bodies and feelings do as they talk about the experience. Our minds can fool us, but our bodies and feelings do not lie.

By way of closing this section and ending this chapter, we provide the "Personal Bill of Rights" from Timmen Cermak's book *A Time to Heal*, material we often share with our clients and their families (1).

1. Life should have choices beyond mere survival.
2. I have a right to say no to anything when I do not feel ready or when it is unsafe.
3. Life should not be motivated by fear.
4. I have a right to all of my feelings.
5. I am probably not guilty.

6. I have a right to make mistakes.

7. There is no need to smile when I cry.

8. I have a right to terminate conversations with people who make me feel diminished and humiliated.

9. I can be healthier than those around me.

10. It's okay for me to be relaxed, playful, and frivolous.

11. I have a right to change and grow.

12. It is important to set limits and to take care of myself.

13. I can be angry with someone I love.

14. I can take care of myself no matter what circumstances I am in.

15. I do not have to be fully healed to be fully worthwhile.

16. I do not have to perfect to be perfectly happy.

17. I do not have to be perfect, period! No one else is!

REFERENCES

1. Cermak, T. (1988). *A time to heal*. Los Angeles, CA: Jeremy P. Tarcher.

2. Alanon Family Group Publication.

3. Brown, S. (1985). *Treating the alcoholic: A developmental model*. New York: Wiley.

4. Black, C. (1982). *It will never happen to me*. Denver, CO: MAC.

5. Woitiz, J. (1983). *Adult children of alcoholics*. Pompano Beach, FL: Health Communications.

6. Howard, G. (1993). Personal communication.

7. Evans, K., & Sullivan, J. M. (1990). *Dual diagnosis: Counseling the mentally ill substance abuser*. New York: Guilford Press.

8. Galanter, M. (1993). *Network therapy for alcohol and drug abuse: A new approach in practice*. New York: Basic Books, HarperCollins.

9. Gorski, T. (1993). False memory syndrome. *The Counselor*, Fall, 10–15.

10. Yapko, M. D. (1994). *Suggestions of abuse: True and false memories of childhood sexual trauma*. New York: Simon & Schuster.

11. Gardner, R. A. (1993). *True and false accusations of child sex abuse*. Crosskill, NJ: Creative Therapeutics.

12. Schaef, A. W., & Fassel, D. (1988). *The addictive organization*. San Francisco, CA: Harper Row.

Afterword: The Dragon Dies, the Child Survives

$\diamond$

Again and again we have seen survivors use the image of a dragon to symbolize their abuse experiences. Often they use this to represent the perpetrator of the abuse. The dragon is dangerous yet fascinating, powerful yet mysterious. One of our survivor clients painted a picture for us representing her experience of recovery from incest. She depicted a dragon asleep on a shore and curled around a pile of beautiful jewels. The jewels represent her innocence, and the dragon represents her stepfather. The powerful dragon robbed her of her jewels. The dragon is lying on sand, with more sand flowing through an hourglass to symbolize the passing of time. On the beach there is also a dresser and mirror. In the mirror the stern face of a woman looks silently out at the viewer, seeing all but saying nothing. In another part of the painting this woman drew herself commanding a magical little ship, square in shape, in which she is sailing back across the sea to reclaim what her stepfather took from her. In her ship are the things that help her feel safe: an artist's easel and paints and books on mythology, psychology, and philosophy. A unicorn is painted on the side of the square little ship, and in the ship is a young child who looks strong and determined. In the sky is the sun in the form of the Tao—yin and yang joined together in integrated wholeness. Empowered, the small girl is ready to conquer the dragon.

The journey that this painting recounts with its rich imagery is both the beginning and the end of our discussion of treating the addicted survivor—with one exception. We want to close this book with a discussion

254

of some issues concerning our own "therapist's PTSD." This is a result of both our own childhood trauma and the trauma that comes from working many hours each day with other survivors. We have found that unless we work our own recovery program, we burn out and become less effective with our clients. We humbly assume that this is an issue for many who do this kind of work and speak from our own experience, strength, and hope to these issues. Our experience working with clients, supervising other therapists, and presenting workshops convinced us that any book on treating addicted survivors would be incomplete without such a section.

TRANSFERENCE AND COUNTERTRANSFERENCE

In previous chapters we explored some of the transference and counter-transference issues that arise when working with addicted survivors and their families. Transference, or the reenactment of client issues in the relationship with the therapist, is inevitable in therapy, especially with survivors. It is also necessary. Effective therapy with survivors requires at least some degree of transference, with the transference that occurs in the therapeutic relationship enabling survivors to work through and heal the wound caused by the trauma. This transference can take many forms. The therapist may become the good mother the client never had or the fairy godmother the client always wished would come and effect a rescue. And in situations involving negative transference the therapist may become the abusive or abandoning parent or family member.

Typically, clients' transference begins in a somewhat positive mode; otherwise, clients are likely to drop out of treatment. Negative transference is likely to arise later in treatment; hopefully, the therapist and client can work this through and resolve the matter. Safely experiencing a "real" and integrated relationship is immensely healing for clients, allowing them to "become present" and to be free of the past.

Countertransference occurs when therapists reenact unresolved issues from their own past in their relationships with clients. Perhaps the critical mother of an adolescent client reminds the therapist too much of his or her own critical parent; if so, the clinician cannot be objective with the adolescent or the family. For therapists who played the role of hero in their family of origin, a common pitfall is to enable or rescue clients. Regardless of whether they follow a more psychoanalytic model of therapist neutrality or an alcohol and drug counseling model geared more toward mentoring through explicit support, challenge, and self-disclosure, therapists must be prepared to manage and cope with both client transference and their own countertransference. The therapeutic relationship with addicted survivors is likely to be highly emotionally charged for all parties.

Being the focus of such intense transference (even if positive) day in and day out can take its toll on the therapist. While the adult part of us knows that survivors' rage is a projection of their angry wounded part and is not really directed against us, our bodies very often still react with a strong fight-or-flight response. Containing our own impulses to strike back or run away goes with the job. However, this generally causes a great deal of stress and can lead to stress-related problems for therapists. We have found that we are susceptible to many viral illnesses when we work too many hours or have too few mental health days off. We both have back problems that tend to flair up when we are under too much stress. We also start waking up in the middle of the night, obsessing over details of our clinic or about specific clients. Katie starts to grind her teeth, and Mike becomes irritable and impatient. When we notice these things happening, we know it is time to take some time off and do something relaxing and fun. We also try to maintain an exercise routine and eat regular, well-balanced meals.

In addition to the physical toll on our bodies, work with addicted survivors often has a strong negative effect on our emotions. Most of us therapists and counselors are sensitive, intuitive human beings who want to help others. We tend to experience things intensely. That is one of the reasons we are in this business and one of the resources necessary to be effective with clients. Our clients depend on our sensitive nature to help them feel understood and supported. Successfully pacing clients also requires that we empathetically join with them. Participating at some level with each client's trauma is a necessary part of this work. If we keep too much emotional distance between ourselves and survivors and their pain, in order to protect ourselves, clients will feel abandoned. But if we join and pace too closely, we will be submerged in and overwhelmed by our clients' trauma and pain. Spending the day doing trauma resolution work often has the effect on us of living and working in an emotional war zone. If we professionals did not have PTSD before we began working with survivors, it is likely that we would have it after working with them.

We have found that crisis and integration stage work are the most stressful times for us. Hospitalizing clients; managing suicidal ideation, self-mutilation, and flooding; and dealing with chemical use relapses as part of the crisis stage and the trauma drama can certainly bring havoc to our day. Couple this with the need to return phone calls, complete paperwork, and talk with reviewers of managed health care companies, and the end of the day cannot come too soon. If more than one client is in crisis at the same time, we sometimes begin to question our choice of career, and running a small deli or managing an espresso cart begins to look like an appealing alternative to clinical practice.

The integration stage, with its intense abreaction and grief work, is another stage of recovery that can leave us drained. Katie's integration work with Rachel, whose story we told in Chapter 2, proved to be very intense. When Katie led Rachel back to the time of her abuse, Rachel vomited repeatedly into the trash can in Katie's office. Katie felt as if she had actually watched a 3-year-old being raped. Mike worked with one male who had been horribly physically abused by his father. In the course of doing integration work with this man, Mike once was working with a part of the client who suddenly began walking toward him with the intent of strangling him. Several very tense minutes ensued, but the strength of the therapeutic alliance and the man's containing skills saved the day.

We have sometimes found ourselves at the end of the day with high levels of free-floating anxiety, feelings of extreme fatigue, or even emotional numbness. We have found ourselves reenacting in our minds details of some our clients' stories or overreacting to reports of abuse in the media. Most troubling for us is the challenge our work brings to our worldview that the world and humans are basically good and well-meaning. All this, incidentally, does not help our relationships with our own family members.

Appropriately, all the concepts and skills we teach clients are useful to us in managing our "therapist's PTSD." We try to practice good self-care and use social support (more than once we have collapsed in each other's office ventilating feelings and reactions that persisted after a particularly difficult session). We constantly use our own feelings containers and the safe place we have established in our mind. We "turn over and let go" of our cares and concerns to our higher power, and we practice observing and shuttling out of PTSD-type trances induced by our work with clients. Remembering that PTSD is a normal response to an abnormal situation helps us refrain from being too critical of ourselves for having these reactions.

THERAPISTS AS SURVIVORS

Working with survivors is enough to induce secondary PTSD. However, we have long known that many members of the helping professions are themselves survivors. This personal dose of trauma is a double-edged sword. If counselors have not addressed their own survivor issues and do not work a recovery program for them, they run an increased risk of countertransference, secondary PTSD, and burnout. If counselors, however, are working through their issues and maintain an active recovery program, they can bring to their therapy work a genuine empathy, an understanding of the issues that is both intellectual and emotional, and a therapeutic potency that comes from "walking the walk" and not merely "talking the talk."

Both of us are survivors of childhood trauma. In addition, Katie is in recovery from addiction and has been working a dual recovery program since 1983. She found that it was essential to begin her survivor and ACOA work at the time of initial sobriety; she felt that her recurrent acute depressions meant that it would be impossible for her to avoid or postpone work on these issues and still maintain her sobriety. Prior to sobriety, Katie never really acknowledged her survivor issues and the effect they had on her. She spent the first 10 years of her career working in mental health and 7 of those years working for children's protective services investigating cases of child abuse and running therapy groups for incest survivors. Katie became known as an implacable and relentless investigator and a pull-out-all-the-stops therapist and advocate. She minimized the effect on her work of being an adult child of an alcoholic and only discussed her rape by a relative at age 16 when she had too much to drink. Katie also thought it was normal to medicate her "job stress" with Valium. In retrospect, she believes that some of her passion for her career reflected her own unresolved issues, a passion that made her work a quest and not a job and that led to chronic burnout. And, not surprisingly, Katie, whose main defense was to be "perfect and in control," was constantly rageful toward perpetrators. Ultimately, her prescription drug addiction led her to treatment and to recovery. After her treatment Katie, now sober, was able to continue her child abuse investigation work for only a year; she found that the nightmares, flooding, and anxiety associated with her work were no longer tolerable and were a threat to her recovery.

Alcoholism and associated ACOA issues run rampant through Mike's extended family. Mike grew up a "lost" child. He felt invisible and tried to avoid drawing attention to himself. At age 11 he was sexually abused by a priest. In response, Mike assumed the role of "hero," partly because a relative (who knew nothing of the abuse) took a special interest in him because of his intelligence. He also repressed memories of the abuse. Although years of compulsive workaholism resulted in external signs of success, Mike never felt that he was good enough. Not surprisingly, he decided early in high school to become a psychologist in order to help people. In retrospect, he knows that he was trying to help himself as well. Every few years Mike, exhausted from his work load and the accumulation of projects—all of which had to be done perfectly—would suffer a nervous breakdown. Although Mike's training included mandatory group therapy, he was too concerned about what his supervisor and peers would think and thus never benefited from this experience. Soon after getting his degree, Mike began to be interested in working with survivors of sexual abuse. This proved both rewarding and very stressful. He felt good helping those "poor survivors" yet found himself drained and constantly angry with the perpetrators and with colleagues who minimized what had happened to his clients. Mike had trouble maintaining intimate relationships through the years. He also had trouble with certain issues and with certain kinds of clients in therapy; perfectly at home with the cognitive–behavior therapies, he had trouble with issues and therapy approaches that dealt with feelings. He would also find his mind beginning to wander in certain therapy sessions and would sometimes miss client dynamics. Teens, in particular, found him "stiff." Another nervous collapse, the end of another relationship, a series of troubling nightmares, and some low-grade panic attacks finally led Mike into therapy. Therapy and publicity about sexual abuse by members of the clergy helped Mike remember his experience of sexual abuse.

We both carry our past with us. Despite years of treatment and ongoing personal work, we still get triggered from time to time in the course of our clinical work and begin to get sucked into our own reenactments. To deal with this, we both try, one day at a time, to practice what we preach. We strive constantly to maintain conditions of safety (both protection and nurturing) in our own lives. Katie regularly attends 12-step meetings and seeks out individual therapy periodically. Mike continues in psychotherapy and works with child advocacy groups. We both have participated in couples counseling. We are both prone to workaholism and constantly have to be on the alert for this. Our office staff have explicit permission to fight with us about scheduling "just one more appointment." We now work a 4-day workweek to allow time for writing and continuing education. We work to eliminate from our lives people who are unkind to us or who make us feel diminished. We strive to make our clinic a healthy work environment, and we openly discuss our clinic's "family problems" as they arise. If one of us gets triggered, we have permission from ourselves and from each other to take a time-out for self-care. Mike does not take referrals for work with offenders and works mainly with survivors in later stages of recovery from addiction. Katie generally refers families to other counselors. We try to keep in mind our limitations and hot spots when working with clients and their families: Mike has to watch out for his response to overprotective mothers or getting angry with distant fathers in family sessions. Katie has to watch out for aligning too closely with an adolescent against a parent and for issues that arise in working with older alcoholics. For example, she transferred one 70-year-old alcoholic female to another clinic for treatment when she discovered that she had countertransference issues with the woman. When Katie noticed that she was beginning to get angry at the woman for relapsing, she realized that the client reminded her too much of her own alcoholic parents. We do joint consultations frequently and sometimes even sit in on each other's sessions (with client permission) for difficult cases. Katie continues to work on her hypersensitivity and her tendency to be too critical of herself and others. Mike continues to work on staying in the present and not getting lost in his head while leaving feelings and the rest of himself behind.

We provide frequent supervision for other therapists in our clinic. We require that all staff recovering from addiction practice a continuous program of recovery, which includes going to both 12-step meetings and therapy, when appropriate. Clinicians with survivor issues need to be aware of them and to be working on their own recovery. Examining these issues and their impact on work with clients is an important and explicit part of our supervision with our staff. Because we try to model openness about dealing with our own issues, staff are very receptive to doing the same.

Both of us were working with survivors prior to our own recovery and trauma-resolution work. We know that our worldview and effectiveness changed after doing our own therapy. We learned that we cannot help our clients to learn lessons we ourselves have not yet mastered, a lesson reflected in the 12-step program message "You can't give away what you don't have." We have worked with many therapists and counselors over the years who were very talented individuals, and we have concluded that they are less effective (and occasionally harmful) if they have not done, and do not continue to do, their own personal work.

PROGRESS, NOT PERFECTION

We all have strengths and weaknesses as both therapists and as human beings. Those of us with a perfection fetish need to remember that perfection is not attainable but that we can make progress in our professional development and personal recovery. We are learning to forgive ourselves and others for mistakes and to accept that things are just the way they are supposed to be. The following passage appears in the Big Book of AA:

> And acceptance is the answer to all my problems today. When I am disturbed it is because some person, place, or thing, some fact of my life, is unacceptable to me; and I can find no serenity until I accept the person, place, thing, or situation as being exactly the way that it is supposed to be at this moment. Nothing, absolutely nothing, happens

in God's world by mistake. Until I could accept my alcoholism, I could not stay sober; unless I can learn to accept life completely on life's terms, I can not be happy. I need to concentrate not so much on what needs to be changed in the world as on what needs to be changed in me and my attitudes.

Relentlessly perfectionistic as we are, this is our favorite passage in the Big Book. We constantly remind ourselves that we are only human and not perfect if we make a remark in a session that is more about our issues than the client's or if we once again schedule too many appointments. We invite you to do the same, and we hope that sharing our own experience, strength, and hope helps you on your journey working with the addicted survivor!

Appendix

DUAL DIAGNOSIS ASSESSMENT TOOL

Client Name _____ Date _____

Section I: Drug/Alcohol Use

1. Have you ever tried to control your use? Y N
2. Has anyone ever criticized your use? Y N
3. Have you ever felt guilty after your use? Y N
4. Have you ever drunk/used first thing in the morning to eliminate a hangover? Y N
5. Have you ever experienced a memory loss when drinking or using drugs? Y N
6. Have you ever missed work/school due to use or hangovers? Y N
7. Have you ever embarrassed yourself due to drug/alcohol use? Y N
8. Have you ever been hospitalized due to or related to your use? Y N
9. Have you ever had any arrests or legal problems related to drug/alcohol use? Y N
10. Has your family expressed concern over your use of chemicals or your behavior when using? Y N
11. Have you ever lied about the amount or the kind of chemicals that you use? Y N
12. Do you ever hide your chemicals in order to protect your supply? Y N
13. Does it take more to get high than it used to? Y N

14. Are you using more often now than before?	Y	N
15. Is there anyone that you are related to who has a problem with alcohol or drugs?	Y	N
16. Have you ever had withdrawal symptoms?	Y	N
17. Have you ever had seizures during withdrawal?	Y	N
18. Have you used any drugs/alcohol in the last 48 hours?	Y	N
19. Do you have any medical problems related to your drinking or drug use?	Y	N

20. List drugs of choice by preference, including alcohol._____

_____

Comment on any yes responses and explain_____

_____

_____

_____

Section II: Mood and Anxiety

21. Have you ever considered committing suicide?	Y	N
22. Have you ever attempted suicide?	Y	N
23. Do you feel as if life is not worth living?	Y	N
24. Have you ever cut yourself or harmed yourself in any other way?	Y	N
25. Do you have trouble sleeping?	Y	N
26. Do you wake up early in the morning, then have trouble falling back to sleep?	Y	N
27. Do you have periods where you do not need sleep for days and feel full of energy?	Y	N
28. Are you afraid to leave your home?	Y	N
29. Does your mind sometimes race so that you have trouble concentrating?	Y	N
30. Do you count objects or have other rituals that you use to help you feel safe?	Y	N
31. Do you have flashbacks of previous traumatic life experiences?	Y	N
32. Do you suffer from nightmares?	Y	N
33. Do you sometimes feel overwhelmed with emotions and unable to manage these feelings?	Y	N
34. Does your heart sometimes pound hard when you think about an unsafe situation?	Y	N

35. Do you find yourself checking out or spacing out when
    you are not drinking or using?   Y   N

36. Do you use drugs or alcohol in an attempt to block out
    or numb the pain?   Y   N

37. Have you ever been prescribed medication to help you
    manage your mood or anxiety?   Y   N

38. Have you ever been hospitalized due to a mood or anxi-
    ety problem?   Y   N

39. Do you have any medical problems that are stress re-
    lated?   Y   N

Comment on any yes responses and explain_____

_____

_____

_____

Section III: Psychosis/Paranoia

40. Have you heard voices from inside or outside your
    head when there was no one there?   Y   N

41. Do you sometimes feel as if people are talking about
    you?   Y   N

42. Do you sometimes find that you are getting special
    messages from the television, radio, or other source?   Y   N

43. Have you ever felt that someone was trying to control
    your thoughts or behavior?   Y   N

44. Have you ever thought that you have special powers
    that other people do not have?   Y   N

45. Do you think that there are people who are purpose-
    fully trying to cause harm to you?   Y   N

46. Do you ever have visions or hallucinations?   Y   N

47. Did you have hallucinations prior to any drug or alco-
    hol use?   Y   N

48. Do you have voices that give you instructions on things
    that you are supposed to do?   Y   N

If yes, do these voices ever tell you to hurt yourself or some-
    one else?   Y   N

49. Does drinking or using drugs help the voices go away? Y   N

50. Does drinking or using drugs make the voices worse?   Y   N

51. Did you hear voices before you ever drank or used
    drugs?   Y   N

52. Does drinking or using drugs make your fear and dis-
    trust increase?   Y   N
53. Do you currently have a plan to hurt yourself or some-
    one else?   Y   N

Comment on any yes responses _____

_____

_____

_____

_____

Scoring

Section I: The presence of three or more "yes" responses indicates chemical
    dependency.

Section II: The presence of two or more "yes" responses indicates a possible
    mood or anxiety problem.

Section III: The presence of two or more "yes" responses indicates a possible
    thought disorder.

Note: A "yes" response to questions 17, 18, 19, 21, 22, 23, 48, or 53 indicates an
    immediate need for further assessment for possible hospitalization for
    safety.

SPECIALIZED STEP WORK FOR THE ANXIOUS SURVIVORS

Step One: "We admitted that we are powerless over our addiction, that our lives had become unmanageable."

Describe three situations where your stress and/or anxiety have caused you a
    problem in your life.

Describe three situations where alcohol or other drugs have harmed you or
    caused you some sort of problem in your life.

Describe a situation where you were embarrassed over your behavior when
    drinking or using drugs.

Describe how you used drugs or alcohol to try to reduce or manage your anxiety.

Describe how alcohol controlled you (e.g., preoccupation with use). Give two
    examples of how you lost control over your use of chemicals.

Describe three problems you have now or have recently had related to your use
    of chemicals.

Describe two ways that drinking or using drugs made your anxiety worse.

Describe three ways you can reduce your stress without drinking or using drugs.

Describe two skills you need to learn to strengthen your recovery program.
Describe how your anxiety makes your life unmanageable.

Step Two: "Came to believe that a power greater than ourselves could restore us to sanity."

Give an example of something that is going better now than before you got clean and sober.
Define who or what you might use as a higher power.
Describe how a belief in this higher power can help your recovery.

Step Three: "We made a decision to turn our will and our lives over to the care of God as we understood him."

Give an example of something that you are currently worrying about, and tell how it might help you to turn this thing over to your higher power.
Describe how you gain control of your life when you let go of trying to control alcohol and other drugs.
Describe how letting go of your stress can help you gain power in your life.
Describe a ritual that you would like to let go of and why.

Step Four: "We made a searching and fearless moral inventory of ourselves."

Describe a situation involving your drinking and using that you still are feeling guilty over.
Describe how by letting go of this guilt your life might be more calm and serene.
List three things that you do well.
List three things that you like about yourself and why.
List two things that you would like to change about yourself.
Describe what you need to do in order to make these changes.
What is one goal that you can work on during the next 6 months that will improve the quality of your recovery and your life?
Describe why taking your medication can be helpful to your recovery program.
Describe why it is important for you to forgive yourself for your past mistakes.
Describe how your protector part helps your recovery program.
Describe how your protector part can hurt your recovery program.
Describe how your nurturing part can help your recovery program.
Describe two ways you can nurture yourself when you are hurting.
Describe how your wounded part can help you in your recovery program.
Describe how your wounded part sometimes jeopardizes your recovery program.

SPECIALIZED STEP WORK FOR THE DEPRESSED SURVIVOR

Step One: "We admitted we were powerless over our addiction and that our lives had become unmanageable."

How did your desire for alcohol and other drugs dominate and preoccupy your thinking?

How did you use alcohol and other drugs to try to manage your feelings or alter your mood?

How did your behavior and personality change when you were under the influence of alcohol and other drugs?

What were some things that you did to get drugs or alcohol that are outside your normal values (e.g., lying about your use, stealing, being unfaithful to a spouse or friend)?

How did you lose control of your behavior when drinking or using drugs?

How were you preoccupied with drinking and using?

How were drugs and alcohol in control of your life instead of you being in control of your life?

How can you get your power back now that you are clean and sober?

How does taking your medication better manage your mood and help your recovery program?

How are you powerless over pain when you are overwhelmed?

What are two things you can do to manage your pain and feel safe other than drink or use drugs?

What are two things you can do to manage your anger other than to drink or use drugs?

Step Two: "Came to believe that a power greater than ourselves could restore us to sanity."

List two ways you feel better now that you have stopped drinking and using drugs.

Give an example of a boundary that you have set on someone; then describe how and why setting boundaries is important to your recovery.

List three people you can call when you are feeling sad or hopeless, and explain how these people could be helpful to you.

Describe one person you know who is also a depressed survivor and for whom the recovery program looks as if it is working. What is this person doing that seems to help him or her succeed?

Give any examples you may have of coincidence or signs that there is a higher power in your life.

Who or what is your higher power?

How can taking your medication assist you in your recovery process?

Step Three: "We made a decision to turn our will and our lives over to the care of God as we understood him."

Give an example of something that you have worried about in the last 30 days. Then describe how you might feel better if you could turn this worry over to your higher power.

Give an example of something that you have tried to control that was out of your control. Describe how you came to see that you were powerless to control this situation.

If you could turn over two negative thoughts or beliefs to help you feel better, what would they be?

Explain your process of "turning things over" or letting something go. Exactly how do you do this (e.g., through prayer or meditation)?

Step Four: "We made a searching and fearless moral inventory of ourselves."

List three talents or gifts that you possess.

Describe two things you have done or experienced that had a positive effect on another person.

List two personality traits you possess that you would like to build on.

Describe two negative things that you beat yourself up about. Explain why it is important for you to stop critiquing yourself about these things.

Describe one thing that you worry a lot about. Then describe how this worrying makes you unhappy.

Describe how you used drugs/alcohol to manage depression.

List two ways you can manage these negative feelings clean and sober.

Describe something you are grateful for and explain why.

Describe how your wounded, sad part is helpful to yourself and others.

Staying Safe Work Sheet

1. When I feel unsafe, I know that I can call _____

2. I need to learn to put my own needs first because _____

   _____

3. I need to be assertive because _____

   _____

4. Something I did recently that I was not very assertive about was _____

   _____

5. It might have gone better if I could have been assertive because _____

   _____

6. An example of an internal boundary I need to set is _____

_____

7. An example of an external boundary I need to set is _____

_____

8. The person I am really angry at is _____

9. I am angry at this person because _____

_____

10. I need to express my anger directly because _____

_____

11. Admitting that I suffer from the disease of addiction helps my recovery
    because _____

_____

12. I know that I am powerless over drugs and alcohol because _____

_____

13. I know that I am also powerless over other people because _____

_____

14. I know that I need to work a recovery program that includes a 12-step
    support group because _____

_____

15. Two ways I have learned to take care of myself are _____

_____

16. An example of how I can be passive–aggressive is _____

_____

17. I know that being direct is a better way to manage my feelings because ___

_____

18. I now know that being able to ask for help is a strength, not a liability, be-
    cause _____

_____

19. I need to ask for help around _____

_____

20. Overcontrolling is a relapse symptom because _____

_____

21. When I am feeling unsafe, a place I can go to is _____

_____

22. When I am flooding with bad feelings, one thing I can do to help myself is _____

   _____

23. When I am having a flashback, one thing I can do to help myself is _____

   _____

24. I like the way I am learning to _____

   _____

SPECIALIZED STEP WORK FOR THE ANGRY ACTING-OUT SURVIVOR

Step One: "We admitted we are powerless over our addiction, that our lives had become unmanageable."

Describe five situations where you suffered negative consequences as a result of drinking or using drugs.

List at least five reasons why drinking or using drugs is unsafe behavior

How does drinking or using drugs interfere with your recovery from PTSD?

List three situations where you did things that were not safe when drinking or using drugs.

Describe how your drug and/or alcohol use was controlling you instead of you controlling it.

Step Two: "Came to believe that a power greater than ourselves could restore us to sanity."

Insanity is making the same mistake and expecting different results. Give two examples of something that you repeated in spite of the fact that it was hurting you.

Describe some behavior related to your drinking and/or using that made you feel insane.

Describe how using drugs and drinking affected the angry part of you, the wounded part of you, and the sad part of you.

Give an example of something that is going better now that you have stopped drinking and using.

Describe your childhood God (skip if you had no beliefs).

Describe how you feel your God has let you down.

Describe how you feel you have let your God down.

Who or what is your higher power?

Describe why faith is so important to recovery.

Step Three: "Made a decision to turn our will and our lives over to the care of God as we understood him."

Describe how you go about turning something over to your higher power.

Give an example of something that you can turn over to your higher power that will help you recover.

Give an example of something that you have already turned over to your higher power; describe how you did that and what happened.

List three things that you need to turn over.

List two resentments that your angry part is holding on to that might be helpful to turn over.

Step Four: "Made a searching and fearless moral inventory of ourselves."

List five things you like about yourself.

List two ways your protector part is helpful.

Describe how your wounded part helps you in recovery.

Describe how your nurturing part can help you in your recovery program.

List four situations where you have been helpful to others.

Describe how things you are currently feeling guilty over relate to your sexual behavior.

List three current resentments that are hurting you in your recovery program.

Describe four current fears you have. Discuss how you might let go of these fears.

Give an example of how you are beginning to have faith in something greater than yourself.

List the people you most trust, and explain why you believe these people to be safe.

Describe how you are better at setting boundaries today than when you were drinking and using drugs.

Describe two ways you now know to nurture yourself when you are feeling unsafe.

A Relapse Exercise for the Acting-Out Survivor: Getting and Staying Safe

1. When I am feeling unsafe, I can go to _____

2. When I feel unsafe, I can always call _____

3. If I cannot reach my first choice, I can also call _____

4. One thing I can do when I feel full of rage is to _____

   _____

5. One thing I can do when I am flooded with fear is to _____

   _____

6. One thing I can do when I am flooded with sadness is _____

_____

7. I know that I need to take care of that wounded part of me because _____

_____

8. I know that hurting myself is not an option because _____

_____

9. I know that drinking and using drugs only make things worse because ___

_____

10. The trigger for my current pain is _____

_____

Forgiving Myself for My Relapse

1. One reason I should forgive myself for relapsing is _____

_____

2. One thing I learned from my relapse is _____

_____

3. In looking back on it I believe that the trigger for my relapse was _____

_____

4. One thing I might have done other than relapse is _____

_____

5. I am going to strengthen my recovery program by _____

_____

Index